Evidence-Based Surgery

Achilles Thoma · Sheila Sprague
Sophocles H. Voineskos
Charles H. Goldsmith
Editors

Evidence-Based Surgery

A Guide to Understanding and Interpreting the Surgical Literature

Springer

Editors
Achilles Thoma
Department of Surgery, Division of Plastic Surgery, Department of Health Research Methods, Evidence and Impact (HEI)
McMaster University
Hamilton, ON, Canada

Sheila Sprague
Department of Surgery, Division of Orthopaedic Surgery, Department of Health Research Methods, Evidence and Impact (HEI)
McMaster University
Hamilton, ON, Canada

Sophocles H. Voineskos
Department of Surgery, Division of Plastic Surgery
McMaster University
Hamilton, ON, Canada

Charles H. Goldsmith
Department of Health Research Methods, Evidence and Impact (HEI)
McMaster University
Hamilton, ON, Canada

Faculty of Health Sciences
Simon Fraser University
Burnaby, BC, Canada

Department of Occupational Science and Occupational Therapy, Faculty of Medicine
The University of British Columbia
Vancouver, BC, Canada

ISBN 978-3-030-05119-8 ISBN 978-3-030-05120-4 (eBook)
https://doi.org/10.1007/978-3-030-05120-4

Library of Congress Control Number: 2018963289

This Springer imprint is published by the registered company Springer Nature Switzerland AG
The registered company address is: Gewerbestrasse 11, 6330 Cham, Switzerland

Preface

The terms Evidence-Based Medicine (EBM) and Evidence-Based Surgery (EBS) are ubiquitous now. With very few exceptions, however, most surgeons who use these terms do not have a good grasp of the meaning of these words. The editors of this book have the privilege of being associated with the institution (McMaster University) where the ideas and concepts of EBM and EBS originated.

The British Medical Journal heralded EBM as one of the top 15 advances in health care in the last 150 years [1]. We have been teaching and writing about EBS for over the last two decades. In our interactions with surgeons of all specialties, we believe that there is a lack of understanding what EBS is all about and how it is applied in one's clinical practice.

Most surgeons, regardless of their specialty, have the surgical skills to perform an operation well. There is, however, a gap in understanding and interpreting what surgeons read in the surgical literature. It is the purpose of this book to fill this gap. Some surgeons may have perceived this gap already; others may not be aware of it. The sooner this gap is bridged the better for you as the surgeon at the individual level and the better for all us collectively as surgical specialties.

Since the late 1970s, we have been witnessing a gradual paradigm shift in the practice of medicine and surgery. The teaching of medicine and surgery by "authority" figures has been largely replaced by the scientific evidence. To paraphrase Pincus and Tugwell, eminence-based surgery camouflaged in the oratorical skills and demeanor of senior surgeons who have been making the same mistakes with increasing confidence over a number of years unchallenged has been supplanted by Evidence-Based Surgery [2].

At conferences, academic rounds, and journal clubs, we hear surgeons frequently quote this or that Randomized Controlled Trial (RCT) to support their argument for their clinical decisions. Although it is true that the RCT is considered the gold standard in examining the efficacy or effectiveness of some novel surgical intervention in comparison to standard care, the majority of our clinical decisions are based on designs other than RCT or meta-analyses of such studies. Furthermore, even if we find an RCT that may seem relevant to our clinical question, how do we know that the conclusions of such study are credible? The term RCT in an article does not give it legitimacy unless it deserves it.

The quality of evidence cannot be decided simply by the hierarchical categorization of the research by study design alone (meta-analysis, RCT, cohort studies, case-control studies, cases series). The reality is that not all published RCTs or systematic reviews or any other study designs are of equal quality. In a series of articles published in Lancet since 2009, it has been estimated that 85% of what is spent on health research is wasteful. Some of the reasons given are as follows: poor study design, unclear reporting (so others cannot interpret them or replicate the research), and finally what is published cannot be applied to patients [3–5].

The surgical literature is expanding year by year. PubMed alone has added between 13,000 and 210,000 surgery-related articles annually since 2008 [6]. More recently, we have seen a surge of not only legitimate surgical journals but also predatory ones [7]. While "legitimate" surgical journals have a supposedly, rigorous a peer-review process, this is currently haphazard. Not all reviewers have research methodology backgrounds and consequently, often, what we read is far from the truth and so, should not be implemented with patients.

The purpose of this book specifically is to teach surgeons (academic or community), surgical fellows and surgical residents regardless of the surgical specialty, the skills to appraise what they read in the surgical literature. Surgeons need to be able to understand what they read before applying the conclusions of a surgical article to their practice. As most surgeons do not have the extra training in health research methodology, understanding how the research was done, how to interpret the results, and finally deciding to apply them to the patient level is indeed a difficult task.

In a series of chapters in this book, we explain the methodological issues pertaining to the various study designs reported in the surgical literature. In most chapters, we will start with a clinical scenario with uncertain course of action with which most surgeons are struggling. The reader will be guided how to search the literature for the best evidence that will answer a surgical problem. Finding the evidence through a correct literature search is as essential as your scalpel at surgery.

An identified article that seems relevant to the problem you are investigating will then be appraised by addressing three key questions:

1. Is the study I am reading valid?
2. What are the results of this study?
3. Can I apply these results to my patients?

The ability to appraise a published surgical article effectively is as important as your surgical skill to complete the operation without harm. Evidence indicates that exposing surgical residents to health research methodology concepts increases research productivity and performance [8].

Therefore, while the primary goal of this book is to teach surgeons how to appraise the surgical literature, a collateral benefit is that the concepts explained here may help research-minded surgeons produce better research.

Hamilton, ON, Canada

Achilles Thoma, MD, M.Sc., FRCSC
Department of Surgery
Division of Plastic Surgery
Department of Health Research Methods
Evidence and Impact
McMaster University

Hamilton, ON, Canada

Sheila Sprague, Ph.D.
Department of Surgery
Division of Orthopaedic Surgery
Department of Health Research Methods
Evidence and Impact
McMaster University

Hamilton, ON, Canada

Sophocles H. Voineskos, MD, M.Sc., FRCSC
Department of Surgery
Division of Plastic Surgery
McMaster University

Hamilton, ON, Canada
Burnaby/Vancouver, BC, Canada

Charles H. Goldsmith, Ph.D.
Department of Health Research Methods
Evidence and Impact, McMaster University
Faculty of Health Sciences
Simon Fraser University
Department of Occupational Science
and Occupational Therapy
Faculty of Medicine
The University of British Columbia

References

1. Kamerow D, editor. Milestones, tombstones and sex education. BMJ. 2007;334:0–a.
2. Pincus T, Tugwell P. Shouldn't Standard Rheumatology Clinical Care be Evidence-Based Rather Than Eminence-Based, Eloquence-Based, or Elegance Based? J Rheumatol. 2007;34:1–4.
3. Glasziou P, Chalmers I. Is 85% of health research really "wasted"? [Internet]: 2016. Available from https://blogs.bmj.com/bmj/2016/01/14/paul-glasziou-and-iain-chalmers-is-85-of-health-research-really-wasted/. Accessed by 16 July 2018.
4. Chalmers I, Glasziou P. Avoidable waste in the production and reporting of research evidence. Lancet. 2009;374(9683):86–9.
5. Glasziou P, Altman DG, Bossuyt P, Boutron I, Clarke M, Julious S, et al. Reducing waste from incomplete or unusable reports of biomedical research. Lancet. 2014;383 (9913):267–76.

6. Corlan AD. Medline trend: automated yearly statistics of PubMed results for any query [Internet]; 2004. Available from http://www.webcitation.org/65RkD48SV. Accessed by 16 July 2018.
7. Rohrich R, Weinstein A. Predator-in-Chief: Wolves in Editors' Clothing. PRS Go. 2018; 6: 2-pe1652.
8. Farrokhyar F, Amin N, Dath D, Bhandari M, Kelly S. Impact of the Surgical Research Methodology Program on surgical residents' research profiles. J Surg Educ. 2014;71: 513–20.

Contents

1 **History of Evidence-Based Surgery (EBS)** 1
Achilles Thoma, Jessica Murphy, Sheila Sprague and Charles H. Goldsmith

2 **The Steps of Practicing Evidence-Based Surgery (EBS)** 9
Achilles Thoma, Sheila Sprague, Luis H. Braga and Sophocles H. Voineskos

3 **Developing a Surgical Clinical Research Question: *To Find the Answer in Literature Search or in Pursuing Clinical Research*** 17
Achilles Thoma, Sheila Sprague, Sophocles H. Voineskos and Jessica Murphy

4 **Finding the Evidence Through Searching the Literature** 23
Laura Banfield, Jo-Anne Petropoulos and Neera Bhatnagar

5 **Hierarchy of Evidence in Surgical Research** 37
Gina Del Fabbro, Sofia Bzovsky, Achilles Thoma and Sheila Sprague

6 **Evaluating Surgical Interventions** 51
Aristithes G. Doumouras and Dennis Hong

7 **A Primer on Outcome Measures for Surgical Interventions** 61
Joy MacDermid

8 **Patient-Important Outcome Measures in Surgical Care** 71
Katherine B. Santosa, Anne Klassen and Andrea L. Pusic

9 **Surrogate Endpoints** 85
Seper Ekhtiari, Ryan P. Coughlin, Nicole Simunovic and Olufemi R. Ayeni

10 **How to Assess an Article that Deals with Health-Related Quality of Life** 93
Achilles Thoma, Jenny Santos, Margherita Cadeddu, Eric K. Duku and Charles H. Goldsmith

11 **Randomized Controlled Trial Comparing Surgical Interventions** 103
Max Solow, Raman Mundi, Vickas Khanna and Mohit Bhandari

12 **How to Assess a Pilot Trial in Surgery** 115
Guowei Li, Gillian A. Lancaster and Lehana Thabane

13 **Non-inferiority Randomized Controlled Trials** 125
Yaad Shergill, Atefeh Noori, Ngai Chow and Jason W. Busse

14 **Expertise-Based Randomized Controlled Trials** 135
Daniel Waltho, Kristen Davidge and Cagla Eskicioglu and for the Evidence-Based Surgery Working Group

15 **The Surgeon's Guide to Systematic Review and Meta-Analysis** 145
Andrea Copeland, Lucas Gallo and Noor Alolabi

16 **Prospective and Retrospective Cohort Studies** 159
Ramy Behman, Lev Bubis and Paul Karanicolas

17 **Case-Control Studies** 171
Achilles Thoma, Jenny Santos, Jessica Murphy, Eric K. Duku and Charles H. Goldsmith

18 **Evaluating Case Series in Surgery** 183
Christopher J. Coroneos and Brian Hyosuk Chin

19 **Quality Improvement and Patient Safety in Surgery** 193
Martin A. Koyle and Jessica H. Hannick

20 **Diagnostic Studies in Surgery** 201
Stuart Archibald, Jessica Murphy, Achilles Thoma and Charles H. Goldsmith

21 **How to Assess a Prognostic Study** 217
Saurabh Gupta, Kevin Kim, Emilie Belley-Côté and Richard P. Whitlock

22 **Decision Analysis and Surgery** 225
Gloria M. Rockwell and Jessica Murphy

23 **Economic Evaluations in Surgery** 239
Achilles Thoma, Feng Xie, Jenny Santos and Charles H. Goldsmith

24 **Studies Reporting Harm in Surgery** 255
Robin McLeod

25 **Evaluating Surveys and Questionnaires in Surgical Research** 265
Brian Hyosuk Chin and Christopher J. Coroneos

26 **Opinion Pieces in Surgery** 277
M. Torchia, D. Austin and I. L. Gitajn

27 Simple Statistical Tests and *P* Values 285
Charles H. Goldsmith, Eric K. Duku, Achilles Thoma and Jessica Murphy

28 Confidence Intervals 301
Jessica Bogach, Lawrence Mbuagbaw and Margherita O. Cadeddu

29 Power and Sample Size 311
Jessica Murphy, Eric K. Duku, Achilles Thoma and Charles H. Goldsmith

30 Subgroup Analyses in Surgery 327
Alexandra Hatchell and Sophocles H. Voineskos

31 Introduction to Clinical Practice Guidelines 337
Christopher J. Coroneos, Stavros A. Antoniou, Ivan D. Florez and Melissa C. Brouwers

Index 347

Contributors

Noor Alolabi Department of Orthopedics, Division of Hand and Microvascular Surgery, Mayo Clinic, Rochester, MN, USA

Stavros A. Antoniou Department of Surgery, Royal Devon and Exeter NHS Foundation Trust, Exeter, UK

Stuart Archibald Department of Surgery, Division of Head and Neck Surgery, McMaster University, Hamilton, ON, Canada

D. Austin Division of Orthopaedics, Dartmouth-Hitchcock, Lebanon, NH, USA

Olufemi R. Ayeni Department of Surgery, Division of Orthopaedic Surgery, McMaster University, Hamilton, ON, Canada; Department of Health Research Methods, Evidence, and Impact, McMaster University, Hamilton, ON, Canada

Laura Banfield Health Science Library, McMaster University, Hamilton, ON, Canada

Ramy Behman Department of Surgery, University of Toronto, Toronto, ON, Canada

Emilie Belley-Côté Department of Health Research Methods, Evidence, and Impact, Department of Medicine, Division of Cardiology & Critical Care, Population Health Research Institute, McMaster University, Hamilton, ON, Canada

Mohit Bhandari Department of Surgery, Division of Orthopaedic Surgery, McMaster University, Hamilton, ON, Canada

Neera Bhatnagar Health Science Library, HSC 2B, McMaster University, Hamilton, ON, Canada

Jessica Bogach Department of Surgery, Faculty of Health Sciences, McMaster University, Hamilton, ON, Canada

Luis H. Braga Department of Surgery, McMaster University, Hamilton, ON, Canada

Melissa C. Brouwers School of Epidemiology and Public Health, University of Ottawa, Ottawa, ON, Canada; Department of Oncology, McMaster University, Hamilton, ON, Canada

Lev Bubis Department of Surgery, University of Toronto, Toronto, ON, Canada

Jason W. Busse Department of Health Research Methods, Evidence, and Impact, McMaster University, Hamilton, ON, Canada; Department of Anesthesia, McMaster University, Hamilton, ON, Canada; Michael G. DeGroote Institute for Pain Research and Care, McMaster University, Hamilton, ON, Canada; Michael G. DeGroote Centre for Medicinal Cannabis Research, McMaster University, Hamilton, ON, Canada

Sofia Bzovsky Department of Surgery, Division of Orthopaedic Surgery, McMaster University, Hamilton, ON, Canada

Margherita Cadeddu Department of Surgery, Division of General Surgery, McMaster University, Hamilton, ON, Canada

Margherita O. Cadeddu Department of Surgery, Faculty of Health Sciences, McMaster University, Hamilton, ON, Canada

Brian Hyosuk Chin Department of Surgery, Division of Plastic Surgery, Faculty of Health Sciences, McMaster University, Hamilton, ON, Canada

Ngai Chow Department of Health Research Methods, Evidence, and Impact, McMaster University, Hamilton, ON, Canada

Andrea Copeland Department of Surgery, Division of Plastic and Reconstructive Surgery, McMaster University, Hamilton, ON, Canada

Christopher J. Coroneos Department of Surgery, Division of Plastic Surgery, Faculty of Health Sciences, McMaster University, Hamilton, ON, Canada

Ryan P. Coughlin Department of Surgery, Division of Orthopaedic Surgery, McMaster University, Hamilton, ON, Canada

Kristen Davidge Department of Surgery, Division of Plastic Surgery, University of Toronto, Toronto, ON, Canada

Gina Del Fabbro Department of Surgery, Division of Orthopaedic Surgery, McMaster University, Hamilton, ON, Canada

Aristithes G. Doumouras Department of Surgery, McMaster University, Hamilton, ON, Canada

Eric K. Duku Offord Centre for Child Studies, Department of Psychiatry and Behavioral Neurosciences, McMaster University, Hamilton, ON, Canada; Department of Health Research Methods, Evidence and Impact, McMaster University, Hamilton, ON, Canada

Seper Ekhtiari Department of Surgery, Division of Orthopaedic Surgery, McMaster University, Hamilton, ON, Canada

Cagla Eskicioglu Department of Surgery, Division of General Surgery, McMaster University, Hamilton, ON, Canada

Ivan D. Florez Department of Pediatrics, University of Antioquia, Medellin, Colombia; Department of Health Research Methods, Evidence and Impact, McMaster University, Hamilton, ON, Canada

Lucas Gallo Department of Surgery, Division of Plastic and Reconstructive Surgery, McMaster University, Hamilton, ON, Canada

I. L. Gitajn Division of Orthopaedics, Dartmouth-Hitchcock, Lebanon, NH, USA

Charles H. Goldsmith Department of Health Research Methods, Evidence and Impact, McMaster University, Hamilton, ON, Canada; Faculty of Health Sciences, Simon Fraser University, Burnaby, BC, Canada; Department of Occupational Science and Occupational Therapy, Faculty of Medicine, The University of British Columbia, Vancouver, BC, Canada

Saurabh Gupta Department of Surgery, Division of Cardiac Surgery, Department of Health Research Methods, Evidence, and Impact, McMaster University, Hamilton, ON, Canada

Jessica H. Hannick Department of Surgery, McMaster University, Hamilton, ON, Canada

Alexandra Hatchell Department of Surgery, Division of Plastic Surgery, McMaster University, Hamilton, ON, Canada

Dennis Hong Department of Surgery, St. Joseph's Healthcare, Hamilton, ON, Canada

Paul Karanicolas Department of Surgery, University of Toronto, Sunnybrook Health Sciences Centre, Sunnybrook Research Institute, Toronto, ON, Canada

Vickas Khanna Department of Surgery, Division of Orthopaedic Surgery, McMaster University, Hamilton, ON, Canada

Kevin Kim Department of Health Research Methods, Evidence and Impact, Hamilton Health Sciences, Hamilton General Hospital, Hamilton, ON, Canada

Anne Klassen Department of Pediatrics, McMaster University, Hamilton, ON, Canada

Martin A. Koyle Department of Pediatric Urology, The Hospital for Sick Children, Toronto, ON, Canada

Gillian A. Lancaster Institute of Primary Care and Health Sciences, Keele University, Keele, UK

Guowei Li Department of Health Research Methods, Evidence, and Impact, McMaster University, St. Joseph's Healthcare Hamilton, Hamilton, Canada

Joy MacDermid Roth|McFarlane Hand and Upper Limb Centre, London, Canada; Western University, London, ON, Canada; School of Rehabilitation Science, McMaster University, Hamilton, ON, Canada

Lawrence Mbuagbaw Department of Health Research Methods, Evidence and Impact, McMaster University, Hamilton, ON, Canada

Robin McLeod Department of Surgery and the Institute of Health Policy, Management and Evaluation, University of Toronto, Toronto, ON, Canada

Raman Mundi Department of Surgery, Division of Orthopaedic Surgery, McMaster University, Hamilton, ON, Canada

Jessica Murphy Department of Surgery, Division of Plastic Surgery, McMaster University, Hamilton, ON, Canada

Atefeh Noori Department of Health Research Methods, Evidence, and Impact, McMaster University, Hamilton, ON, Canada

Jo-Anne Petropoulos Health Science Library, McMaster University, Hamilton, ON, Canada

Andrea L. Pusic Department of Surgery, Brigham Health, Boston, MA, USA

Gloria M. Rockwell Department of Surgery, Division of Plastic Surgery, University of Ottawa, Ottawa, ON, Canada

Jenny Santos Department of Surgery, Division of Plastic Surgery, McMaster University, Hamilton, ON, Canada

Katherine B. Santosa Department of Surgery, University of Michigan, Ann Arbor, MI, USA

Yaad Shergill Department of Health Research Methods, Evidence, and Impact, McMaster University, Hamilton, ON, Canada

Nicole Simunovic Department of Surgery, Division of Orthopaedic Surgery, McMaster University, Hamilton, ON, Canada

Max Solow St. George's University School of Medicine, St. George's, West Indies, Grenada

Sheila Sprague Department of Surgery, Division of Orthopaedic Surgery, McMaster University, Hamilton, ON, Canada; Department of Health Research Methods, Evidence and Impact, McMaster University, Hamilton, ON, Canada

Lehana Thabane Department of Health Research Methods, Evidence, and Impact, McMaster University, St. Joseph's Healthcare Hamilton, Hamilton, Canada

Achilles Thoma Department of Surgery, Division of Plastic Surgery, McMaster University, Hamilton, ON, Canada; Department of Health Research Methods, Evidence and Impact, McMaster University, Hamilton, ON, Canada

M. Torchia Division of Orthopaedics, Dartmouth-Hitchcock, Lebanon, NH, USA

Sophocles H. Voineskos Department of Surgery, Division of Plastic Surgery, McMaster University, Hamilton, ON, Canada

Daniel Waltho Department of Surgery, Division of Plastic Surgery, McMaster University, Hamilton, ON, Canada

Richard P. Whitlock Department of Surgery, Division of Cardiac Surgery, Department of Health Research Methods, Evidence, and Impact, McMaster University, Population Health Research Institute, Hamilton, ON, Canada

Feng Xie Faculty of Health Sciences, McMaster University, Hamilton, ON, Canada; Department of Health Research Methods, Evidence, and Impact, McMaster University, Hamilton, ON, Canada

1 History of Evidence-Based Surgery (EBS)

Achilles Thoma, Jessica Murphy, Sheila Sprague and Charles H. Goldsmith

Evidence-based surgery (EBS) as a paradigm shift in surgical practice evolved from its precursor, evidence-based medicine (EBM), a term first coined by Gordon Guyatt in the early 1990s [1]. Before the development of "science-based medicine", physicians from the time of Hippocrates learned the craft of medicine, on experience. The art and knowledge of surgery was passed from teacher to student.

The EBM movement was introduced to address this gap, with a goal to ensure that patients were treated based on evidence, not the word of authorities [2]. While EBM, as a movement, is relatively new to the medical community, clinical trials have been taking place in some form since the 1500s. It has been reported that the first clinical trial was conducted, accidentally, by Ambroise Pare while treating military soldiers [3]. When the supply of oil, the standard treatment for wounds was sparse, he mixed a digestive of egg yolks, rose oil, and turpentine. Pare reported the differences between the two treatments, with those receiving the new treatment experiencing little pain and decreased swelling [3]. The first physician-conducted controlled clinical trial within the modern era was recorded 200 years later by James Lind. Lind planned a trial comparing cures for scurvy using 12 patients at sea [3]. From this study, it was discovered that citrus fruits could treat scurvy; however, it wasn't until 50 years later that the British Navy made lemon juice a part of sailors' diets [3].

Notable events that occurred since then leading the development of science-based surgery and medicine overall included: (1) The careful documentation of surgical interventions and results by Billroth and Halstead [4]; (2) the publication of the Flexner report in the early twentieth century, cementing "scientific inquiry as the bedrock of American medicine" [5]; and (3) the US FDA Kefauver-Harris Act in the

A. Thoma (✉) · J. Murphy
Department of Surgery, Division of Plastic Surgery, McMaster University, Hamilton, ON, Canada
e-mail: athoma@mcmaster.ca

J. Murphy
e-mail: murphj11@mcmaster.ca

S. Sprague
Department of Surgery, Division of Orthopaedic Surgery, McMaster University, Hamilton, ON, Canada
e-mail: sprags@mcmaster.ca

A. Thoma · S. Sprague · C. H. Goldsmith
Department of Health Research Methods, Evidence and Impact, McMaster University, Hamilton, ON, Canada
e-mail: cgoldsmi@sfu.ca

C. H. Goldsmith
Faculty of Health Sciences, Simon Fraser University, Burnaby, BC, Canada

C. H. Goldsmith
Department of Occupational Science and Occupational Therapy, Faculty of Medicine, The University of British Columbia, Vancouver, BC, Canada

A. Thoma et al. (eds.), *Evidence-Based Surgery*,
https://doi.org/10.1007/978-3-030-05120-4_1

1960s, demanding rigorous empirical testing of clinical trials in humans leading to the established claims regarding drug efficacy and safety of new pharmaceutical innovations [5].

The "experiential" nature of the development of surgery in modern times was highlighted by Meakins [6]. He believed that surgical training was performed "in a hierarchical environment" where the professor or chief likely defined the way clinical situations were to be managed, and how the operation was to be done [6].

Sometime within the 1970s and 80s a paradigm shift occurred in which evidentiary rules changed the hierarchical system mentioned above by Meakins; this new paradigm placed a higher value on evidence than authority. The protagonists in this paradigm shift were a group of clinical epidemiologists, including David Sackett (considered by most, the father of EBM), David Eddy, Archie Cochrane, and others. They highlighted the need for strengthening the empirical evidence of medicine [5–11]. They proposed the initial evidentiary rules for guiding clinical decisions, and shortly after, published the first of a series of articles in the Canadian Medical Association Journal (CMAJ) advising physicians how to appraise the medical literature [12]. This series of articles was followed by the well-known article series, Users' guides to the medical literature, first published in JAMA in 1993 [13].

Some may argue that the seeds of the EBM movement started with the publication of a rudimentary form of levels of evidence by the Canadian Task Force on Periodic Health Examination in 1976 as a result of a joint effort of the Deputy Health Ministers across the ten Canadian provinces [7]. This Task Force proposed an evidence rating system with four levels of evidence (LOE) and the corresponding types of evidence (see Fig. 1.1). This LOE rating system which is central to the philosophy of EBM and EBS was improved by Sackett to include five levels (see Fig. 1.2) [8]. These early LOE rating scales have been since modified and made more stringent to take into account a study's methodological quality [14].

The advent of the EBM movement in the early 1980s was slowly adopted by surgery, likely because the fathers of this paradigm shift were primarily internists. Their publications on the concepts of EBM focused on clinical scenarios in internal medicine that were not considered relevant to surgeons.

To introduce the principles of EBM into surgery, the definition of EMB was slightly altered to EBS by a group of surgeons and methodologists at McMaster University [15]. Evidence-Based Surgery (EBS) is thus defined as the integration of best research evidence, patients' preferences/values, health resource availability, clinical setting, and ultimately our surgical expertise. This group of surgeons and methodologists, including mentees and colleagues of David Sackett, published a series of articles in the Canadian Journal of Surgery with the goal to teach surgeons of all subspecialties the skills of appraising a surgical article before applying the conclusions of the article to their practice [15–35]. Gradually some surgical subspecialties encouraged their members to adopt the principles of EBS [36, 37]. There is an impression that the increase and quality of surgical research seen since 2000 in these specialties is due to the adoption of the EBM and EBS philosophies.

In practicing evidence-based surgery, we base our decisions on the five pillars shown in Fig. 1.3. First, we consider our patient's preferences and actions. Second, we consider the healthcare resources available to us. Third, we consider the best available evidence. Fourth, we consider the clinical setting we are practicing (e.g., academic, community, developing nation, war zone, etc.), finally we integrate these with our own surgical skills.

Since the introduction of EBM and EBS, numerous surgical training programs across North American have started to integrate evidence-based training and research into their core curriculum. Duke University's surgical departments are associated with the Duke Clinical Research Institute (DCRI). Here, surgical residents have the opportunity to receive training, participate, and lead clinical research projects [39]. The DCRI strives to create meaningful and realistic clinical trials that can shape patient care, and then integrate the results into practice [39]. Similarly, Stanford University has a Center for

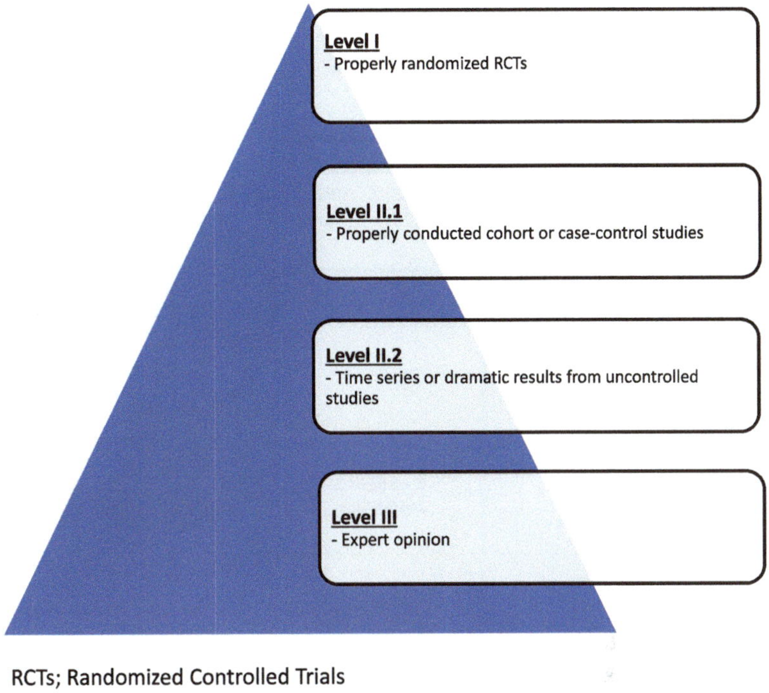

Fig. 1.1 CTFPHE's examination's levels of evidence. Adapted from the CTFPHE [7]

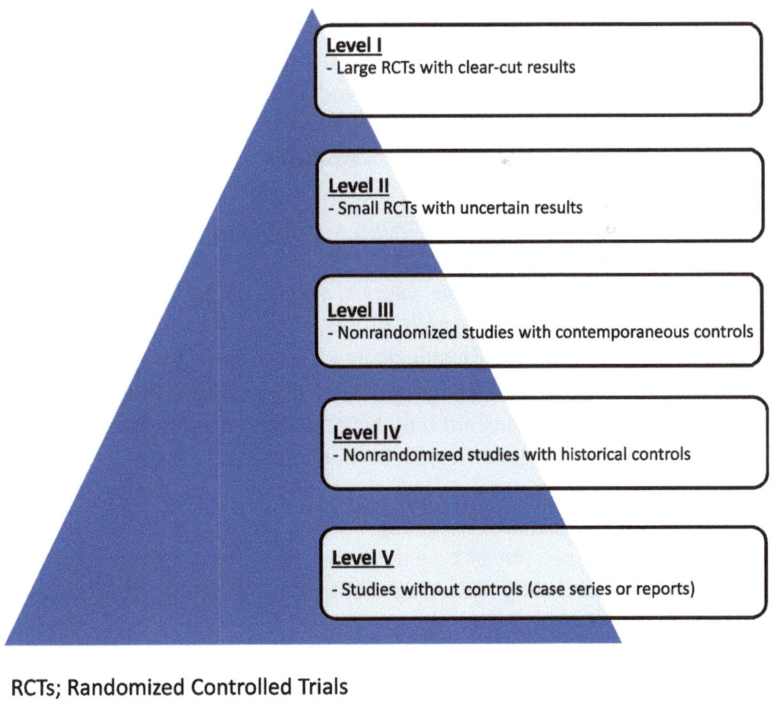

Fig. 1.2 David Sackett's levels of evidence. Adapted from Sackett et al. [8]

Fig. 1.3 Model for surgical decisions. Adapted from Haynes et al. [38]

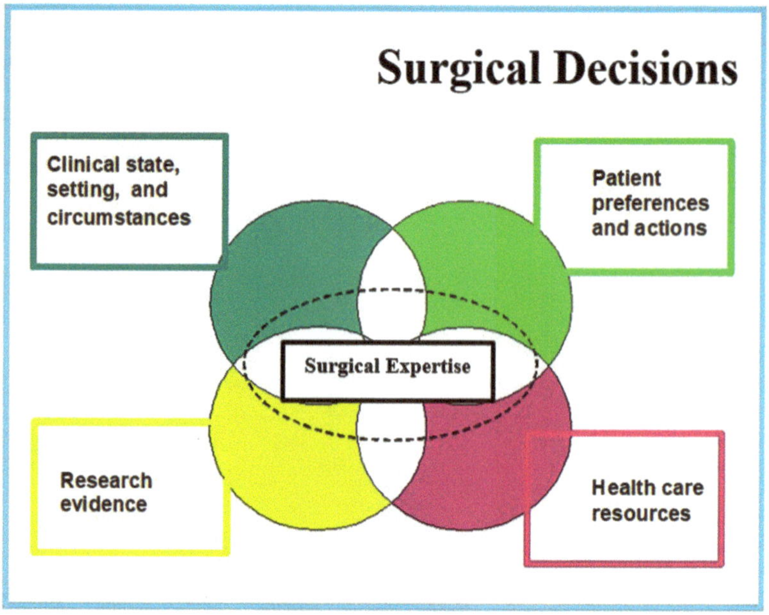

Clinical Research (SCCR) that focuses on research collaboration, innovation, and evidence-based operations [40]. The SCCR integrates educational sessions into their program with past sessions on clinical research education, good clinical practice, and the informed consent process [40]. McMaster University has included very similar programming into their core surgical curriculum by incorporating a Surgical Research Methodology (SRM) course [41]. Through this course, residents learn critical thinking and the appreciation for statistical interpretation [41]. The success of these programs can be shown through the increases in research productivity and performance in surgical residents among all disciplines [40]. It is believed that the implementation of such programs not only benefits the future careers of surgical residents but also encourages evidence-based patient care [41].

Included in many research-training courses is the introduction of research guidelines that standardize the reporting and measurement of outcomes. One of the earliest initiatives to improve outcome measurement was OMERACT (Outcome Measurements in Rheumatology) [42]. OMERACT is an independent initiative of healthcare professionals that was introduced in the early 1990s [42]. OMERACT continues to develop and validate clinical and radiographic measures in rheumatic diseases [42]. Every 2 years OMERACT organizes meetings to continuously develop outcome measure consensus among panel members within the context of musculoskeletal and autoimmune diseases [42]. Information on the OMERACT group can be found at their website, www.omeract.org.

The introduction of OMERACT was closely followed by GRADE (Grading of Recommendations Assessment, Development and Evaluation). GRADE was developed by an international panel of experts in the area of evidence-based practice [43]. The aim of GRADE was to create an easy to follow and transparent guide to rating the quality/certainty of evidence and strength of recommendations in systematic reviews and guideline development [43]. From this initiative came the development of the GRADEpro and its corresponding phone application that can be used as an all-on-one tool for summarizing and presenting information for decision-making in health care [43]. More information can be found at their website www.gradeworkinggroup.org.

GRADE was adopted by the Cochrane Collaboration to evaluate the quality of evidence from systematic reviews and further, to summarize the findings and present the evidence to decision makers [44]. The Cochrane Collaboration (named in honor of Archie Cochrane) is an independent network of researchers, professionals, healthcare workers, and patients, which was formed in the mid-2000s [45]. Its goal is to improve healthcare decisions and transform the way decisions are made in health care. To accomplish this goal, Cochrane gathers and summarizes the best evidence to help the professional make informed treatment decisions [45]. As of 2018, there are 37,000 contributors from over 130 countries working together to create a source of credible and accessible health information, free of commercial sponsorship or conflict of interest [45]. The contributors include leaders in the fields of medicine, health policy, research methodology, and consumer advocacy. The work of Cochrane is necessary as access to health evidence, and the subsequent risk of misinterpreting data increases [45]. More information on Cochrane can be found at www.cochrane.org.

To regulate the methodological quality of health measurement, the COSMIN (COnsensus-based Standards for the selection of health Measurement INstruments) initiative was developed [46]. In 2006, this group published an appraisal tool for evaluating the quality of studies based on measurement properties of health measurement instruments [46]. The checklist, which was developed in an international Delphi study, focuses on health-related patient-reported outcomes and is also useful in evaluating studies on performance-based tests or clinical rating scales [46]. More information on the COSMIN initiative, as well as their checklist, can be found at www.cosmin.nl.

The EQUATOR (Enhancing the QUAlity and Transparency Of health Research) Network is a well-known international initiative that aims to improve reliability and value of health research [47]. To accomplish this goal, the EQUATOR Network has created stringent guidelines to be used for reporting, based on study type [47]. The EQUATOR Network provides information pertaining to all of their guidelines at their website www.equator-network.org. Table 1.1 lists the guidelines and their respective study types.

While the abovementioned guidelines from the EQUATOR network outline proper reporting in the health research literature, the COMET (Core Outcome Measures in Effectiveness Trials) initiative focuses on the development and application of agreed-upon standardized outcome sets or "core outcome sets" [48]. This initiative outlines the minimum that should be both measured and reported within a clinical trial in regard to a specific condition [48]. This outlines the expectation that the identified core outcomes will be collected and reported for each respective condition, allowing results from many trials to be compared and combined [48]. The COMET handbook is available at their website: www.comet-initiative.org.

Regulating the quality of both health measurement and health reporting is incredibly important for the standardization of the clinical literature. However, maintaining public transparency of methods, anonymized results, and adverse events is potentially just as important for the overall quality of clinical research. In 1997, the Food and Drug Administration (FDA) established an up-to-date and monitored database of clinical trials [49]. This government-led website, made public in 2000, provides resources on publicly and privately supported clinical trials for patients, family members, and healthcare professionals [49]. Maintained by the National Library of Medicine (NLM) from the National Institutes of Health (NIH), this database is updated and strictly monitored to ensure up to date information [49]. This registry is a government website and therefore does not host, receive funding or advertise any commercial entities or content [49]. As of March 2018, there are over 268,000 study records on the ClinicalTrials.gov database that are being conducted in all 50 States and 203 countries [49]. The registry is a great way to stay current on developments in the various fields of medicine, find collaborating partners and identify gaps within specific areas of interest. Anyone can search this database, without registering, by visiting www.clinicaltrials.gov/ct2/home.

Researchers can also register systematic reviews with PROSPERO, the International prospective registrar of systematic reviews [50]. PROSPERO was produced by the Centre for

Table 1.1 Reporting guideline by study type

Study type	Suggested guideline	Secondary guideline
Randomized trials	CONSORT	
Observational studies	STROBE	
Systematic reviews	PRISMA	
Case reports	CARE	
Qualitative research	SRQR	COREQ
Diagnostic/prognostic studies	START	TRIPOD
Quality improvement studies	SQUIRE	
Economic evaluations	CHEERS	
Animal preclinical studies	ARRIVE	
Study protocols	SPIRIT	PRISMA-P
Clinical practice guidelines	AGREE	RIGHT

Note Information in this is taken from the EQUATOR network [47]

Reviews and Dissemination at York University and funded by the NIH [50]. This international database contains detailed information about systematic review protocols in numerous areas including health and social care, welfare, public health, and education [50]. Key features from each review protocol are recorded and maintained to provide a comprehensive list of registered systematic reviews to help avoid duplication and reduce the opportunity for reporting bias [50]. Cochrane protocols are also included in PROSPERO with links to the full protocol found on the Cochrane Library. Readers can learn more about PROSPERO by visiting: www.crd.york.ac.uk/prospero.

The application of the abovementioned guidelines helps to address the many areas of failure that can occur during the research process [51]. The EQUATOR Network guidelines, COMET handbook, and COSMIN tool are critical in the design, implementation, and reporting of clinical and observational trials; GRADE can be applied in systematic reviews, meta-analyses, and guideline development [51]. Through the integration of the recommendations of the EQUATOR guidelines, surgeons will advance reporting and transparency of surgical research; similarly, by applying COSMIN, surgical research will be more efficient. All of these initiatives will thus advance the overall philosophy of EBS. Future challenges to EBS that need to be addressed are Knowledge Translation of new advances in surgery into practice. With so many journals and information being published in both legitimate and predatory journals, the "true signal" of surgical advances may be lost in the "noise". The new generation of surgeons should be trained in appraisal skills and informed of important pre-appraised information such as systematic reviews or clinical practice guidelines. Utilizing the EQUATOR Network, COMET, COSMIN, and GRADE guidelines can help surgeons appraise and be aware of clinically important literature within their subspecialties.

References

1. Guyatt GH. Evidence-based medicine. ACP J Club. 1991; A-16:114.
2. Smith R, Rennie D. Evidence based medicine—an oral history. BMJ. 2014;348:371–3.
3. Bhatt A. Evolution of clinical research: a history before and beyond James Lind. Perspect Clin Res. 2010;1(10):6–10.
4. Imber G. Genius on the edge: the bizarre double life of Dr. William Steweard Halsted. New York: Kaplan Publishing; 2011.
5. Djulbegovic B, Guyatt GH. Progress in evidence-based medicine: a quarter century on. Lancet. 2017;290(10092):415–23.
6. Meakins JL. Innovation in surgery. Am J Surg. 2002;183:399–405.

7. Canadian Task Force on the Periodic Health Examination (CTFPHE). The periodic health examination. Can Med Assoc J. 1979;121(9):1193–254.
8. Sackett DL. Rules of evidence and clinical recommendations on the use of antithrombotic agents. Chest. 1989;95(Supp 2):2S–4S.
9. Eddy DM, Billings J. The quality of medical evidence: implications for quality of care. Health Aff (Millwood).1988;7(1):19–32.
10. Cochrane AL. Effectiveness and efficiency: random reflections on health services. London: Nuffield Provincial Hospitals Trust; 1972.
11. Eddy DM. Guidelines for the cancer related checkup: recommendations and rationale. CA: Cancer J Clin. 1980;30:3–50.
12. Sackett DL. How to read clinical journals: I. Why to read them and how to start reading them critically. Can Med Assoc J. 1981;124(5):555–8.
13. Oxman AD, Sackett DL, Guyatt GH. Users' guides to the medical literature. I. How to get started. The evidence-based medicine working group. JAMA. 1993;270(17):2093–95.
14. Oxford Centre for Evidence-based Medicine. Levels of evidence (March) 2009. http://www.cebm.net/oxfordcentre-evidence-based-medicine-levels-evidence-march-2009. Accessed 8 Aug 2014.
15. Archibald S, Bhandari M, Thoma A. Evidence based surgery series. Users' guide to the surgical literature: how to use an article about a diagnostic test. Can J Surg. 2001;44(1):17–23.
16. Urschel J, Tandan V, Miller J, Goldsmith CH. Users' guide to evidence-based surgery: how to use an article evaluating surgical interventions. Can J Surg. 2001;44(2):95–100.
17. Thoma A, Sprague S, Tandan V. Users' guide to the surgical literature: how to use an article on economic analysis. Can J Surg. 2001;44:347–55.
18. Hong D, Tandan V, Goldsmith CH, Simunovic M. Users' guide to the surgical literature: how to use an article reporting population-based volume-outcome relationships in surgery. Can J Surg. 2002;45(2): 109–15.
19. Birch D, Eady A, Robertson D, De Pauw S, Tandan V. Users' guide to the surgical literature: how to perform a literature search. Can J Surg. 2003;46(2):136–41.
20. Bhandari M, Devereaux PJ, Montori V, Cinà C, Tandan V, Guyatt GH. Users' guide to the surgical literature: how to use a systematic literature review and meta-analysis. Can J Surg. 2004;47(1):60–7.
21. Thoma A, Farrokhyar F, Bhandari M, Tandan V. The evidence-based surgery working group. Users' guide to the surgical literature: how to assess a randomized controlled trial in surgery. Can J Surg. 2004;47 (3):200–8.
22. Birch D, Goldsmith CH, Tandan V. Users' guide to the surgical literature: self audit and practice appraisal for surgeons. Can J Surg. 2005;48(1):57–62.
23. Mastracci TM, Thoma A, Farrokhyar F, Tandan VR, Cina CS. Users' guide to the surgical literature: how to use a decision analysis. Can J Surg. 2007;50 (5):403–9.
24. Thoma A, Cornacchi S, Lovrics P, Goldsmith CH. Users' guide to the surgical literature: how to assess an article on health-related quality of life. Can J Surg. 2008;51(3):215–24.
25. Cadeddu M, Farrokhyar F, Thoma A, Haines T, Garnett A, Goldsmith CH. Users' guide to the surgical literature: how to assess power and sample size. Can J Surg. 2008;51(6):476–82.
26. Hansebout R, Cornacchi SD, Haines T, Goldsmith CH. Users' guide to the surgical literature: how to use an article on prognosis. Can J Surg. 2009;52(4):328–36.
27. Dijkman B, Kooistra B, Bhandari M. Users' guide to the surgical literature: how to work with a subgroup analysis. Can J Surg. 2009;52(6):515–22.
28. Thoma A, Cornacchi SD, Farrokhyar F, Bhandari M, Goldsmith CH. Users' guides to the surgical literature: how to assess a survey in surgery. Can J Surg. 2011;54(6):394–402.
29. Cadeddu M, Farrokhyar F, Levis C, Cornacchi, Haines T, Thoma A. For the evidence-based surgery working group. Users' guide to the surgical literature: understanding confidence intervals. Can J Surg. 2012;55(3):207–11.
30. Coroneos CJ, Voineskos SH, Cornacchi SD, Goldsmith CH, Ignacy TA, Thoma A. Users' guide to the surgical literature: how to evaluate clinical practice guidelines. Can J Surg. 2014;57(4):280–6.
31. Waltho D, Kaur MN, Haynes RB, Farrokhyar F, Thoma A. Users' guide to the surgical literature: how to perform a high-quality literature search. Can J Surg. 2015;58(5):349–58.
32. Thoma A, Kaur MN, Farrokhyar F, Waltho D, Levis C, Lovrics P, Goldsmith CH. Users' guide to the surgical literature: how to assess an article about harm in surgery. Can J Surg. 2016;59(5):351–7.
33. Gallo L, Eskicioglu C, Braga L, Farrokhyar F, Thoma A. Users' guide to the surgical literature: how to assess an article using surrogate outcomes. Can J Surg. 2017;60(4):280–7.
34. Thoma A, Farrokhyar F, Waltho D, Braga LH, Sprague S, Goldsmith CH. Users' guide to the surgical literature: how to assess a noninferiority trial. Can J Surg. 2017;60(6):426–32.
35. Gallo L, Murphy J, Braga L, Farrokhyar F, Thoma A. Users' guide to the surgical literature: how to assess a qualitative study. Can J Surg. Accepted for publication October 2017.
36. Thoma A. Evidence-based plastic surgery: design, measurement and evaluation. Toronto Ontario: Clin Plastic Surg. 2008;35(2):ix.
37. Bhandari M, editor. Evidence-based orthopedics. Oxford: Wiley-Blackwell; 2012.
38. Haynes RB, Devereaux PJ, Guyatt GH. Clinical expertise in the era of evidence-based medicine and patient choice. BMJ Evid-Based Med. 2002;7:36–8.
39. Duke University. Duke Clinical Research Institute: from thought leadership to clinical practice—about

us [Internet]. Duke University; 2017 [cited 13 Mar 2018]. Available from https://www.dcri.org/about/who-we-are/.
40. Stanford University. Stanford Center for Clinical Research (SCCR) [Internet]. Stanford University; 2018 [cited 13 Mar 2018]. Available from http://med.stanford.edu/sccr.html.
41. Farrokhyar F, Amin N, Dath D, Bhandari M, Kelly S, Kolkin AM, et al. Impact of the surgical research methodology program on surgical residents' research profiles. J Surg Educ. 2014;71(4):513–20.
42. OMERACT Outcome Measures in Rheumatology. Welcome to OMERACT [Internet]. OMERACT [cited 19 Mar 2018]. Available from http://www.omeract.org.
43. GRADE Working Group. GRADE: welcome to the grade working group—from evidence to recommendations—transparent and sensible [Internet]. GRADE working group [cited 13 Mar 2018]. Available from http://www.gradeworkinggroup.org/.
44. McMaster University Mac GRADE Centre. About GRADE [Internet]. McMaster University [cited 29 Mar 2018]. Available from https://cebgrade.mcmaster.ca/aboutgrade.html.
45. Cochrane. About Us [Internet]. Cochrane group [cited 29 Mar 2018]. Available from http://www.cochrane.org/about-us.
46. VU University Medical Center. COSMIN [Internet]. VU University [cited 13 Mar 2018]. Available from http://www.cosmin.nl/.
47. The EQUATOR Network. Equator network—about us [Internet]. The EQUATOR network [cited 13 Mar 2018]. Available from http://www.equator-network.org/about-us/x.
48. COMET Initiative. The COMET initiative [Internet]. COMET [cited 13 Mar 2018]. Available from http://www.comet-initiative.org/.
49. National Institute of Health (NIH). Clinicaltrials.gov [Internet]. NIH [cited 20 Mar 2018]. Available from http://www.clinicaltrials.gov.
50. University of York Centre for Reviews and Dissemination—PROSPERO. About PROSPERO [Internet]. York [cited 29 Mar 2018]. Available from https://www.crd.york.ac.uk/prospero/#aboutpage.
51. Innes N, Schwendicke F, Lamont T. How do we create, and improve the evidence? Br Dent J. 2016;220(12):651–5.

2 The Steps of Practicing Evidence-Based Surgery (EBS)

Achilles Thoma, Sheila Sprague, Luis H. Braga and Sophocles H. Voineskos

In Chap. 1, we explained the historical development of the Evidence-Based Medicine (EBM) and Evidence-Based Surgery (EBS) and paradigm shifts of practicing medicine and surgery to the present era. EBS is defined as an approach of practicing surgery in which the surgeon is aware of the best evidence in support of practice and the strength of that evidence.

In 2008, the *British Medical Journal (BMJ)* hailed this paradigm shift as one of the 15 most important milestones in medicine in the last 150 years [1]. The experiential and authoritarian approach to learning and practicing medicine and surgery in the past has been supplanted by the evidence-based approach [2]. Many surgeons, however, are not familiar with the concepts of EBS and how they can be applied. We hope that this book will help close that gap.

This chapter will show you step by step how to adopt an evidence-based approach to your surgical practice. There are five distinct steps in the process of systematically finding, appraising, and using the contemporaneous research findings as the basis for clinical decisions [3].

These steps need to be followed precisely in their correct order (see Table 2.1). They will become clearer as you read the following chapters of the book, which go into more detail and also explain the methodological issues of the various study designs.

STEP 1. Construct a relevant, answerable **question** from a clinical scenario.

The construction of a clinically relevant, answerable question from a surgical case that you encounter in your clinical practice is the first step. This step is important for both the "Users" of clinical research, i.e., those who want to know, like most of us surgeons but also other stakeholders such as other clinicians, patients, patients' families, policy decision-makers, administrators, and general public. It is also necessary for the "Doers", such as investigator surgeons, who intend to find the answer to a surgical question through clinical research.

An example of a relevant clinical question is described below.

A. Thoma (✉)
Department of Surgery, Division of Plastic Surgery, Department of Health Research Methods, Evidence and Impact, McMaster University, Hamilton, ON, Canada
e-mail: athoma@mcmaster.ca

S. Sprague
Department of Surgery, Division of Orthopaedic Surgery, Department of Health Research Methods, Evidence and Impact, McMaster University, Hamilton, ON, Canada
e-mail: sprags@mcmaster.ca

L. H. Braga
Department of Surgery, McMaster University, Hamilton, ON, Canada

S. H. Voineskos
Department of Surgery, Division of Plastic Surgery, McMaster University, Hamilton, ON, Canada
e-mail: Sophocles.voineskos@medportal.ca

A. Thoma et al. (eds.), *Evidence-Based Surgery*,
https://doi.org/10.1007/978-3-030-05120-4_2

Table 2.1 Steps to evidence-based surgery

1	Construct a relevant, answerable **question** from a clinical scenario (see Chap. 3)
2	Plan and carry out a literature **search** for best external evidence (see Chap. 4)
3	Critically **appraise** the literature for validity and applicability (see Chaps. 6, 10 and 11)
4	**Apply** the evidence to your clinical practice (see resolution of scenarios in Chaps. 6, 10 and 11)
5	**Evaluate** your performance

Scenario

At the weekly general surgery rounds, a senior surgeon challenged a newly appointed colorectal surgeon when he claimed that the incidence of ureteral injury is lower with a laparoscopic approach rather than with open surgery because of better visibility.

This is a plausible scenario that can generate enough controversy to create a research question. The answer to this question may not be readily available. To find it, we proceed as suggested in Step 1, developing a clinically relevant and answerable question from this scenario. The question is structured in such a way as to identify the **P**opulation or **P**atients, **I**ntervention, **C**omparative Intervention, **O**utcome, and **T**ime Horizon. These terms can be remembered by the acronym **PICOT** [4, 5].

For the abovementioned scenario, the proper research question using the structure of PICOT would be, "In colorectal cancer patients, does laparoscopic, as compared to open surgery, result in less ureteral injury 30 days following surgery?"

As a rule of thumb, we ask such questions in one breath. If you cannot ask such PICOT formatted question in one breath, it means that your question is convoluted. Try practicing "one breath PICOT questions until you become an expert".

The structure and formulation of the research question are discussed in more detail in Chap. 3.

STEP 2. Plan and carry out a **search** of the literature for best external evidence.

For the literature search conducted in this step, we select key words using our PICOT formulation, which as you remember is generated from our clinical scenario/problem. Such key words will include "colon cancer", "laparoscopic surgery", "open Surgery", and "ureter injury".

These key words are then first entered into a filtered electronic database to see if any articles address the research question. Filtered databases, such as the Cochrane Database, include articles pre-appraised by methodological experts. If there are no hits obtained on this database, an unfiltered database could be used. Unfiltered databases are ones in which articles go through the usual review process; examples of unfiltered database are Medline or Embase.

The literature search is an important step and all surgeons should be familiar with it; for more detailed information on how to perform and evaluate a literature search please see Chap. 4.

STEP 3. Critically **appraise** the literature for validity and applicability.

The appraisal of a surgical article involves answering three important questions:

Question #1: Is the study presented in the article valid?
Question #2: If valid, what were the results?
Question #3: Can the results be applied to my patients or practice?

Depending on the study design we are examining, each of these three main questions may have additional subsidiary questions. These questions will be a recurrent theme in the chapters to follow. If on reading the article, in particular the methods section, you do not believe it is valid, do not waste your time reading the article in its' entirety. If on the other hand, you believe it is valid, then you should proceed and examine the results and what they may mean for the study group in the article and potentially, your own patients. Chapter 6 explains how to interpret the results of surgical interventions. This book contains chapters dedicated to explaining how to appraise properly, the evidence, based on the specific content or methodology used in a study.

STEP 4. Apply the evidence to your clinical practice.

If you believe that the investigators have used correct methods in their study and on assessing their results, you find that the novel intervention shows better results than the standard approach you are using, then you need to decide if you can apply them to your practice.

This decision will be made if you believe that the patients examined in the article you read are similar to your patients. If, for example, the study was done in pediatric patients, but your patients are adults, the study's results may not be applicable to your practice. You may also consider the clinical resources available to you as you may be working in a rural hospital, where you may not have access to the latest technological advances (e.g., robotic surgery, single-port laparoscopic instrumentation).

STEP 5. Evaluate your effectiveness and efficiency in carrying out Steps 1–4.

(A) Evaluate your performance in asking answerable questions.
(B) Evaluate your performance in searching and finding external evidence through electronic database searching.
(C) Evaluate your performance in critical appraisal.
(D) Evaluate your performance in integrating evidence and patients' values into your practice.

Make sure to conduct an ongoing evaluation, ideally with the help of a mentor, of the effects the implementation of this new evidence has made in your practice.

How to Apply Steps 1–5

An example of how to apply the abovementioned steps into your practice is shown below. For this example, the following scenario will be used:

> At the weekly general surgery rounds, a senior surgeon challenged a newly appointed colorectal surgeon (who just completed his fellowship) when the young surgeon claimed that the incidence of ureteral injury is lower with the laparoscopic technique than the open technique during colorectal surgery. He claimed that the laparoscopic method because of better visualization is less likely to lead to damage of the ureter. The head of the Division asks the Minimal Access Surgery Fellow in the Service to review the surgical literature and report whether this is true or not at next week's rounds.

STEP 1. Construct a relevant, answerable **question** from a clinical scenario.

Using the PICOT as a guide, your clinical question would include the following:

Population: Patients undergoing colorectal surgery.
Intervention: Laparoscopic surgery.
Comparison Intervention: Open-technique surgery.
Outcome: Ureteral injury.
Time Horizon: Up to 30 days following surgery.

Therefore, the finalized research question would be: *In patients undergoing colorectal surgery, is laparoscopic surgery less likely to result in damage to the ureter than open-technique surgery, 30 days post-surgery?*

STEP 2. Plan and carry out a **search** of the literature for best external evidence.

Using your search tool of chose, whether filtered or unfiltered, the PICOT elements would be entered in order to find the best evidence for your question. For example, to find articles related to the above-stated research question, we would want to use the following search terms: *Colorectal Cancer* AND *Ureteral Injury* AND *Laparoscopic Surgery* AND *Open*.

Below is an example of how you would perform a literature search using The Cochrane Library (Fig. 2.1a and b).

As an appropriate article was not found using the Cochrane database, a search in PubMed can be used (Fig. 2.2a and b).

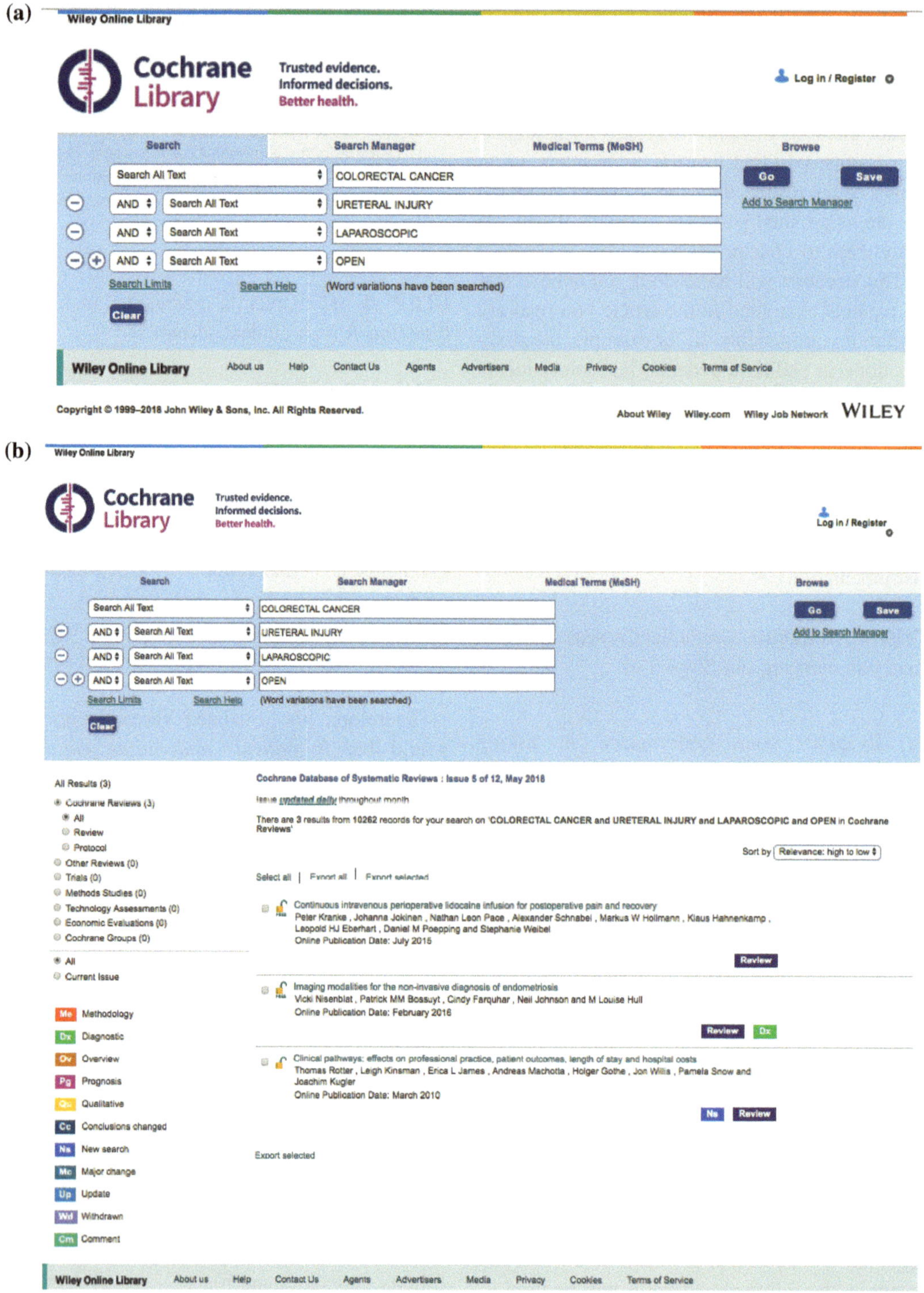

Fig. 2.1 **a** Search terms from your research questions are entered. **b** A list of appropriate articles

(a)

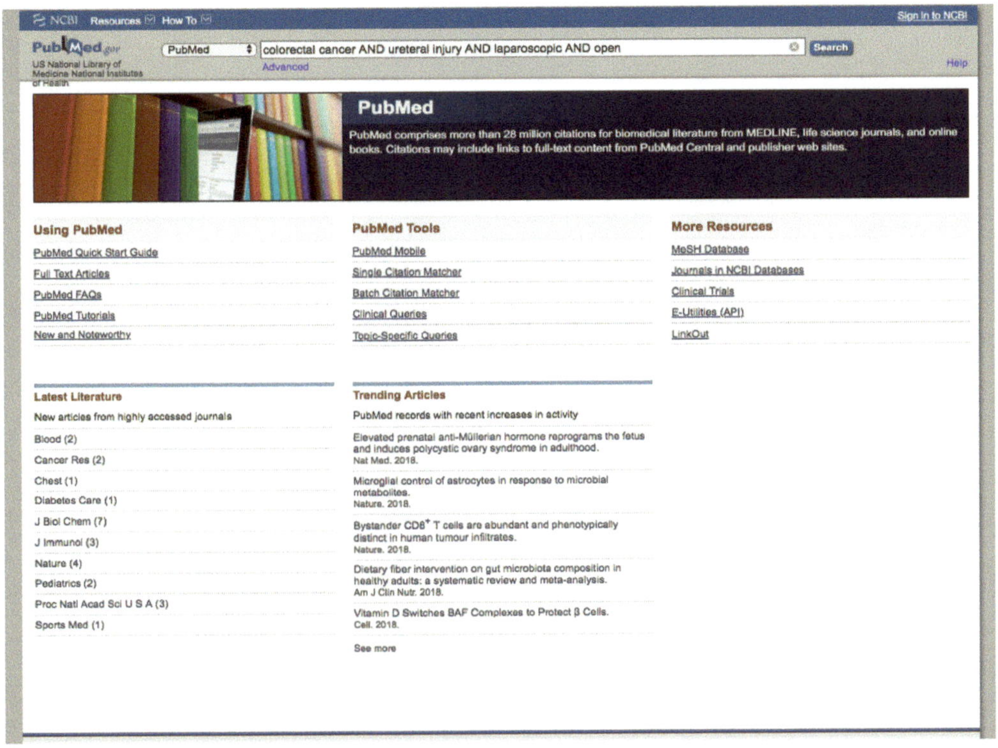

(b)

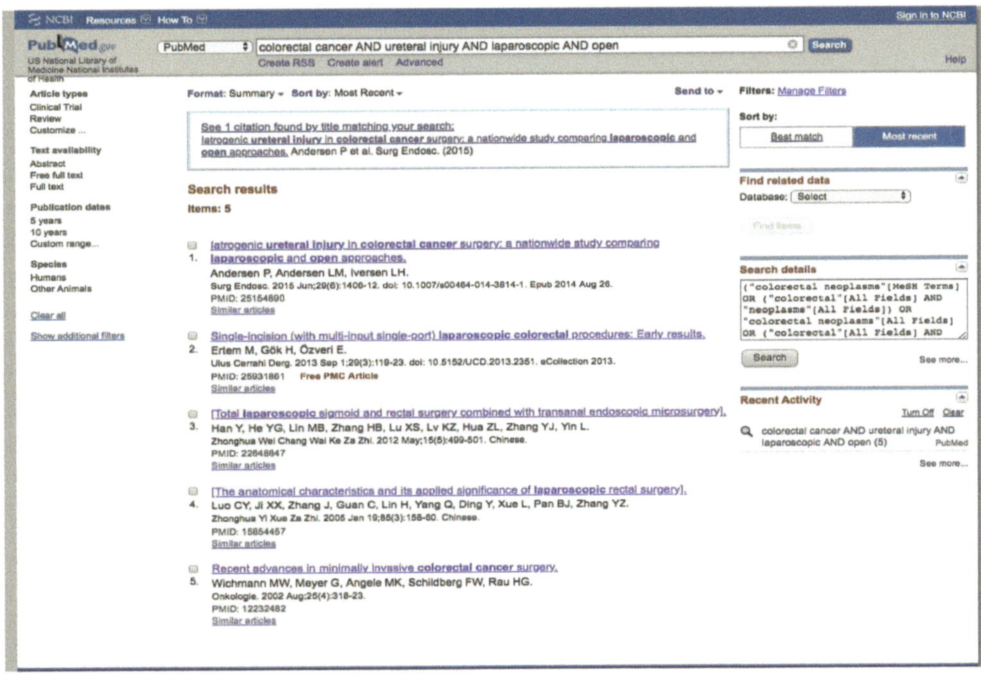

Fig. 2.2 **a** Search terms from your research question are entered. **b** A list of appropriate articles for your research question is listed

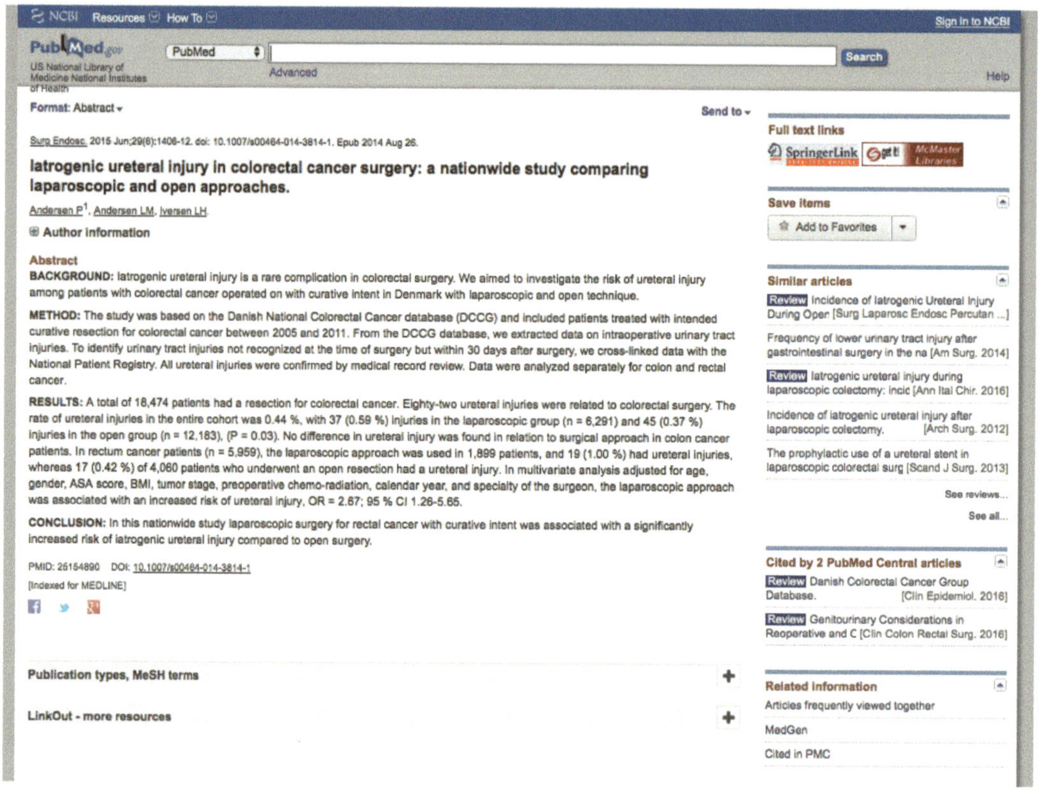
NCBI Resources How To Sign in to NCBI

PubMed.gov US National Library of Medicine National Institutes of Health | PubMed | Search | Advanced | Help

Format: Abstract Send to

Surg Endosc. 2015 Jun;29(6):1406-12. doi: 10.1007/s00464-014-3814-1. Epub 2014 Aug 26.

Iatrogenic ureteral injury in colorectal cancer surgery: a nationwide study comparing laparoscopic and open approaches.

Andersen P[1], Andersen LM, Iversen LH.

Author information

Abstract

BACKGROUND: Iatrogenic ureteral injury is a rare complication in colorectal surgery. We aimed to investigate the risk of ureteral injury among patients with colorectal cancer operated on with curative intent in Denmark with laparoscopic and open technique.

METHOD: The study was based on the Danish National Colorectal Cancer database (DCCG) and included patients treated with intended curative resection for colorectal cancer between 2005 and 2011. From the DCCG database, we extracted data on intraoperative urinary tract injuries. To identify urinary tract injuries not recognized at the time of surgery but within 30 days after surgery, we cross-linked data with the National Patient Registry. All ureteral injuries were confirmed by medical record review. Data were analyzed separately for colon and rectal cancer.

RESULTS: A total of 18,474 patients had a resection for colorectal cancer. Eighty-two ureteral injuries were related to colorectal surgery. The rate of ureteral injuries in the entire cohort was 0.44 %, with 37 (0.59 %) injuries in the laparoscopic group (n = 6,291) and 45 (0.37 %) injuries in the open group (n = 12,183), (P = 0.03). No difference in ureteral injury was found in relation to surgical approach in colon cancer patients. In rectum cancer patients (n = 5,959), the laparoscopic approach was used in 1,899 patients, and 19 (1.00 %) had ureteral injuries, whereas 17 (0.42 %) of 4,060 patients who underwent an open resection had a ureteral injury. In multivariate analysis adjusted for age, gender, ASA score, BMI, tumor stage, preoperative chemo-radiation, calendar year, and specialty of the surgeon, the laparoscopic approach was associated with an increased risk of ureteral injury, OR = 2.67; 95 % CI 1.26-5.65.

CONCLUSION: In this nationwide study laparoscopic surgery for rectal cancer with curative intent was associated with a significantly increased risk of iatrogenic ureteral injury compared to open surgery.

PMID: 25154890 DOI: 10.1007/s00464-014-3814-1

[Indexed for MEDLINE]

Publication types, MeSH terms

LinkOut - more resources

Full text links: SpringerLink | McMaster Libraries

Save items: Add to Favorites

Similar articles
- Review Incidence of Iatrogenic Ureteral Injury During Oper [Surg Laparosc Endosc Percutan ...]
- Frequency of lower urinary tract injury after gastrointestinal surgery in the na [Am Surg. 2014]
- Review Iatrogenic ureteral injury during laparoscopic colectomy: incic [Ann Ital Chir. 2016]
- Incidence of iatrogenic ureteral injury after laparoscopic colectomy. [Arch Surg. 2012]
- The prophylactic use of a ureteral stent in laparoscopic colorectal surg [Scand J Surg. 2013]

See reviews... See all...

Cited by 2 PubMed Central articles
- Review Danish Colorectal Cancer Group Database. [Clin Epidemiol. 2016]
- Review Genitourinary Considerations in Reoperative and C [Clin Colon Rectal Surg. 2016]

Related information
- Articles frequently viewed together
- MedGen
- Cited in PMC

Fig. 2.3 Abstract review of chosen article

Using PubMed, using the same search terms, five articles, which were better suited to answer the research question, were found. After reviewing the available articles, you choose the article that best addresses your research question, in this example, the selected article is iatrogenic ureteral injury in colorectal cancer surgery: a nationwide study comparing laparoscopic and open approaches by Andersen et al. [6]. This article appears to be a possibly relevant article to give answer your research question. You then proceed to read the abstract shown in Fig. 2.3. If it looks promising we then proceed to read the whole article.

STEP 3. Critically **appraise** the literature for validity and applicability.

Question 1: Is the study valid?

The validity of the chosen study will be judged in different ways based on the methodology and focus of the article. For example, with this article, we may look at if patients in the two groups were similar in regard to prognostic factors known to be associated with the outcome. In this particular example, Andersen et al. [6] explained that the two groups were comparable in gender; however, there were significant differences, including but not limited to age, body mass index, and tumor stage. A second question regarding validity may be to look at if follow-up time was sufficiently completed. In the article of Andersen et al. [6], patients were included if they had surgery between January 2005 and December 2011, the database used had a completeness rate of over 96% and it followed patients up to 30 days after surgery. Therefore, it would be acceptable to state that follow-up was sufficient.

Question 2: What were the results?

When listing the results of Andersen et al. [6], one could look at the association between the exposed and the outcome. For example, those patients who had open surgery, 0.37% suffered ureteric injury; 0.59% experienced ureteric injury in the laparoscopic group. The authors claimed that, for the whole cohort, laparoscopic surgery was significantly associated with an increased risk of iatrogenic ureteral injury; an odds ratio of 1.64 and 95% Confidence Interval of 1.02–2.63, $p = 0.04$ was given. An odds ratio greater than 1 indicates a higher risk of harm in the exposed group (the laparoscopic group). The odds ratio was calculated using a multivariable analysis to control for the differences in risk factors between groups.

Question 3: Can the results be applied to my patients or practice?

When answering question three, one needs to consider if the patients in the study were similar to patients in your practice, if the exposure is similar to what might occur in your patients, the magnitude of the risk, and any possible benefits associated with the exposure. In this example article, the patients in the study were from Denmark; therefore, this may be something to consider when applying results to your patients.

STEP 4. Apply the evidence to your clinical practice.

If you believe that the patients and the technique and magnitude of risk and benefits described in the article are all similar to yours, you should consider applying the evidence to your practice.

STEP 5. Evaluate your performance.

The final step in EBS practice is the continuous assessment of your performance in implementing all the steps mentioned above. You may want to approach a mentor and ask him/her to provide you with feedback on whether you mastered the skills of (a) constructing answerable questions on the PICOT format (b) performing successful literature searches to find the best evidence (c) appraising what you read and are capable of separating "the chaff from the wheat" and (d) implementing what you found in your practice.

References

1. Kamerow D. Milestones, tombstones, and sex education. BMJ. 2007;334:0–a.
2. Meakins JL. Innovation in surgery: the rules of evidence. Am J Surg. 2002;183(4):399–405.
3. Sackett DL, Strauss SE, Richardson WS, Rosenberg W, Haynes RB. Evidence-based medicine: how to practice and teach EBM. 2nd ed. Edinburgh, Scotland: Churchill Livingston; 2000.
4. Richardson WS, Wilson MC, Nishikawa J, Hayward RS. The well-built clinical question: a key to evidence-based decisions. ACP J Club. 1995;123(3):A12–3.
5. Nollan R, Fineout-Overhold E, Stephenson P. Asking compelling clinical questions. In: Melnyk BM, Fineout-Overhold E, editors. Evidence-based practice in nursing and healthcare: a guide to best practice. 2nd ed. Philadelphia, PA: Lippincott Williams & Wilkins; 2005.
6. Andersen P, Andersen LM, Iversen LH. Iatrogenic ureteral injury in colorectal cancer surgery: a nationwide study comparing laparoscopic and open approaches. Sur Endosc. 2015;39:1406–12.

3 Developing a Surgical Clinical Research Question: *To Find the Answer in Literature Search or in Pursuing Clinical Research*

Achilles Thoma, Sheila Sprague, Sophocles H. Voineskos and Jessica Murphy

Abbreviations

FINER Criteria	F: Feasible; I: Interesting; N: Novel; E: Ethical; R: Relevant
PICOT Format	P: Population; I: Intervention; C: Comparison Intervention; O: Outcome; T: Time Horizon
QOL	Quality of Life
DIEP	Deep Inferior Epigastric Perforator
NIH	National Institute of Health
TAP Blocks	Transverse Abdominal Plane Blocks
ECTR	Endoscopic Carpal Tunnel Release
OCTR	Open Carpal Tunnel Release

In clinical practice, we are faced with clinical questions on a daily basis by our medical students, surgical residents, colleagues or patients. While we frequently know, and can readily provide an answer, sometimes this is not the case and we must proceed to find it through a literature search. In such cases, we suggest utilizing the approach to literature searches described by Banfield et al. in Chap. 4. If we do not know the answer and we cannot find it in the surgical literature, we may decide to find it by performing a clinical research project.

Whether it is to find the evidence through a literature search or via a clinical experimentation, the structure of the research question follows the same format. This chapter will explain how to properly form a research question, as it is the foundation of clinical evidence and proper clinical research. To understand and interpret the findings of a surgical article, or to design one's own clinical research project, a surgeon must master the art of formulating "the clinical research question". The posing of the research question should be automatic in a surgeon's daily practice just like driving. The same applies to the surgeon-investigator; however, in this case, prior knowledge on the subject must be identified through a literature search. Being familiar with the current knowledge in an area is also known as understanding the "boundary of knowledge"; this must be done prior to forming the research question [1].

A. Thoma (✉)
Department of Surgery, Division of Plastic Surgery, Department of Health Research Methods, Evidence and Impact, McMaster University, Hamilton, ON, Canada
e-mail: athoma@mcmaster.ca

S. Sprague
Department of Surgery, Division of Orthopaedic Surgery, Department of Health Research Methods, Evidence and Impact, McMaster University, Hamilton, ON, Canada
e-mail: sprags@mcmaster.ca

S. H. Voineskos · J. Murphy
Department of Surgery, Division of Plastic Surgery, McMaster University, Hamilton, ON, Canada
e-mail: Sophocles.voineskos@medportal.ca

J. Murphy
e-mail: murphj11@mcmaster.ca

A. Thoma et al. (eds.), *Evidence-Based Surgery*,
https://doi.org/10.1007/978-3-030-05120-4_3

There are two types of clinical questions that are frequently asked in surgery: (1) background questions and (2) foreground questions [2, 3]. The background questions are the ones usually asked by medical students, surgical interns, and other learners early in their training. These types of questions ask for general knowledge about a surgical problem and have two essential components: (1) a question root (what, who, when, where, how, why) with a verb and (2) a surgical problem. Examples of such questions are: (1) What causes ileus after laparotomy? (2) Why do some thin mastectomy skin flaps undergo necrosis? (3) When should a temporary ileostomy be reversed?

The foreground questions, on the other hand, should be asked by senior surgical residents, surgical fellows, and surgeons. These questions ask about the management of patients with surgical problems.

It is important for a research question to be persuasive and clear. A compelling and concise research question helps guide and create a successful study, and is appealing to both grant agencies and institutions.

This chapter will focus on two tools that can be used to help form a proper research question: (1) The FINER (Feasible, Interesting Novel, Ethical, Relevant) Criteria [4–6] and (2) The PICOT (Population, Intervention, Comparative intervention, Outcomes, Time Horizon) formulation [7, 8].

The FINER Criteria

The FINER criteria, (Table 3.1) have been proposed as important preconditions to develop a good research question [4–6]. These criteria, outlined further below, help to highlight the aspects that should be addressed to increase the chances of success in a research project.

Feasible

This aspect focuses on whether or not there are (1) an adequate number of patients (participants);

Table 3.1 The FINER criteria

Criteria	Definition
Feasible	Is the research question manageable? (i.e., enough participants, expertise, time, and money)
Interesting	Do the investigator and the target audience find the research question to be clinically important?
Novel	Does the research question contribute new information to the literature?
Ethical	Is the question ethical? (a clinical research question should be investigated when it is ethical to do so; it requires approval by an Ethics Review Board)
Relevant	Will the research question make an impact, guide further research, or influence practice?

Adapted from Hulley et al. [4]

(2) technical expertise; (3) resources (time, support staff, and money); and (4) a proper study design, to make the project manageable [4–6]. There are numerous barriers that may arise from each research project.

For example, a study with the following research question: *"Does the supramicrosurgical periumbilical abdominal flap provide better Quality of Life (QOL) as compared to the deep inferior epigastric perforator (DIEP) flap in breast reconstruction after mastectomy?"* may experience the following technical barriers: (1) We do not know how to transfer a flap with a 0.8 mm luminal diameter of the vascular pedicle and (2) We do not have the required super delicate microsurgical instruments. Additionally, there is the following study design barrier (3) QOL scales may not be sensitive enough to capture the difference. Therefore, the research question may need to be reassessed based on feasibility.

Interesting

This aspect asks whether or not the outcomes of your study will be of interest to your peers, including other surgeons, healthcare providers, and patients [4–6]. Hulley et al. [4] recommend speaking with mentors, potential funding agencies and experts in the area to determine if your proposed research question will be of interest to a large audience.

For example, the use of suprafascial perforator flaps for postmastectomy reconstruction would be of great interest to patients. With this technique of harvesting autogenous tissue to reconstruct a breast, the patient will not worry about the potential of abdominal hernia or abdominal bulge as the abdominal muscles are not interfered with.

Novel

This variable asks if your research will provide new information, or if it will refute, confirm or extend previous findings. An important aspect of each research project is explaining why this project is important in light of what is already known [4–6]. Additionally, a research question can be novel, while at the same time not being completely original. The novelty of your research question can be established with a literature search, which can help identify gaps and remaining questions in your research area. For example, recreating a previous study but reducing past limitations, or focusing on a new population, could also be considered novel [4].

For example, the suprafascial periumbilical perforator flaps for postmastectomy reconstruction is a novel technique for harvesting autogenous tissue for reconstruction and extends the boundary of microsurgical instrumentation and skills [9].

Ethical

While there is a certain level of risk associated with most research projects, one must ensure that the proposed research project will be amendable to approval by the local research ethics board [4–6]. If an original research question poses unacceptable risks to patients/participants, it may be possible to utilize a different study design to find the appropriate answer. Although the Randomized Control Trial design with a narrow Confidence Interval would provide the highest level of evidence in a question of effectiveness, this study design would not be deemed ethical if the research question is about harm. For a question of Harm in surgery, a better study design is a case–control study [10].

Relevant

Lastly, this aspect asks whether or not the issue that is under consideration in a project is clinically relevant to physicians/surgeons, patients, health policymakers, and other researchers. This aspect also focuses on if the issue being researched is timely [4–6]. The National Institutes of Health (NIH), in the United States of America, emphasizes the importance of a research question. By importance, we mean how the results, will improve knowledge, and how results will impact clinical services, methods, and concepts [4].

For example, the use of the suprafascial periumbilical perforator flap will be deemed relevant and timely to the stakeholders mentioned above. An older technique for breast reconstruction such as a regional pedicled skin flap would be considered a "historical" method of reconstruction and not currently relevant.

While the FINER criteria justify a planned research project, The PICOT format helps in the development of a specific research question [6] which will help us find the answer through the literature search if we are "Users" of surgical research. If we are "Doers" of surgical research, it will help us formulate our research question before we submit it to the local ethics committee or a granting agency.

The PICOT Format

The sooner a surgeon adopts the PICOT format the earlier he/she becomes able to search the literature and find the answer to a clinical problem. For the surgeon-investigator, a clinical question posed in the PICOT format will guide research. Once a systematic review is complete and the "boundary of knowledge" is understood, the question can be formed.

The PICOT format, summarized in Table 3.2, includes the following components: (1) patient or population, (2) intervention, (3) comparative intervention, (4) outcome, and (5) time horizon [3, 5–8]. For the surgeon-investigator a clinical question posed in the PICOT format will guide research. The PICOT format is outlined in more detail in the following text, which demands clarification for each of its components.

Patient or Population

For the first component, *Patient* or *Population*, the type of patient or patient population we are dealing with must be clarified [3, 5–8] Having a clear definition of the patient or patient population allows one to identify if the patient(s) referenced in an article we read are similar enough to the patient or population for whom we need the answer. For example, in the case of an appendicitis patient or population, does our patient have acute appendicitis or chronic appendicitis? In the case of inguinal hernia, does our patient have a stable inguinal hernia or an acute strangulated one?

Table 3.2 The PICOT format

Component	Definition
Patient or population	The patient population of interest
Intervention	What is being done for/to the patient
Comparison intervention	What is the intervention being compared to? Often what is currently being done or the "gold standard"
Outcome	What is being measured? What are you hoping to improve/see change in?
Time horizon or time frame	How long following the intervention do you measure the outcome?

This table was formed using information from [3, 5–8]

Intervention

In the second component of the PICOT formula, *Intervention*, we would like to know, as precisely as possible, what the main intervention is [3, 5–8]. For example, if we are comparing laparoscopic versus open cholecystectomy, the laparoscopic procedure could be identified as the main intervention. In this case, we would want to know if the main intervention is a four-port laparoscopic approach or a single port laparoscopic intervention.

Comparative Intervention or Control

Using the same reasoning for the *Comparative Intervention*, we would like to know, again precisely, what this comparative intervention was [3, 5–8]. The Comparative Intervention is often either a control group or the best current standard procedure for the respective condition. Using the example of laparoscopic versus open cholecystectomy where the laparoscopic procedure was the main intervention, the comparative intervention would be the open cholecystectomy. For the open cholecystectomy, we may want to know how extensive the incision was; was it a Kocher incision? Was it a midline incision from the xiphoid to the suprapubic area? Or was it just limited to the epigastric area (above the umbilicus)?

Outcome

With regard to the Outcome component of the PICOT, we would like to know what was hoping to be measured, accomplished, improved or affected [3, 5–8]. Is it a critical outcome such as mortality, was it a QOL outcome or was it something minor such as a rash around the incision? The outcomes can be variable and may include, but not be limited to: (1) a critical outcome (mortality), (2) a QOL outcome, (3) pain, (4) hospitalization days, or (5) ability to return to work. The primary outcome of a study should be succinctly stated as it has implications in the study design, sample size, and power of the study. These issues will be discussed later in Chap. 29.

Time Horizon

The final component of the PICOT formulation should address the *Time Horizon* of the study. The time horizon describes when the outcome was measured in reference to the intervention/event [4]. For example, was the outcome measured 1-month post-procedure or 1 year? The time horizon of a study will depend on the nature of the surgical problem we are exploring. Nobody will take us seriously if we reported our survival results of laparoscopic versus open colon cancer resection at 6 months after surgery. On the other hand, this time horizon may be quite appropriate after acute appendectomy. There may be occasions, for example, when measuring pain, where an intermediate follow-up period, in addition to a long-term follow-up is relevant. Even if there is no difference in survival after colon resection with open vs. laparoscopic approaches, there may be a difference in pain levels or length of time hospitalized. It is important for investigators or authors of published reports or clinical trials to justify the time horizon used [11].

When all components are combined, they form a clear and searchable research question. Examples of such foreground questions with their equivalent PICOT formulation are:

1. In patients undergoing laparoscopic surgery for colorectal cancer, does the use of ultrasound-guided transversus abdominis plane (TAP) blocks reduce pain up to 72 h following surgery?

P Population: patients with colorectal cancer undergoing laparoscopic surgery
I Intervention: ultrasound-guided TAP blocks
C Comparative Intervention: no TAP block
O Outcome: pain
T Time Horizon: up to 72 h following randomization.

2. In patients undergoing prostatectomy for prostate cancer, is robotic-assisted prostatectomy more likely to allow patients to maintain erectile function than traditional open approach, at 1 year post-surgery?

P Population: patients with prostate cancer undergoing prostatectomy
I Intervention: robotic-assisted prostatectomy
C Comparative Intervention: open prostatectomy
O Outcome: erectile function
T Time Horizon: 1 year.

3. In patients 65 years or older who experience a hip fracture, does accelerated surgery (surgery within 6 h) decrease all-cause mortality compared to usual care within 30 days following surgery?

P Population: patients 65 years or older with a hip fracture
I Intervention: accelerated surgery (surgery within 6 h)
C Comparative Intervention: standard surgical care
O Outcome: all-cause mortality
T Time Horizon: 30 days from surgery.

4. In patients with carpal tunnel syndrome, is the Endoscopic Carpal Tunnel Release (ECTR) technique more cost-effective than the Open Carpal Tunnel Release (OCTR) technique at 1 year post-surgery?

P Population: patients with clinical symptoms of carpal tunnel syndrome confirmed with electromyography and nerve conduction studies
I Intervention: ECTR
C Comparative Intervention: OCTR
O Outcome: cost-effectiveness (dollars per natural unit)
T Time Horizon: 1 year.

The development of a research question could be seen as the most important step in a research project. In this chapter, we explained two tools that can be used to ensure the formation of a clear and concise clinical research question: The FINER criteria and the PICOT format (Tables 3.1 and 3.2). A strong research question lays the foundation of a well-designed research project. When structured properly, a research question will make your literature search more efficient through minimizing the results you encounter. Furthermore, a well-formed research question lays a strong foundation and provides direction for the surgeon-investigator throughout all stages of the research project, from study design to publication.

References

1. Haynes RB, Sackett DL, Guyatt GH, Tugwell P. Clinical epidemiology: how to do clinical practice research. 3rd ed. Philadelphia, PA: Lippincott Williams & Wilkins; 2006.
2. Sackett D, Richardson WS, Rosenburg W, Haynes RB. How to practice and teach evidence based medicine. 2nd ed. London, England: Churchill Livingstone; 1997.
3. Thoma A, McKnight L, McKay P, Haines T. Forming the research question. Clin Plast Surg. 2008;35 (2):189–93.
4. Hulley SB, Cummings SR, Browners WS, Grady DG, Newman TB. Conceiving the research question and developing the study plan. In: Gaertner R, editor. Designing clinical research. 4th ed. Philadelphia, PA: Lippincott Williams & Wilkins, a Wolters Kluwer business; 2013. p. 14–22.
5. Thabane L, Thomas T, Ye C, Paul J. Posing the research question: not so simple. Can J Anesth. 2009;56:71–9.
6. Farrugia P, Petrisor BA, Farrokhyar F, Bhandari M. Research questions, hypotheses and objectives. Can J Surg. 2010;53(4):278–81.
7. Richardson WS, Wilson MC, Nishikawa J, Hayward RS. The well-built clinical question: a key to evidence-based decisions. ACP J Club. 1995;123(3): A12–3.
8. Nollan R, Finout-Overhold E, Stephenson P. Asking compelling clinical questions. In: Melnyk BM, Fineout-Overhold E, editors. Evidence-based practice in nursing and healthcare: a guide to best practice. Philadephia, PA: Lippincott Williams & Wilkings; 2005.
9. Koshima I, Yamamoto T, Narushima M, Mihara M, Ilda T. Perforator flaps and supermicrosurgery. Clin Plast Surg. 2010;37:683–9.
10. Thoma A, Kaur MN, Farrokhyar F, Waltho D, Levis C, Lovrics P, Goldsmith CH. Users' guide to the surgical literature: how to assess an article about harm in surgery. Can J Surg. 2016;59(5):351–7.
11. Mowakket S, Karpinski M, Gallo L, Gallo M, Banfield L, Murphy J, et al. Reporting time horizons in randomized controlled trials in plastic surgery: a systematic review. Plastic Reconst Surg. 2018; (in press).

4 Finding the Evidence Through Searching the Literature

Laura Banfield, Jo-Anne Petropoulos and Neera Bhatnagar

Introduction

Questions often arise that require finding evidence to inform clinical decisions. However, not all clinicians seek answers to all questions [1, 2]. Clinician reasons for not seeking answers include: lack of time, questions lack urgency, importance, or are forgotten, perception that an appropriate or relevant answer does not exist, questions are patient specific and non-generalizable, and challenges in using the resources [1–7]. "Because of the increasing volume and speed of new research, finding useful evidence efficiently remains challenging" [8]. PubMed alone has added between 130,000 and 210,000 surgery related articles annually since 2008, reinforcing the necessity to be efficient when seeking information [9]. As stated by Waltho et al. [10], "[s]urgeons must always ensure that the care they provide is rooted in the best available evidence" [10]. This chapter will equip surgeons with knowledge and skills to locate the best evidence to inform their practice.

L. Banfield (✉) · J.-A. Petropoulos · N. Bhatnagar
Health Science Library, HSC 2B, McMaster University, Hamilton, ON, Canada
e-mail: banfie@mcmaster.ca

A. Thoma et al. (eds.), *Evidence-Based Surgery*,
https://doi.org/10.1007/978-3-030-05120-4_4

Clinical Scenario

A 67-year-old female is seen in the bariatric program with morbid obesity and hypertension. Her height is 5 ft., 6 in. Her weight is 360 lbs. She was not able to reduce her weight with dieting over the last decade. She finally decided to proceed with bariatric surgery. Her bariatric surgeon recommended Roux-en-Y surgery. Her best friend however had a sleeve gastrectomy and was happy with the results. She is not certain which procedure to undergo. She is willing to undergo the procedure which is likely to help her lose at least 50% of her weight over the long term (>5 years). As the surgeon, you decide to review the literature to determine which of the two options will best meet the patient's goal. However, you are unsure of how to search the literature.

Clinical Question

As outlined in Chap. 3, *Clinical Question*, a number of different questions may arise from any one scenario or clinical encounter. Remember, "a well-designed research question addresses several components of the clinical scenario", often in the form of PICO(T)—P as the population affected, I as the intervention, C as the comparator, comparison intervention or standard of care, O as the outcome of interest, and T as either time or type of study [10]. For example, in this scenario, the clinical question you developed is: in patients with morbid obesity and BMI >40, does Roux-en-Y, in contrast to sleeve gastrectomy, lead to more weight loss that persists at greater than 5 years?

P morbidly obese patients with BMI >40
I Roux-en-Y bariatric surgery
C sleeve gastrectomy
O loss of 50% weight
(T) greater than 5 years

Importance of the Question

A well formulated clinical question plays a crucial role in efficiently and effectively finding the evidence. When written well, a clinical question can inform what to search (i.e., concepts) and where to search (i.e., resources).

Clinical questions can be further broken down into background and foreground questions. Background questions typically begin with who, what, when, where, and how (e.g., the pathophysiology of a disease, explanation of a surgical procedure). These questions can be answered in textbooks or reference books. Foreground questions seek to address a specific clinical problem (e.g., causal or risk factors, prognosis, treatment effectiveness as it pertains to a specific patient or patient population). The answers to these questions can be found through effective use of resources supporting Evidence-Based Medicine such as those within the Pyramid of EBM Resources or 6S Pyramid (see Choosing Appropriate Resources) [8, 11]. Although some of the resources found within the pyramids can be used to find background information, the focus of this chapter will be on how to use them to find evidence to support clinical decisions and research.

We acknowledge that even a well-written clinical question may not have an answer. Potential reasons could include: "no feasible study design or measurement tools exist that investigators could use to resolve an issue", or "no one has conducted and published the necessary study" [8]. In these instances, you will need to reevaluate your question (see Chap. 3).

Developing a Search Strategy

This section describes the core principles for developing a search strategy. As mentioned previously, a key step to an efficient search is formulating a well-written question. This is followed by identifying search concepts and their related search terms, and then combining them using the Boolean operators; "[h]erein lies the art to efficient searching" [12].

Identifying Concepts

Begin with identifying concepts from your question. This is important for developing an effective search strategy. Concepts can be more easily identified once the clinical question has been written using the format of PICO(T). Each of the components of PICO(T) become your concepts (Table 4.1).

Table 4.1 Clinical question broken into PICO(T) concepts

Concept A	Concept B	Concept C	Concept D	Concept E
P	I	C	O	T
Morbidly Obese Patient (BMI > 40kg/m^2)	Roux-en-Y Bariatric Surgery	Sleeve Gastrectomy	Weight Loss	> 5 years

Identifying Search Terms

After you have identified your concepts, think of alternative terms, known as keywords or text words, for each concept. Keywords are individual words or phrases that may appear in the title, abstract, author-supplied keywords, or the body of the text depending on the nature of the resources being searched. Consider including synonyms or related terms relevant to each concept. Be sure to incorporate variations of the root words as part of your list of keywords (e.g., anesthesia, anaesthesia, anesthetic, anaesthetic). An efficient way to include these variations is by adding an asterisk (*), known as a truncation symbol or a wildcard (e.g., anesthes*, anaesthes*) (Table 4.2). Be mindful of which words you apply the asterisk to as it may result in capturing words you may not have intended (e.g., stud* will retrieve stud or studs or study or studies or student or students). Some resources also allow you to include a form of internal truncation, sometimes referred to as wildcards. The purpose of internal truncation is to allow for variation in spelling (e.g., an?esthesia)—a question mark (?) or a number sign (#) may be used depending on the database.

Advanced Search Tip: Generating Additional Search Terms

To generate more search terms, take a known article and look at the title and abstract for words related to your concepts and the author-supplied keywords at the bottom of the abstract.

Another strategy is to look up the article in a database (e.g., PubMed) to identify relevant controlled vocabulary.

Controlled Vocabulary

Some resources offer alternatives to keyword only searches; this is referred to as searching with controlled vocabulary (e.g., subject headings, descriptors). Controlled vocabulary are predefined terms (labels) set by the databases to facilitate finding information. These terms are used to describe the contents of an article and are helpful when authors use different terms to describe a particular concept. For example, an author might refer to one of the following terms to describe our concept of gastric bypass surgery:

Table 4.2 Search concepts and search terms

Concept A	Concept B	Concept C	Concept D	Concept E
P	I	C	O	T
Morbidly Obese Patient (BMI > 40kg/m^2)	**Roux-en-Y Bariatric Surgery**	**Sleeve Gastrectomy**	**Weight Loss**	**> 5 years**
Obese	Gastric Bypass	Gastric Sleeve Surgery	Weight Reduc*	
Over weight	Gastroileal Bypass		Decrease* Weight	

Table 4.3 Controlled vocabulary term for Gastric Bypass in PubMed (MeSH term) and related terms covered by Gastric Bypass

MeSH	Gastric Bypass
Coverage	Bypass, Gastric Roux-en-Y Gastric Bypass Bypass, Roux-en-Y Gastric Gastric Bypass, Roux-en-Y Roux-en-Y Gastric Bypass Greenville Gastric Bypass Gastric Bypass, Greenville Gastroileal Bypass Bypass, Gastroileal Gastrojejunostomy Gastrojejunostomies

Advanced Search Tip: Controlled Vocabulary

Not all databases include controlled vocabulary. For those that do, there is no single universal controlled vocabulary. Rather, there are many sets of controlled vocabulary; some are unique to the database (e.g., Emtree for Embase) and some are used by more than one database (e.g., MeSH [**Me**dical **S**ubject **H**eading] is used by MEDLINE®, PubMed, and Cochrane Database of Systematic Reviews).

gastric bypass or gastroileal bypass or gastrojejunostomy or Roux-en-Y gastric bypass (Table 4.3). Controlled vocabulary recognizes that these terms are all referring to the same concept. Instead of searching on every single term, you can search on the controlled vocabulary term to retrieve articles that use one of the four terms in our example. It is important to note that a comprehensive search should include a combination of keywords and controlled vocabulary terms.

Boolean Operators

You can now begin to create a search strategy. Boolean operators can be used to logically organize concepts and keywords. The primary Boolean operators are AND, OR, and NOT (Fig. 4.1). In general, the AND operator is used to combine search concepts (Table 4.4). It allows you to retrieve evidence containing two or more concepts. For example, a search using

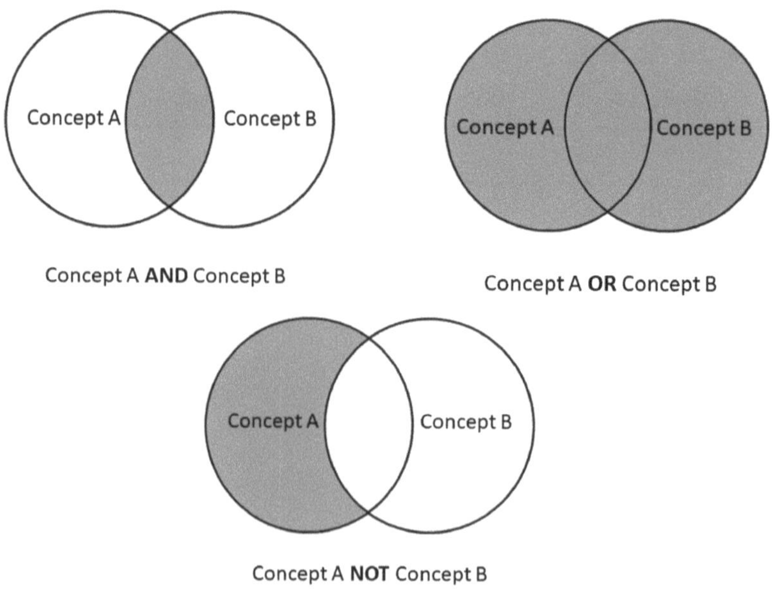

Fig. 4.1 Boolean operators. *Note* Shading indicates the result set when concepts are combined using AND OR NOT.

Table 4.4 Applying Boolean operators to search concepts and search terms

Concept A	Concept B	Concept C	Concept D	Concept E
P AND	I AND	C AND	O AND	T
Morbidly Obese Patient (BMI > 40kg/m^2)	**Roux-en-Y Bariatric Surgery**	**Sleeve Gastrectomy**	**Weight Loss**	**> 5 years**
Obes* OR	Gastric Bypass OR	Gastric Sleeve Surgery	Weight Reduc* OR	
Over weight OR	Gastroileal Bypass OR		Decrease* Weight	
Overweight	Greenville Gastric Bypass OR			
	Gastrojejunostomies			

Obesity AND Gastric Bypass will retrieve evidence containing both concepts. The OR operator is most often applied when combining related keywords within a search concept. Using the OR operator will retrieve evidence containing any of the keywords in isolation or where they may show up together (Table 4.4). For example, a search using Surgery OR Gastric Bypass will retrieve evidence containing either or both keywords related to the same concept. In contrast, the NOT operator will explicitly exclude articles containing those terms from the result set. For example, a search using NOT animals will eliminate all articles with a reference to animals. The NOT operator should be used with caution as it could eliminate relevant articles that incidentally mention the term you are excluding. Using the same example, NOT Animals will also eliminate articles that reference both animals and humans (i.e., studies that incorporate human and animal models).

Using either the AND or the NOT operators will narrow the scope of the search and decrease the number of articles retrieved (see Limits section); also referred to as specificity. On the other hand, the OR operator will broaden the scope of the search and increase the number of articles retrieved, also referred to as sensitivity.

Advanced Search Tip: Applying Boolean Operators

Typically, search concepts are combined using the AND operator. However, there are circumstances in which they can be combined using the OR operator (e.g., Intervention (Roux-en-Y bariatric surgery) OR Comparator (Sleeve gastrectomy). This is particularly applicable to surgical questions.

Within each concept, the alternative terms and controlled vocabulary are usually combined using the OR operator.

Creating a Search Strategy

For the purposes of this section, we have identified two approaches to searching: simple and complex. These approaches can be applied to the sources of evidence identified in the Pyramid of EBM Resources and 6S Pyramid (see Choosing Appropriate Resources). The nature of the resource will dictate the approach to searching. See Table 4.5 for a list of resources in which these search strategies can be applied.

Simple Search Strategy (i.e., Basic)

A simple search strategy can be applied to any resource using one or two concepts, one term per concept (Fig. 4.2). However, it is best applied at the top levels in both pyramids (e.g., specifically DynaMed Plus, UptoDate®).

Using the concepts from our PICO(T) (Table 4.1), the search strategy could be any one of the following but not limited to:

Table 4.5 List of resources for simple search and complex search

Resource	Website	Simple Search	Complex Search
ACCESSSS	https://www.accessss.org/	✔	
ACP Journal Club¶	http://annals.org/aim/journal-club	✔	
BMJ Best Practice¶	https://bestpractice.bmj.com/	✔	
CINAHL Database¶	https://health.ebsco.com/products/the-cinahl-database/allied-health-nursing	✔	✔
Cochrane Central Register of Controlled Trials (CENTRAL)¶	http://www.cochranelibrary.com/about/central-landing-page.html	✔	✔
Cochrane Database of Systematic Reviews (CDSR))¶	http://www.cochranelibrary.com/cochrane-database-of-systematic-reviews/	✔	✔
DynaMed Plus¶	http://www.dynamed.com/	✔	
Embase¶	https://www.elsevier.com/solutions/embase-biomedical-research	✔	✔
Epistemonikos	https://www.epistemonikos.org/	✔	✔
Essential Evidence Plus¶	https://www.essentialevidenceplus.com/	✔	
LILACS	http://lilacs.bvsalud.org/en/	✔	✔
MEDLINE®¶	https://www.nlm.nih.gov/bsd/medline.html	✔	✔
OrthoEvidence™¶	https://myorthoevidence.com/	✔	
PEPID¶	https://www.pepidconnect.com/	✔	
PsycINFO®¶	http://www.apa.org/pubs/databases/psycinfo/	✔	✔
PubMed	https://www.ncbi.nlm.nih.gov/pubmed/	✔	✔
Scopus¶	https://www.elsevier.com/solutions/scopus	✔	✔
TRIP⁺	https://www.tripdatabase.com/	✔	✔
UpToDate®¶	https://www.uptodate.com/contents/search	✔	
CMA CPG Infobase⁺	https://www.cma.ca/En/Pages/clinical-practice-guidelines.aspx	✔	
International Guideline Library	https://www.g-i-n.net/library/international-guidelines-library/international-guidelines-library	✔	✔
NICE Guidance	https://www.nice.org.uk/	✔	
SIGN Guidelines	http://www.sign.ac.uk/our-guidelines.html	✔	
WHO Guidelines	http://www.who.int/publications/guidelines/en/	✔	

¶fee-based

⁺premium or extra features with additional fee

Note Access to fee-based resources may be provided through your professional, academic, clinical, and hospital affiliations

Fig. 4.2 Applying a simple search to UpToDate®. (used with permission)

1. Obesity
2. Roux-en-Y bariatric surgery
3. Sleeve gastrectomy
4. Obese AND Sleeve gastrectomy

Advanced Search Tip: Searching for Clinical Practice Guidelines

Searching for guidelines can be achieved through meta-search tools such as TRIP, association or organization websites, or through the article databases. The TRIP database allows you to construct a simple search as above using the search function or to use the PICO tool. In either instance, you will use the limits on the result screen to look at guidelines specifically. Known associations and organizations (professional, health) are good starting points for guidelines and may have them listed in the documents or publications sections of their websites. Alternately, guidelines may be published in journals and thus it may be more effective to search the article databases and include guideline as a concept.

When searching with one or two concepts, you scan or scroll the summary to obtain more detailed information incorporating the other aspects of your PICO(T). For many resources within these levels, you may apply a similarly simple search. However, there are some exceptions, specifically, searching for guidelines.

Complex Search Strategy (i.e., Advanced)

A complex search strategy can be applied to many of the highlighted resources related to the Pyramid of EBM Resources and 6S Pyramid and to other resources outside of it. This type of strategy involves two or more concepts and may also involve more than one term, including controlled vocabulary, per concept. It is best applied when searching for syntheses and studies (i.e., Non-preappraised or Syntheses and Studies levels).

Again, using the concepts from our PICO(T), the search strategy could be any one of the following but not limited to:

1. (Obes* OR overweight OR over-weight) AND (sleeve gastrectomy OR gastric band* OR lap-band)
2. (sleeve gastrectomy OR gastric band* OR lap-band) AND (Roux-en-Y bariatric surgery OR RYGB)
3. (bariatric surg*) AND (weight loss or weight reduc*) (Table 4.6)

Table 4.6 Sample of a Complex Search using OVID MEDLINE®

Line	Search terms
1	Obesity/
2	obes*.mp.
3	over weight.mp.
4	overweight.mp.
5	1 or 2 or 3 or 4
6	sleeve gastrectom*.mp.
7	Gastric Bypass/
8	roux-en-y bariatric surgery.mp.
9	7 or 8
10	5 and 6 and 9

Note The / indicates use of controlled vocabulary (MeSH) and.mp. indicates use of keywords. Line 5 illustrates the combining of terms used to describe the population. Line 6 illustrates the comparison, while Line 9 illustrates the combining of terms used to describe the intervention. Line 10 is the combining of all 3 concepts by applying AND. This search could be built upon through the addition of more related terms and concepts

Advanced Search Tip: Selecting Search Concepts

In PICO(T) a comparator (C) or time period/type of study (T) may not always be part of your search strategy. These can be very helpful when reviewing your search results. The more concepts you search on, the more specific your search is, and the narrower your results become.

Advanced Search Tip: Limits as a Search Concept

A helpful strategy is to treat a limit as a search concept. This will increase the sensitivity of the search by allowing you to use more terms to describe it (e.g., Randomi?ed Controlled Trial* or RCT* or blind* or conceal*…). This advanced approach can also involve using controlled vocabulary in addition to keywords.

Limits and Search Filters

Most resources enable you to limit or narrow your search results. The limit options available vary across the resources. Examples of limits include: publication date, language, age, and publication type. It is best to apply these limits one at a time, and at the end of your search. This will allow you to see the impact that each of the limits will have on narrowing your results. In some circumstances, it may be necessary to revisit the limits you have chosen based on your preliminary results. This is easier to do if the limits have been applied one at a time.

Filters, also known as hedges, are combinations of predefined search terms used to retrieve results on a particular topic (e.g., cancer), with a particular study design (e.g., randomized controlled trials or cohort), or using a particular study methodology (e.g., prognosis or therapy). Filters are applied to improve the quality of the result set by reducing the number of irrelevant results and increasing the number of relevant results [13–17]. These filters are added to the search terms being used for the content.

PubMed, Ovid MEDLINE®, Embase, and PsycINFO®, and EBSCO CINAHL and MEDLINE®, have all adopted the search filters (clinical hedges) developed by Health Information Research Unit (HiRU) at McMaster University [18, 19]. The HiRU hedges, known as Clinical Queries, are found under the Additional Limits in Ovid® and are found within the Edit feature in the search history and Refine Results section of EBSCO CINAHL. In PubMed, the link to Clinical Queries is located in the PubMed Tools section on the homepage. The common clinical queries filters cover the following categories: therapy, diagnosis, etiology, prognosis, and clinical prediction guides. Additional HiRU hedges include reviews, economics, qualitative, and costs [19].

Advanced Search Tip: Additional search filters

Not all filters are created equally. It should be noted that not all filters have been developed using a rigorous methodology nor have all been validated. As a result, you should look critically at those available before selecting one that best suits your needs.

HiRU Search Filters
https://hiru.mcmaster.ca/hiru/HIRU_Hedges_home.aspx

Scottish Intercollegiate Guidelines Network (SIGN)
http://www.sign.ac.uk/search-filters.html

InterTASC Information Specialists' Sub-Group (ISSG) Search Filter Resource
https://sites.google.com/a/york.ac.uk/issg-search-filters-resource/

Strings attached: CADTH database search filters
https://www.cadth.ca/resources/finding-evidence/strings-attached-cadths-database-search-filters

Choosing Appropriate Resources

"As a surgeon using EBM [Evidence-Based Surgery] at point of care, it is critical for you to ensure you are taking advantage of the best resources for making clinical and surgical decisions" [10]. This section will provide an overview of selected resources and the differences between them. Strengths and weaknesses of the resources will not be discussed as such assessments are partially based on personal preferences, availability, and access. However, it is worth noting that many of these may not have comprehensive coverage of surgical content.

There are many ways to describe and organize sources of evidence. Two of the more common ways are: Pyramid of EBM Resources and 6S hierarchy of evidence-based resources Pyramid [8, 11].

Pyramid of EBM Resources

The Pyramid of EBM Resources divides resources into three categories: summaries and guidelines, preappraised research, and non-preappraised research.

Summaries and Guidelines

Summaries and guidelines are rarely limited to a specific clinical question. Instead, they are topic or condition driven, often integrating background and foreground information to inform clinical decision making [8]. These resources rate the strength of the recommendations based on either or both internally defined criteria and externally defined criteria (eg. GRADE). Examples of these resources include UptoDate®, DynaMed Plus, BMJ Best Practice, and clinical practice guidelines.

Preappraised Research

Preappraised research represents a single page synopsis of a systematic review or single study. The synopsis includes an evaluation of the quality of the methods, clinical relevance, and expert commentary. [8] Examples include ACP Journal Club and OrthoEvidence™.

Non-preappraised Research

Non-preappraised research refers to primary studies with no evaluation [8]. Examples include articles found in PubMed, Embase, MEDLINE®, and Cochrane Central Register of Controlled Trials (CENTRAL).

6S Pyramid

The 6S Pyramid takes a slightly different approach to organizing the sources of evidence, yet the similarities between the two are evident (Fig. 4.3). Both pyramids place studies at the bottom and move up towards more clinically driven resources. The key differences include the addition of a Systems layer at the top and the apparent subdivision within the preappraised research and non-preappraised research categories in the 6S Pyramid.

Systems

Systems represent an ideal situation in which the best available evidence informing clinical decision making is integrated with the information unique to each patient through the electronic medical record [11]. To our knowledge, there are few in existence. We recognize their role in and potential to contribute to evidence-based patient care, but we will not explore them further.

Summaries

As with the Summaries and Guidelines level from the Pyramid of EBM Resources, this level provides "a comprehensive view of the body of evidence at a topic level" [8]. Examples of these resources include UptoDate®, DynaMed Plus, BMJ Best Practice, Essential Evidence Plus, Micromedex®, PEPID, and clinical practice guidelines.

Synopses of Syntheses

Synopses of syntheses are typically one-page structured summaries that provide an appraisal of a systematic review. They are explicit in their assessment of the quality and will often note newsworthiness and relevance to clinical practice and research. Examples of resources relevant to surgery in this category include OrthoEvidence™, ACP Journal Club, and Cochrane evidence summaries.

Syntheses

Commonly referred to as a systematic review, a synthesis is a comprehensive summary of all the

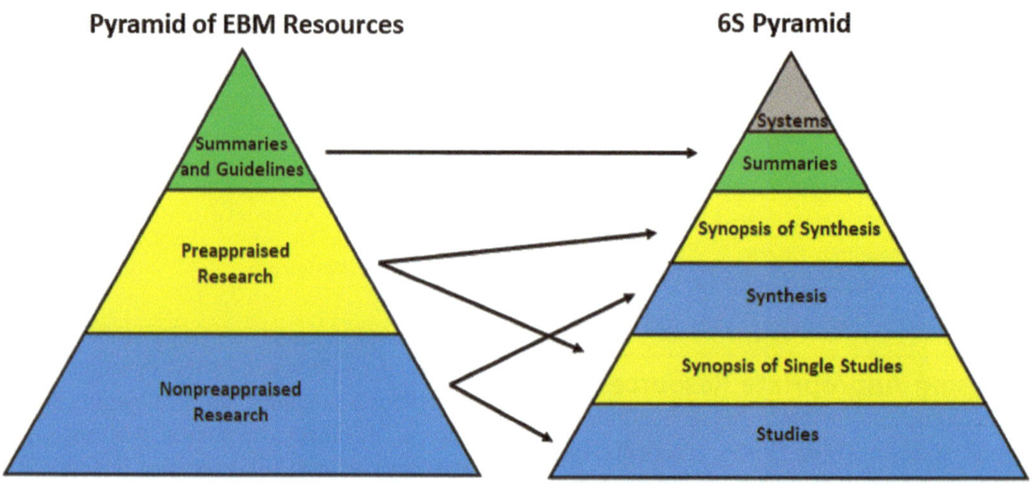

Fig. 4.3 Relationship of the Pyramid of EBM Resources to the 6S Pyramid (Used with permission)

evidence surrounding a particular research question. Examples of where systematic reviews can be found include individual journals and through the Cochrane Database of Systematic Reviews, PubMed, MEDLINE®, and Embase.

Synopses of Single Studies

Synopses of original studies are typically one-page structured summaries that provide an appraisal of single studies. Similar to synopses of synthesis, they are explicit in their assessment of the quality of the study and will often note newsworthiness and relevance to clinical practice and research. Examples of resources include OrthoEvidence™, ACP Journal Club, and BMJ Evidence-based Medicine.

Studies

Studies are single articles reporting on original research. Unlike the resources above, the responsibility for critically appraising or assessing the quality of the evidence falls to the reader. Examples of where studies can be found include individual journals and through databases including PubMed, MEDLINE®, Embase, and Cochrane Register of Controlled Trials (CENTRAL).

Other Resources

After reviewing the resources described, it is common to question the necessity of searching multiple resources. If your purpose in searching is emerging out of a clinical situation to which you need a more immediate answer, the preappraised and summaries resources are likely to be your best starting point (Fig. 4.3). However, if you are undertaking a systematic review, clinical practice guideline, or other form of knowledge synthesis, you are more likely to be working with the non-preappraised resources (synthesis and studies). Before beginning your search consider why you are searching, what resources you have access to, and how much time you have.

Federated Search Tools

These are resources that search across multiple sources of evidence simultaneously are referred

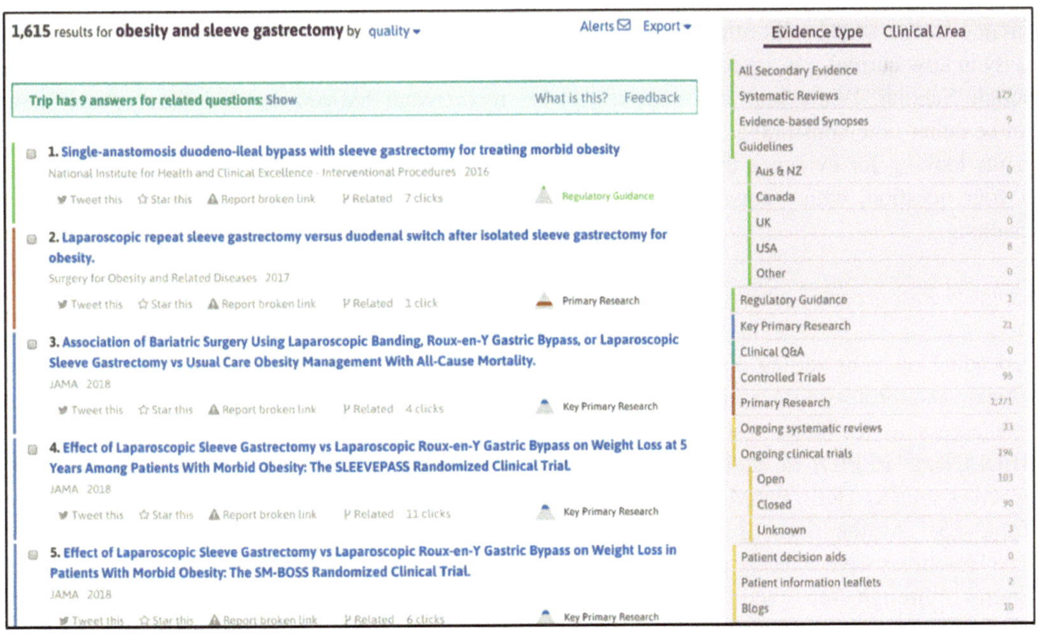

Fig. 4.4 Result set from TRIP database (Used with permission)

to as federated or meta-search tools. The search results from a number of resources are displayed together and may be broken up into categories depending on the organization of the tool (Fig. 4.4). Examples include: TRIP database, Epistemonikos, ACCESSSS, SumSearch.

Google and Google Scholar

A few words on Google and Google Scholar: both are powerful, convenient, and easy to use search tools. Google can be very helpful in identifying information about rare conditions, procedures, and emerging trends and outbreaks, as well as in identifying reports and policy statements from governmental and nongovernmental organizations and agencies, research institutes and think tanks. Google Scholar is helpful in identifying research literature across disciplines and articles in press.

However, they should be used with caution. Google searches across a wide range of information and web-based communication, not all of which is scientific, evidence-driven or without some form of bias (e.g., personal opinion, commercially driven). It is not easy to determine the good from the bad without employing strong skills in critical appraisal. The lack of transparency in the search algorithm and the uncertainty in how current it is are some concerns with Google Scholar. While both are easy to use, it can be rather time-consuming sifting through the results looking for evidence that can be applied to your question, which outweighs the ease of searching.

Access to Resources

Depending on your setting and your academic, clinical, and professional affiliations, you may have access to fee-based resources (e.g., Ovid MEDLINE®, PEPID) in addition to the "free" resources such as TRIP, PubMed, Epistemonikos (Table 4.5). At the time of writing, some of "free" resources were offering premium and extra features through an additional fee (e.g., TRIP PRO provides images, videos, greater search refinement, etc.).

Keeping Current

Staying current with the latest evidence keeps you informed of what others in your field are doing, assists in contextualizing your work and helps with identifying research and knowledge gaps. Many of the previously mentioned resources will allow you to stay current with the latest evidence. Depending on the resource, you can create: table of contents alerts, search alerts, and alerts informed by predefined categories (e.g., discipline, topic, profession) (Fig. 4.5.). These alerts can be customized to frequency and timing of delivery, number of results, and format of the alert (e.g., email, RSS, citation management software compatible).

Resolution of the Clinical Scenario

You are now ready to resolve the clinical scenario by applying what you have learned in this chapter. The approach you take will be informed by your purpose in searching, what you have access to, and the amount of time you have. These factors together with either of the pyramids discussed will help to identify which resources are more appropriate to search given your circumstances.

If the purpose is to inform patient care, we recommend that you start with the resources at the top of the pyramid and work downwards until you find a suitable answer. Alternatively, if the purpose is to engage in research, we recommend that you start with the resources at the bottom of the pyramid and take into account existing synthesis.

Applying a simple search (e.g., roux-en-y, sleeve gastrectomy) in DynaMed Plus leads to the evidence summary entitled Bariatric Surgery [20]. Resources at the summaries level, such as DynaMed Plus, tend to be topic or concept driven. They contain both background and foreground information and require you to read within the entry to find the evidence.

Building upon the complex search strategy from Ovid Medline (Table 4.6) and adding limits for age and humans, a 2017 article comparing sleeve gastrectomy to Roux-en-Y in older adults

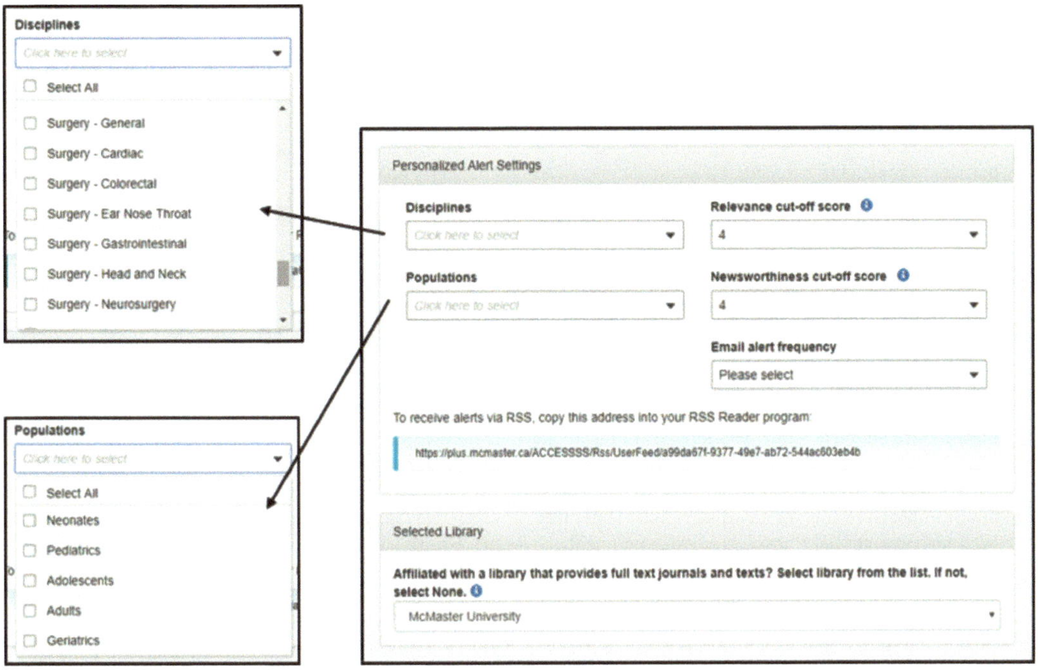

Fig. 4.5 Alert settings from ACCESSSS (Used with permission)

by Casillas et al. is found [21]. As this is a prospective cohort study, you will need to apply the critical appraisal skills discussed in Chap. 16.

Conclusion

Surgeons encounter questions that require them to search for evidence to inform a clinical decision or research process. There are many sources of information available and different search strategies that can be applied. This chapter has covered the core principles for developing a search strategy from identifying concepts, search terms, and controlled vocabulary (if applicable), to combining concepts and terms using Boolean operators, and selecting resources. However, no single resource will be sufficient to address all of your information needs and it may be necessary to search multiple sources. Federated search tools, such as TRIP and ACCESSSS, can be invaluable especially when time is a factor.

Medical and health sciences librarians are also a key resource in assisting you with developing your searching skills and with searching for complex topics or difficult to answer questions. We encourage you to reach out, they will be happy to help you.

Paraphrasing Glasziou, Burls, and Gilbert, the ability to effectively search the literature is as essential as the stethoscope to a clinician's practice or the scalpel to a surgeon [22].

References

1. Del Fiol G, Workman TE, Gorman PN. Clinical questions raised by clinicians at the point of care: a systematic review. JAMA Intern Med. 2014;174(5):710–8.
2. Brassil E, Gunn B, Shenoy AM, Blanchard R. Unanswered clinical questions: a survey of specialists and primary care providers. J Med Libr Assoc. 2017;105(1):4–11.
3. Cook DA, Sorensen KJ, Linderbaum JA, Pencille LJ, Rhodes DJ. Information needs of generalists and specialists using online best-practice algorithms to answer clinical questions. J Am Med Inform Assoc. 2017;24(4):754–61.
4. Ely JW, Osheroff JA, Chambliss ML, Ebell MH, Rosenbaum ME. Answering physicians' clinical questions: obstacles and potential solutions. J Am Med Inform Assoc. 2005;12(2):217–24.

5. Ely JW, Osheroff JA, Ebell MH, Chambliss ML, Vinson DC, Stevermer JJ, et al. Obstacles to answering doctors' questions about patient care with evidence: qualitative study. BMJ. 2002;324(7339):710.
6. Green ML, Ruff TR. Why do residents fail to answer their clinical questions? A qualitative study of barriers to practicing evidence-based medicine. Acad Med. 2005;80(2):176–82.
7. Bennett NL, Casebeer LL, Zheng S, Kristofco R. Information-seeking behaviors and reflective practice. J Contin Educ Health Prof. 2006;26(2):120–7.
8. Agoritsas T, Vandvik PO, Neumann I, Rochwerg B, Jaeschke R, Hayward R et al. In: Guyatt GH, Rennie D, Meade MO, Cook DJ, editors. Finding the best evidence. Users' guides to the medical literature: a manual for evidence-based clinical practice. 3rd ed. New York: McGraw-Hill Education; 2015. p. 29–49.
9. Corlan AD. Medline trend: automated yearly statistics of PubMed results for any query, 2004 [Internet]. Web resource at URL: http://dan.corlan.net/medline-trend.html. Accessed: 2012-02-14. Available at: Archived by WebCite at http://www.webcitation.org/65RkD48SV.
10. Waltho D, Kaur MN, Haynes RB, Farrokhyar F, Thoma A. Users' guide to the surgical literature: how to perform a high-quality literature search. Can J Surg. 2015;58(5):349–58.
11. DiCenso A, Bayley L, Haynes RB. ACP Journal Club. Editorial: Accessing preappraised evidence: fine-tuning the 5S model into a 6S model. Ann Intern Med. 2009;151(6):JC3-2, JC3-3.
12. Herbert R, Jamtvedt G, Hagen KB, Mead J. Practical evidence-based physiotherapy. 2nd ed. Edinburgh: Elsevier/Churchill Livingstone; 2011.
13. McKibbon KA, Wilczynski NL, Haynes RB, Hedges Team. Retrieving randomized controlled trials from medline: a comparison of 38 published search filters. Health Info Libr J. 2009;26(3):187–202.
14. McKibbon KA, Lokker C, Wilczynski NL, Haynes RB, Ciliska D, Dobbins M, et al. Search filters can find some but not all knowledge translation articles in MEDLINE: an analytic survey. J Clin Epidemiol. 2012;65(6):651–9.
15. Lokker C, Haynes RB, Wilczynski NL, McKibbon KA, Walter SD. Retrieval of diagnostic and treatment studies for clinical use through PubMed and PubMed's Clinical Queries filters. J Am Med Inform Assoc. 2011;18(5):652–9.
16. Shariff SZ, Sontrop JM, Haynes RB, Iansavichus AV, McKibbon KA, Wilczynski NL, et al. Impact of PubMed search filters on the retrieval of evidence by physicians. CMAJ. 2012;184(3):E184–90.
17. EBSCO Help. CINAHL Clinical Queries [Internet]. [cited 2018 June 28]. Available from: https://help.ebsco.com/interfaces/CINAHL_MEDLINE_Databases/CINAHL/CINAHL_Clinical_Queries. Accessed 28 June 2018.
18. Scottish Intercollegiate Guidelines Network (SIGN). Search filters [Internet]. [cited 2018 June 25]. Available from: http://sign.ac.uk/search-filters.html.
19. Health Information Research Unit, McMaster University. Hedges [Internet]. [cited 2018 May 11]. Available from: https://hiru.mcmaster.ca/hiru/hiru_hedges_home.aspx.
20. DynaMed Plus [Internet]. Ipswich (MA): EBSCO Information Services. 1995. Record No. 483434, Bariatric surgery; [updated 2018 Jul 18, cited July 20, 2018]; [about 62 screens]. Available from http://www.dynamed.com/login.aspx?direct=true&site=DynaMed&id=483434. Registration and login required.
21. Casillas RA, Kim B, Fischer H, Zelada Getty JL, Um SS, Coleman KJ. Comparative effectiveness of sleeve gastrectomy versus Roux-en-Y gastric bypass for weight loss and safety outcomes in older adults. Surg Obes Relat Dis. 2017;13(9):1476–83.
22. Glasziou P, Burls A, Gilbert R. Evidence based medicine and the medical curriculum. BMJ. 2008;337:a1253.

Hierarchy of Evidence in Surgical Research

5

Gina Del Fabbro, Sofia Bzovsky, Achilles Thoma and Sheila Sprague

Introduction

When answering a clinical question and applying the principles of evidence-based surgery, critical evaluation of the available evidence is of vital importance. The first step in this process is to determine where the study falls on the hierarchy of evidence. Multiple versions of the hierarchy of evidence tables have been developed since the advent of evidence-based medicine and evidence-based surgery. The Levels of Evidence (LOE) were first introduced by the Canadian Task Force on Periodic Health Examination founded in 1976 at the request of the Conference of Deputy Ministers of Health across Canada [1]. Their proposal of an evidence rating system was later improved upon by David Sackett, who is considered the father of evidence-based medicine and developed the five LOE [2]. Since then, a more rigorous and complex LOE has been developed by the Centre for Evidence-Based Medicine in Oxford, United Kingdom, which ranks articles according to the study design used to answer the primary research question (see Appendix) [3]. Multiple journals and groups have adapted this table or a variation of it for their specialities. The Journal of Bone and Joint Surgery (JBJS) first published their version of the LOE in 2003, basing their system off of an earlier version of the Center for Evidence-Based Medicine's LOE scheme [4]. JBJS has since published an updated version of their LOE, which has been found to be responsive to surgical publications and highly relevant, as it addresses multiple areas of research [5]. Although we chose to utilize the JBJS scheme, this information is applicable to all surgical specialties. In this chapter, we review the hierarchy of evidence for therapeutic research, prognostic research, diagnostic test evaluation, and economic research, as described in JBJS [6].

Levels of Evidence for Therapeutic Research

Therapeutic research evaluates the effect of different treatments on one or more outcomes of interest. Simply stated, therapeutic research addresses questions, such as *does this treatment help* and *what are the harms*? [4]. Figure 5.1 shows the hierarchy of evidence for therapeutic

G. Del Fabbro · S. Bzovsky · S. Sprague
Department of Surgery, Division of Orthopaedic Surgery, McMaster University, Hamilton, ON, Canada

A. Thoma
Department of Surgery, Division of Plastic Surgery, McMaster University, Hamilton, ON, Canada
e-mail: athoma@mcmaster.ca

A. Thoma · S. Sprague (✉)
Department of Health Research Methods, Evidence and Impact, McMaster University, Hamilton, ON, Canada
e-mail: sprags@mcmaster.ca

A. Thoma et al. (eds.), *Evidence-Based Surgery*,
https://doi.org/10.1007/978-3-030-05120-4_5

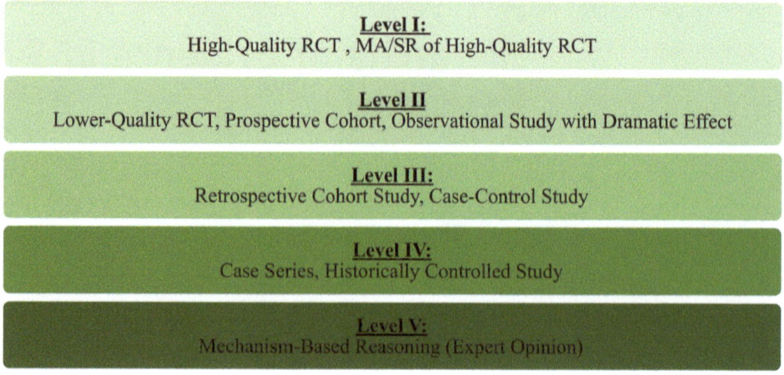

Fig. 5.1 Levels of evidence and their associated study designs for therapeutic research. *RCT* randomized controlled trial; created using information from JBJS [4] and Elsevier [6]

research [4]. High-quality randomized controlled trials (RCTs), as well as systematic reviews (SR) and meta-analyses (MA) of well-conducted RCTs, are considered the highest LOE for therapeutic research. Randomized controlled trials, in which patients are randomly allocated to an intervention group or a comparison group, are considered the highest LOE because they offer the best protection against bias (Fig. 5.2a). Randomization is an effective method of reducing bias as it balances the treatment groups with respect to both known and unknown prognostic factors [7, 8]. Randomized controlled trials are discussed more in Chaps. 12–15. MAs and SRs of properly conducted RCTs also represent Level I evidence. An SR is an investigation of relevant literature related to a specific research question. SRs are conducted according to a protocol that details the search strategy, eligibility criteria for included studies, as well as data abstraction and analysis plans [7–9]. An MA is an SR that uses quantitative methods or statistical techniques to pool the data found in the literature, increasing the effective sample size [7, 8]. For both SRs and MAs, a comprehensive search is necessary to identify all relevant results, including published, unpublished, and gray literature. The more complete the search, the greater the potential for a high-quality study. SRs and MAs are discussed in more detail in Chap. 16.

A lesser quality RCT, defined as an RCT with less than 80% follow-up, no blinding, or improper randomization, is considered Level II evidence when assessing therapeutic research [10]. Although high-quality RCTs represent the highest LOE, they are not suitable for addressing every surgical research question. When RCTs are unethical, impractical, or adequate resources are not available, researchers may elect to conduct an observational study (e.g., prospective comparative study, case-control study etc.) [4]. A prospective cohort study for therapeutic research identifies a group of patients who have received the treatment of interest and compares them with a group of patients who received an alternative treatment (Fig. 5.2b). Patients in both groups are followed for a specified period of time to determine their outcomes [10]. These studies are similar to the RCT in that the criteria for inclusion, the outcomes of interest, and timeframe for follow-up are determined prior to the occurrence of any events/outcomes. However, in contrast to RCTs, the treating surgeon, patient, or both parties, determine which treatment the patient receives, thus introducing a potential source of bias. When a large effect is observed and there are no other considerations for downgrading the quality of the study, the evidence of an observational study is considered satisfactory for Level II. MAs and SRs may also be categorized under Level II evidence if the studies included in the analysis or review are considered Level II evidence, or if the included studies represent Level I evidence but demonstrate inconsistent results [4].

Retrospective cohort studies comparing two or more treatments are commonly encountered in the surgical literature and are classified as Level III evidence. In a retrospective cohort study, the research study is initiated after both the

Fig. 5.2 **a** RCT study design for therapeutic studies. **b** Prospective cohort design for therapeutic studies. **c** Retrospective cohort design for therapeutic studies. **d** Case-control design for therapeutic studies. **e** Case series design for therapeutic studies

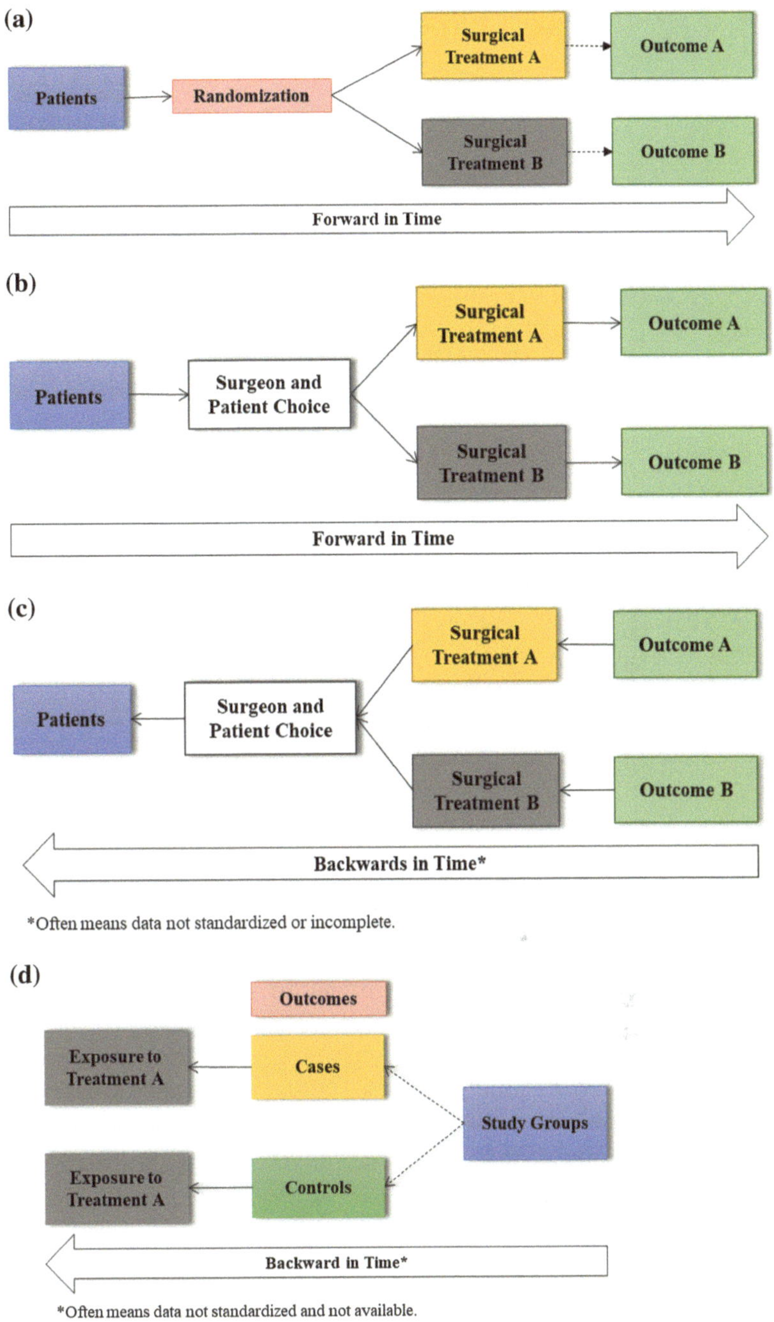

Fig. 5.2 (continued)

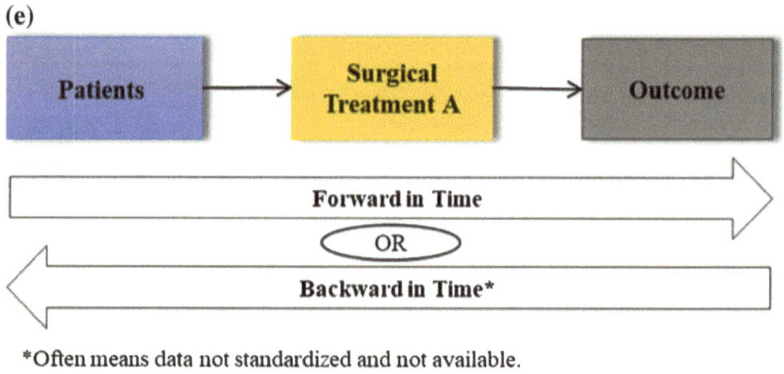

intervention and outcomes have occurred. Researchers review previously recorded data (e.g., from medical records or a registry) to identify patients who received the treatments of interest and then compare their outcomes (Fig. 5.2c) [4]. A case-control study, also at Level III on the hierarchy, compares patients who have the disease or outcome of interest (cases) with controls (patients who do not have the disease or outcome of interest) and looks back in time to compare how frequently the exposure to a risk (e.g., fracture and vitamin D deficiency) is present in each group to determine the relationship between the risk factor and the disease (Fig. 5.2d). However, the status may not have been recorded in the past, and therefore, the presence or absence of the risk factor cannot be determined. Case-control studies are described in greater detail in Chap. 18.

Case series are frequently reported in the surgical literature and are classified as Level IV evidence [4]. A case series is an expansion of an individual case report to include a group of patients with the outcome of interest (Fig. 5.2e). A case series does not involve a comparison group; however, may be valuable at making observations about a rare surgical case or describing a new surgical technique [4]. A case series is also beneficial in developing hypotheses that are to be tested with analytic studies; however, it is not possible to make causal inferences about the relationship between risk factors and the outcome of interest [8, 11]. Similar to case-control studies, in a case series, the status may not have been recorded in the past, so the presence or absence of risk factors cannot be determined. Lastly, case series may not be generalizable, as they often focus on a single surgeon or center's experiences [8]. Case series are very common in the surgical literature as they are relatively easy and inexpensive to do (Please see Chap. 19: Case Series).

A historically controlled study is another study design that constitutes Level IV evidence. This study design includes a control and a treatment group who share the same disorder. The treatment group is comprised of individuals who are currently receiving the treatment of interest and the control group consists of individuals who received an alternative treatment in the past. This design allows researchers to investigate the effects of a new treatment quickly and inexpensively. However, this study design is vulnerable to bias and requires that the selection of historical controls be sufficiently similar to that of the treatment group [12]. Lastly, since the status may not have been recorded in the past, the presence or absence of the risk factor cannot be determined.

Lowest on the hierarchy of evidence for therapeutic research is mechanism-based reasoning [4]. Mechanism-based reasoning is based on expert opinion and is intended to generate hypotheses or interpret evidence from other sources. This LOE relies on the knowledge of underlying mechanisms to predict what the relevant effect of a therapy (or diagnostic test or prognosis, depending on the area of research) will be for the patient [13]. This LOE has the greatest potential for error and is, therefore, the lowest on the hierarchy. Evaluating Level V evidence is described in more detail in Chap. 26.

Level I through Level IV evidence can be graded downward based on study quality, imprecision, indirectness, or inconsistency between studies or when the effect size is very small. Similarly, these studies can be graded upward if there is a dramatic effect size [10].

Clinical Example

An example of a Level I evidence study is, "The Fixation using Alternative Implants for the Treatment of Hip Fractures trial (FAITH)" RCT, which is appraised in Chap. 11.

Levels of Evidence for Diagnostic Research

Diagnostic research evaluates the ability of a diagnostic test to determine the presence or absence of the condition in question. Research questions that diagnostic research addresses include *"Is this (early detection) test worthwhile?"* and *"Is this diagnostic or monitoring test accurate?"* The appraisal of a diagnostic test is explained in Chap. 20. The hierarchy of evidence for diagnostic research is listed in Fig. 5.3.

Similar to therapeutic research, RCTs are considered to be Level I evidence. Diagnostic RCTs are randomized comparisons of two diagnostic interventions (one standard and one experimental) with identical therapeutic interventions based on the results of the competing diagnostic interventions (for example, disease: yes or no) and with the study outcomes being clinically important consequences of diagnostic accuracy (Fig. 5.4a) [14]. Additionally, testing of previously developed diagnostic criteria, using a cohort study design with consecutive patients, consistently applied reference standards, and blinding is also considered to be Level I evidence [4]. In these prospective diagnostic accuracy cohort studies, patients with suspected disease or condition undergo both the diagnostic intervention or criteria being evaluated and the diagnostic reference standard (Fig. 5.4b) [14]. Diagnostic accuracy or the performance of the previously developed experimental diagnostic intervention or criteria is measured using a 2 × 2 table [14]. Diagnostic tests with three or more levels allow for likelihood ratios to be computed, but not sensitivity and specificity. Therefore, diagnostic tests should include likelihood ratios and not sensitivity and specificity, as they go in the wrong direction. While diagnostic cohort studies

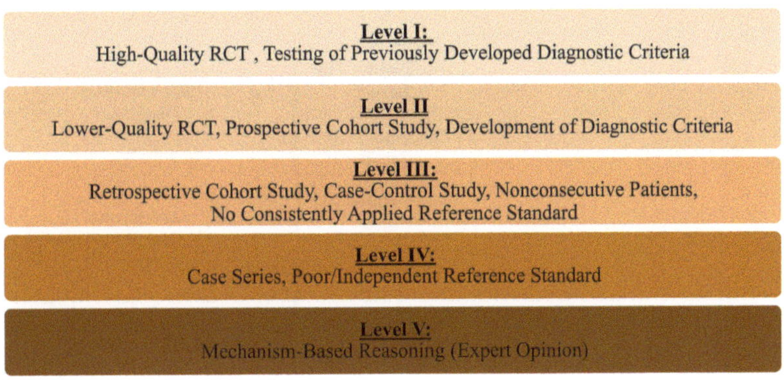

Fig. 5.3 Levels of evidence and their associated study designs for diagnostic research. *RCT* randomized controlled trial; Created using information from JBJS [4] and Elsevier

Fig. 5.4 **a** RCT study design for diagnostic studies. **b** Prospective cohort design for diagnostic studies. **c** Retrospective cohort design for diagnostic studies. **d** Case-control design for diagnostic studies. **e** Case series design for diagnostic studies

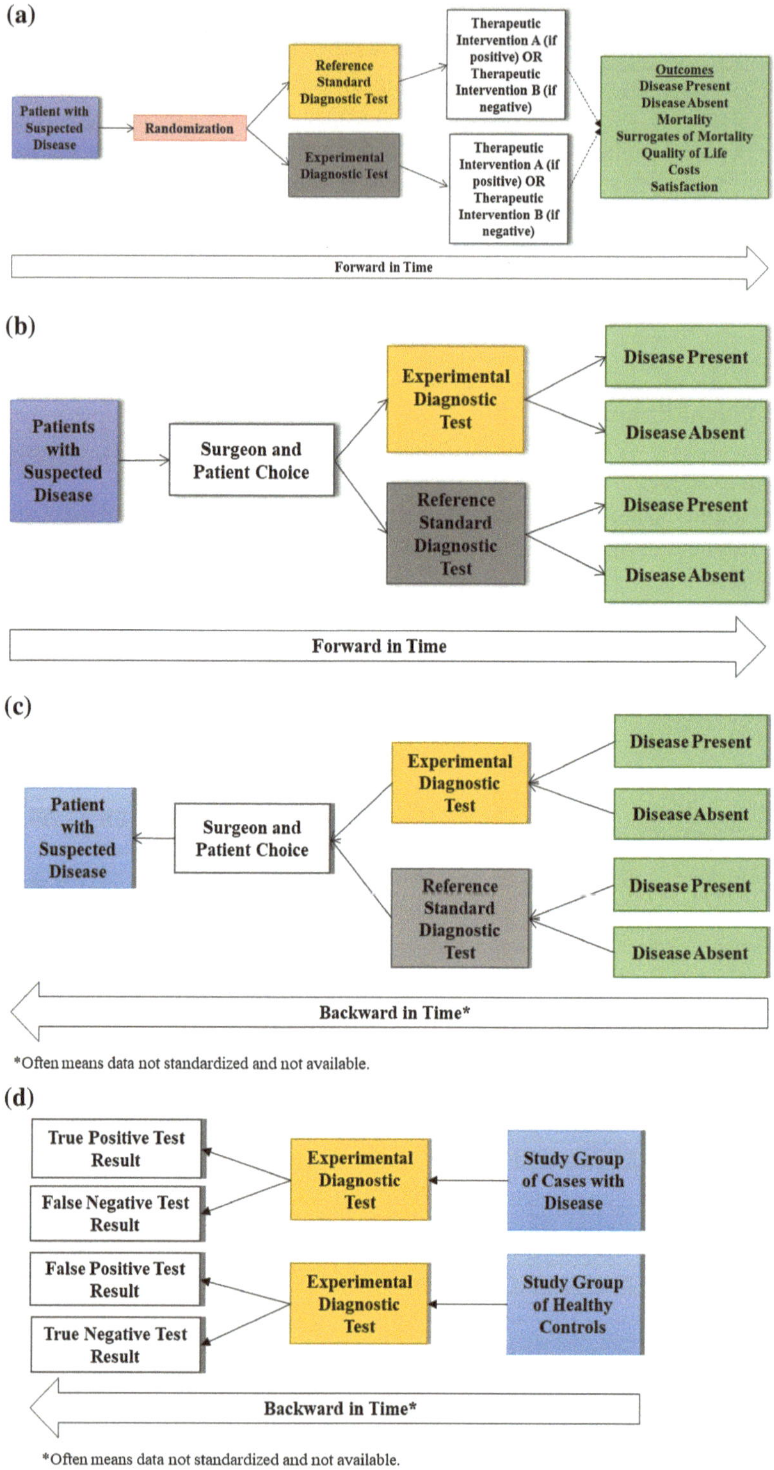

Fig. 5.4 (continued)

(e)

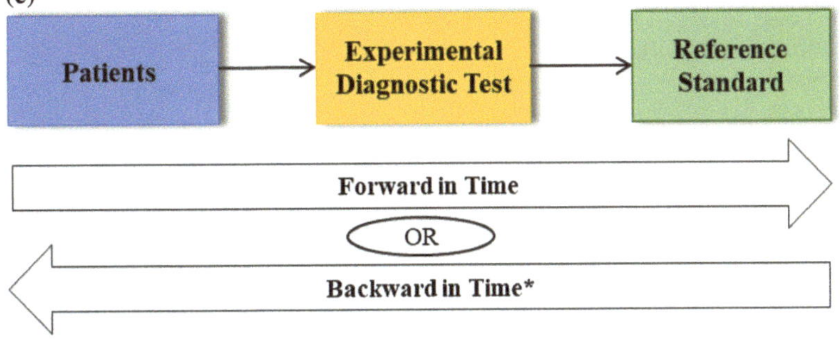

*Often means data not standardized and not available.

inform us about the relative accuracy of an experimental diagnostic intervention compared to a reference standard, they do not inform us about whether the differences in accuracy are clinically important, or the degree of clinical importance (in other words, the impact on patient outcomes) [14].

Level II evidence includes a prospective cohort study, as described above, evaluating a new diagnostic test or diagnostic criteria. Additionally, studies that describe the development of a new diagnostic test or criteria, that include consecutive patients with consistently applied reference standards and blinding, are also considered Level II evidence.

Level III study designs, include retrospective cohort studies. These studies are similar to the cohort studies described above, however, data are collected retrospectively (Fig. 5.4c). Diagnostic case-control studies are also considered to be Level III evidence (Fig. 5.4d). Additionally, prospective cohort studies that includes nonconsecutive patients and does not include a consistently applied reference standard are also considered to be Level III evidence, and, therefore, may not be present in records.

As with therapeutic research, case series describing a diagnostic test or diagnostic criteria are considered to be Level IV evidence (Fig. 5.4 e). When case series, case-control, or retrospective studies look back in time, the included data may not be standardized, or the data are unavailable and were not recorded in the past, resulting in a lower quality of evidence. Additionally, prospective cohort studies that have a poor or nonindependent reference standard are also considered to be Level IV evidence. Lastly, therapeutic studies using mechanism-based reasoning are considered to be Level V evidence.

Clinical Example

An example of a Level II evidence study is the "Prospective validation of the ultrasound based TIRADS (Thyroid Imaging Reporting And Data System) classification: results in surgically resected thyroid nodules" which is appraised in Chap. 20.

Levels of Evidence for Prognostic Research

Prognostic research estimates the risk of future outcomes in individuals based on clinical and nonclinical characteristics [15]. It addresses questions regarding the natural history of the disease. By identifying prognostic studies involving patients with a similar clinical presentation, an attending surgeon is able to inform their patients about their expected clinical course and make better-informed decisions on treatment [15]. Typically, prognostic research consists of prospective, observational studies that aim to assess the causes of disease progression, prediction of risk in individuals, and individual response to treatment [16]. As it is not possible to randomly assign these factors, one usually cannot conduct an RCT to address a prognostic research

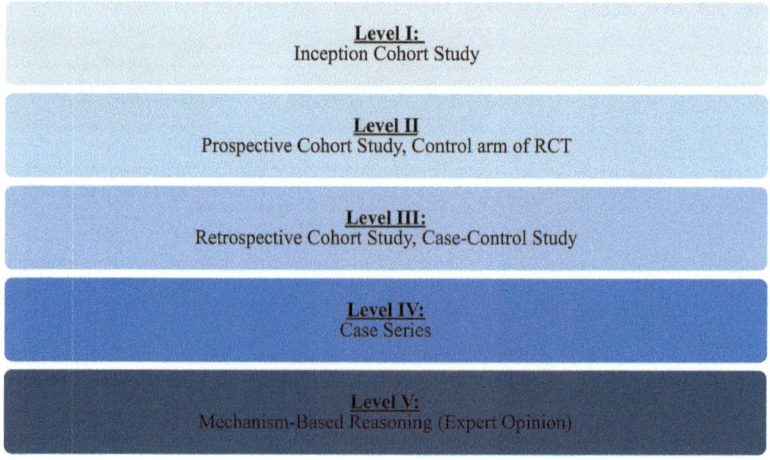

Fig. 5.5 Levels of evidence and their associated study designs for prognostic research

question. Therefore, compared to therapeutic and diagnostic research, prognostic research studies follow different criteria in determining LOE (Fig. 5.5) [17].

Inception cohort studies represent the highest LOE in prognostic research. In an inception cohort study, all patients are enrolled at a common time early in the development of their disease or condition (near the onset of symptoms, soon after diagnosis, or at detection of a clinically important pathological event), and are followed thereafter [18]. Outcomes and factors associated with patient outcomes are then reported (Fig. 5.6a).

Level II evidence includes a prospective cohort study (as described above) in which patients are enrolled at different points of their disease (Fig. 5.6b). Additionally, the use of data from a control arm of a RCT to determine prognostic outcomes is also considered Level II evidence. Retrospective cohort studies (Fig. 5.6 c) and case-control studies (Fig. 5.6d) reporting on prognostic measures are considered Level III evidence.

Similar to therapeutic and diagnostic research, case series are considered to be level IV evidence in prognostic research (Fig. 5.6e) and mechanism-based reasoning is considered to be Level V evidence in prognostic research [7].

Clinical Example

An example of a prognostic study deemed Level III evidence is the "Mechanical or Biologic Prostheses for Aortic-Valve and Mitral-Valve Replacement" retrospective cohort study, which is appraised in Chap. 22.

Levels of Evidence for Economic Research

Economic research evaluates whether or not the intervention or treatment offers the greatest benefit for the amount of dollars spent [4]. All LOE for economic research include computer simulation models (CSM), using Monte Carlo simula-

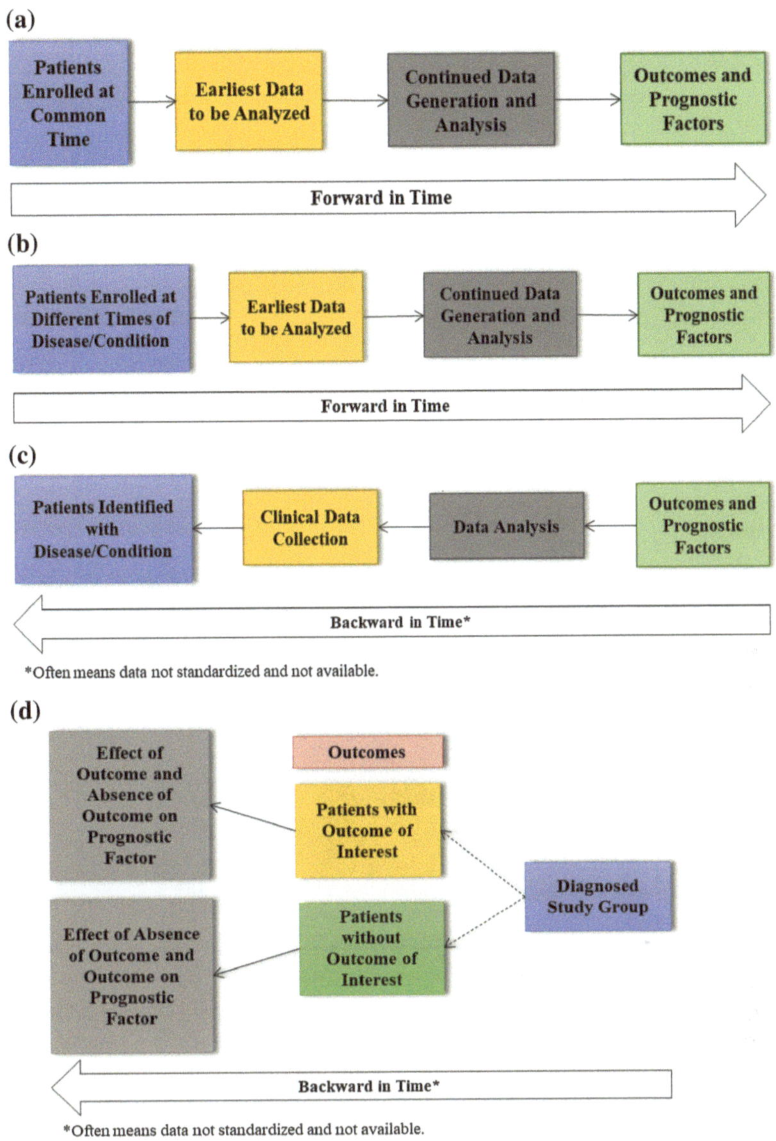

Fig. 5.6 **a** Inception cohort design for prognostic studies. **b** Prospective cohort study design for prognostic studies. **c** Retrospective cohort design for prognostic studies. **d** Case-control design for prognostic studies. **e** Case series design for prognostic studies

tion or Markov models. The inputs for each LOE differs. For Level I evidence, inputs should be derived from Level I studies, as well as include lifetime time duration, outcomes expressed in dollars per quality-adjusted life years (QALYs), and uncertainty examined using probabilistic sensitivity analyses [4].

Level II evidence consists of computer simulation from Level II studies, including lifetime time duration, outcomes expressed in QALYs

Fig. 5.6 (continued)

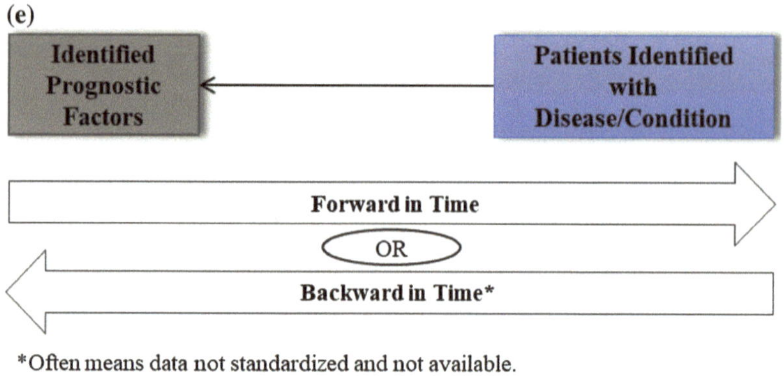

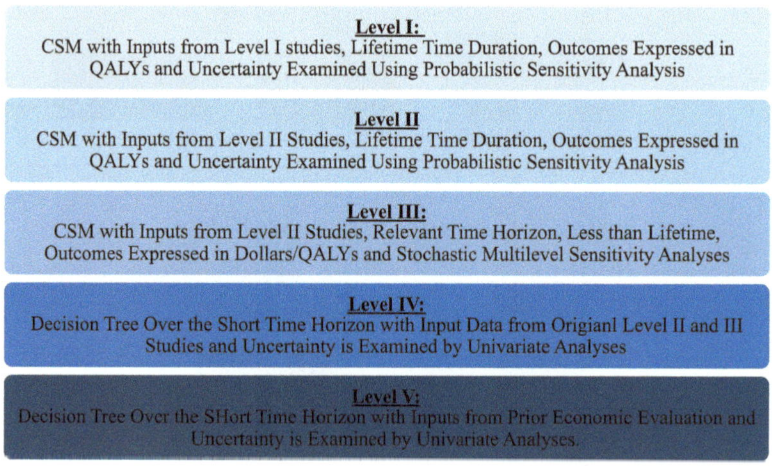

Fig. 5.7 Levels of evidence and their associated study designs for economic research. *CSM* computer simulation model; created with information from JBJS

and uncertainty examined using probabilistic sensitivity analyses. Level III evidence also uses inputs derived from Level II studies, however, differs as it uses a relevant time horizon, less than a lifetime, and outcomes expressed in dollars per QALYs and stochastic multilevel sensitivity analyses [4].

Level IV and V on the hierarchy of evidence for economic research uses a decision tree over the short-time horizon. Level IV uses input data from original Level II and III studies and uncertainty is examined by univariate sensitivity analyses. Level V differs as it uses input data informed by prior economic evaluation and uncertainty is examined by univariate sensitivity analyses [4]. Figure 5.7 summarizes the LOE for economic research and Chap. 23 provides guidance on how to critically appraise economic evaluations.

Clinical Example

An example of a Level I evidence study is the "Cost effectiveness analysis of arthroscopic surgery compared with non-operative management for osteoarthritis of the knee" economic evaluation, which is appraised in Chap. 23.

Summary

To effectively practice evidence-based surgery, a clear understanding of the hierarchy of evidence is necessary. In this chapter, we discussed the hierarchy of evidence as it applies to therapeutic, diagnostic, prognostic, and economic research. Of note, SRs and MAs of high-level clinical studies are suitable for evaluating all clinical questions. Questions about therapy and diagnostics are best addressed with high quality, definitive randomized controlled trials. Inception cohort studies are the highest available evidence for prognostic studies, while a computer simulation model with inputs derived from Level I studies represent the best available evidence for economic analyses.

Concluding Remarks

The LOE are a vital component of evidence-based surgical practice. The hierarchy of evidence provides a valuable tool by which surgeons are able to understand and rank the surgical literature by study design. One, however, should not be dismissive of the lower LOE. Early in their infancy novel interventions progress from a case report, to case series, to comparative cohort studies. Once such innovations are adopted widely, they are then compared in RCTs or meta-analyses. The problem arises when in the face of higher LOE surgeons choose to base their practice on lower LOE because they lack the skills to distinguish the two. When faced with multiple sources and variable LOE, the surgeon should be able to separate the "chaff from the wheat." Later chapters in this book will discuss the next steps of critical appraisal which is specific to each study design.

Appendix 1: Oxford Centre for Evidence-Based Medicine 2011 Levels of Evidence [3]

	Question						
	How common is the problem?	Is this diagnostic or monitoring test accurate	What will happen if we do not add a therapy?	Does this intervention help?	What are the common harms?	What are the rare harms?	Is this (early detection) test worthwhile?
		Diagnosis	Prognosis	Treatment benefits	Treatment harms		Screening
Step 1 (Level 1[a])	Local and current random sample surveys (or censuses)	SR of crosssectional with consistently applied reference standard and blinding	SR of inception cohort studies	SR of randomized trials or *n-of-1* trials	SR of randomized trials, SR of nested case-control studies, *n-of-1* trial with the patient you are raising the question about, or observational study with dramatic effect	SR of randomized trials or *n-of-1* trials	SR of randomized trials
Step 2 (Level 2[a])	SR of surveys that allow matching to local circumstances[b]	Individual cross sectional with consistently applied reference standard and blinding	Inception cohort studies	Randomized trial or observational study with dramatic effect	Individual randomized trial or (exceptionally) observational study with dramatic effect	Randomized trial or (exceptionally) observational study with dramatic effect	Randomized trial
Step 3 (Level 3[a])	Local non-random sample[b]	Non-consecutive, or studies without consistently applied reference standards[b]	Cohort study or control arm of randomized trial[a]	Non-randomized controlled cohort/follow-up study[b]	Non-randomized controlled cohort/follow-up study (post-marketing surveillance) provided there are sufficient numbers to rule out a common harm. (For long-term harms the duration of follow-up must be sufficient)		Nonrandomized controlled cohort/followup study[b]
Step 4 (Level 4)	Case-series[b]	Case-control, or poor or nonindependent reference standard[b]	Case-series or case-control studies, or poor quality prognostic cohort study[b]	Case-series, casecontrol or historically controlled studies[b]	Case-series, case-control, or historically controlled studies[b]		
Step 5 (Level 5)	–	Mechanism-based reasoning	–	Mechanism-based reasoning			

SR Systematic review

[a]Level may be graded down on the basis of study quality, imprecision, indirectness (study of PICO does not match question PICO), because of inconsistency between studies, or because the absolute effect size is very small. Level may be graded up if there is a large or very large effect size

[b]A systematic review is generally better than an individual study

References

1. Canadian Task Force on the Periodic Health Examination. The periodic health examination. Can Med Assoc J. 1979;121(9):1193–1254. https://www.ncbi.nlm.nih.gov/pmc/articles/PMC1704686/pdf/canmedaj01457-0037.pdf. Accessed 27 June 2018.
2. Sackett DL. Rules of evidence and clinical recommendations on the use of antithrombotic agents. Chest. 1989;95(Supp 2):2S-4S.
3. OCEBM Levels of Evidence Working Group. The Oxford 2011 levels of evidence. http://www.cebm.net/index.aspx?o=5653. Accessed 11 June 2018.
4. JBJS. Journals Level of Evidence. J Bone Joint Surg. https://journals.lww.com/jbjsjournal/Pages/Journals-Level-of-Evidence.aspx (Published 2015).
5. Wright JG, Swiontkowski MF, Heckman JD. Introducing levels of evidence to the journal. J Bone Jt Surg. 2003;85(1):1–3.
6. Elselvier. Levels of evidence. http://cdn.elsevier.com/promis_misc/Levels_of_Evidence.pdf (2005). Accessed May 23, 2018.
7. Sprague S, McKay P, Thoma A. Study design and hierarchy of evidence for surgical decision making. Clin Plast Surg. 2008;35:195–205. https://doi.org/10.1016/j.cps.2007.10.007.
8. Petrisor B, Bhandari M. The hierarchy of evidence: levels and grades of recommendation. Indian J Orthop. 2007;41(1):11–5.
9. Fineout-Overholt E, Melnyk BM, Stillwell SB, Williamson KM. Evidence based practice step by step: critical appraisal of the evidence: Part I. Source Am J Nurs. 2010;110(7):47–52. http://www.jstor.org/stable/pdf/25684627.pdf?refreqid=excelsior%3Aadf45c2c61b6114a9a7283ab8269142e. Accessed 24 May 2018.
10. Wupperman R, Davis R, Obremskey WT. Level of evidence in spine compared to other orthopedic journals. Spine (Phila Pa 1976). 32(3):388–393.
11. Brighton B, Bhandari M, Tornetta P, Felson DT. Hierarchy of evidence: from case reports to randomized controlled trials. Clin Orthop Relat Res. 2003;413(413):19–24. https://doi.org/10.1097/01.blo.0000079323.41006.12.
12. Viele K, Berry S, Neuenschwander B, et al. Use of historical control data for assessing treatment effects in clinical trials. Pharm Stat. 2014;13(1):41–54. https://doi.org/10.1002/pst.1589.
13. Howick J, Chalmers I, Glasziou P et al. Explanation of the 2011 Oxford Centre for evidence-based medicine (OCEBM) levels of evidence (background document). Oxford Centre for Evidence-Based Medicine; 2011.
14. Rodger M, Ramsay T, Fergusson D. Diagnostic randomized controlled trials: the final frontier. Trials. 2012;13(1):137. https://doi.org/10.1186/1745-6215-13-137.
15. Moons KGM, Royston P, Vergouwe Y, Grobbee DE, Altman DG. Prognosis and prognostic research: what, why, and how? BMJ. 2009;338:b375. https://doi.org/10.1136/BMJ.B375.
16. Hemingway H, Riley RD, Altman DG. Ten steps towards improving prognosis research. BMJ. 2009;339:b4184. https://doi.org/10.1136/BMJ.B4184.
17. Devries JG, Berlet GC. Understanding Levels of Evidence for Scientific Communication. Foot Ankle Spec. 2010;3(4):205–9.
18. Porta M, Greenland S, Hernán M, dos Santos Silva I, Last J. For the International Epidemiological Association. A dictionary of epidemiology. 6th ed. New York, NY: Oxford University Press; 2014.

Evaluating Surgical Interventions

6

Aristithes G. Doumouras and Dennis Hong

Clinical decision-making in surgery has evolved dramatically in the past several years. Traditionally, surgeons coalesced anecdotal evidence, previous experience, expert opinion, and extrapolation of basic science into clinical decision-making. While this often served patients well, it is also possible that this decision-making process led to suboptimal treatment. To combat this, a plethora of surgical research has been ongoing for the past several decades, and the utilization and understanding of this evidence are vital to surgical practice in the twenty-first century [1]. The evidence itself can vary greatly in quality and therefore several grading systems have been developed to assess quality [2, 3]. Regardless of the grading system, the general hierarchy of evidence remains the same and is based on the propensity of a certain study type to introduce bias into its conclusions. Bias, specifically, refers to any systematic deviation from the truth, which could result in an underestimation or overestimation of the true effect of an intervention [4].

The lowest level of evidence after expert opinion consists of retrospective case series which present outcomes without comparison, and retrospective cohorts, which often are used to compare two or more therapies (see Chap. 5). While uncomplicated to design, the retrospective nature of these studies does not allow for the collection of all potential confounding factors. This limits the ability to infer causation from the conclusions. The next level of evidence consists of prospective, nonrandomized controlled trials. While the prospective nature of these studies allows for better data collection, the lack of randomization can still lead to an imbalance within groups for unmeasured variables that would not be accounted for fully with statistical analyses. Properly designed and conducted randomized trials provide a high level of internal validity to their conclusions but can be limited by their generalizability [3]. Accordingly, the highest level of evidence is when several randomized trials looking at the same topic can be combined into a meta-analysis [5, 6]. Meta-analyses combine the results of several trials in an effort to boost statistical power and minimize false negative results. However, one should be cautious of meta-analyses of observational data as *a meta-analysis of biased data is still biased* though these types of studies may be useful in summarizing the current observational evidence for a topic. Ideally, surgeons can evaluate the evidence they have for the clinical problem at hand and provide optimal care based on this assessment.

A. G. Doumouras
Department of Surgery, McMaster University, Hamilton, ON, Canada
e-mail: aristithes.doumouras@medportal.ca

D. Hong (✉)
Department of Surgery, St. Joseph's Healthcare, Hamilton, ON, Canada
e-mail: dennishong70@gmail.com

A. Thoma et al. (eds.), *Evidence-Based Surgery*,
https://doi.org/10.1007/978-3-030-05120-4_6

Clinical Scenario

You are a general surgeon on a surgical mission to a low-income country. In the course of an inguinal hernia repair requiring mesh, the junior resident who accompanied you on the trip asks you why you are using a sterilized mosquito net rather than polypropylene mesh, the mesh you use back home. You inform her that the typical mesh back home is very expensive and the mission hospital cannot afford it. After the case, you challenge her to review the literature and find out if there is a difference in effectiveness between these two approaches for the major outcomes of inguinal hernia repair such as complication rates and recurrence.

Search Strategy

Your search is designed to cast a wide net and include all relevant articles while ultimately trying to focus on a few number of key articles. Accordingly, you search MEDLINE with a broad strategy that includes both the Medical Subject Headings (MeSH) "Herniorrhaphy," "Hernia" and "Costs and Cost Analysis" and non-MeSH keywords "mesh" and "low-cost." Using non-MeSH terms ensures the inclusion of all relevant abstracts. These search terms are combined with the "OR" Boolean function to create the initial database. From this, abstracts can be reviewed individually or, if still too numerous, the Boolean "AND" function can be used to narrow down the choices and create a more relevant set. For practical purposes, we can also limit it to the English language though this may introduce bias into systematic reviews. To further narrow down the list, we can also look directly for clinical trials (see Chap. 4). In doing this, we get four hits, and of these hits, one is a randomized trial with the desried clinical outcomes by Löfgren et al. [7]. The purpose of this chapter is to assist the reader to interpret the results/data presented in a surgical article. Therefore, we will appraise the Lofren et al. [7] article and find if the authors' conclusions are supported by the data they provide. The evaluation of surgical interventions follows the framework shown in Table 6.1.

When considering the evidence, there are three main aspects of a study that should be assessed: internal validity, the results, and external validity (Table 6.1). We will discuss each of these points individually and how to assess them. We will scrutinize the results of the Löfgren et al. [7], which, are presented in Table 6.2.

Table 6.1 How to appraise an article evaluating surgical interventions [8]

Question	Appraisal
Are the results valid?	– Was patient assignment randomized, and the randomization process "concealed"? – Were study personnel "blinded" to treatment and apart from the experimental intervention, were the groups treated equally? – Were all patients who entered the trial accounted for and was follow-up adequate? – Were patients analyzed according to the "intention to treat" principle? – Was the study large enough to detect a difference?
What are the results?	– What are the outcomes and how were they measured? – How large was the treatment effect? – How precise was the estimate of the treatment effect?
Are the results applicable to my patients?	– Were the study patients similar to my patients? – Were the measured outcomes clinically relevant? – Are my surgical skills similar to those of the study surgeons?

Table 6.2 Primary outcomes and mortality among study participants [7]

	Outcome	Low-cost mesh (*n* = 143)	Commercial mesh (*n* = 148)	Absolute difference		*p*-value
				Percentage points	95% CI	
Primary outcomes	*Hernia recurrence*	1 (0.7)	0	0.7	(−1.2 to 2.6)	1.0
	Any postoperative complication	44 (30.8)	44 (29.7)	1.0	(−9.5 to 11.6)	1.0
Distribution of Postoperative outcomes	*Hematoma or swelling in groin or scrotum*	35 (24.5)	35 (23.6)	0.8	(−9.0 to 10.7)	1.0
	Superficial infection	4 (2.8)	6 (4.1)	1.3	(−5.6 to 3.1)	0.38
	Seroma	1 (0.7)	0	0.7	(−1.2 to 2.6)	1.0
	Impaired wound healing	5 (3.5)	8 (5.4)	1.9	(−6.8 to 3.0)	0.29
	Severe pain	2 (1.4)	0	1.4	(−0.9 to 3.7)	1.0
	Other complications	2 (1.4)	4 (2.7)	1.3	(−4.8 to 2.2)	0.34
Death		2 (1.4)	3 (2.0)	0.6	(−3.9 to 2.6)	1.0

Appraisal of an Article: Are the Results Valid?

Internal validity refers to the soundness of the methodology of the study and relates directly to our ability to infer causation from the results. In observational studies, the correlations presented in the results may not actually represent a true causal relationship and therefore using their conclusions without proper scrutiny may lead to unnecessary or potentially harmful patient care. Two types of errors can threaten internal validity [9]. Type I errors, or false positives, occur when calling a treatment useful when it is not. Type II errors, or false negatives, occur when concluding a treatment has no effect when it is actually useful (see Chap. 29). There are numerous examples of observational study conclusions that turned out to be equivocal or even harmful when examined in a randomized setting. Randomized trials provide the most sound experimental design and results that are most likely to be causal. This section will highlight some of the important points to look for when assessing the internal validity of a study. Importantly, some of this information may actually be in the study protocol rather than the paper itself.

Was Patient Assignment Randomized, and was the Randomization Process "Concealed"?

Relationships between outcomes predictors of interest are subject to confounding. Confounding is the potential for a third variable to influence the relationship between the outcome and predictor thus limiting our ability to infer direct causation (see *Chapter 32: Confounding Factors and Interactions*). For observational studies, many of these confounders can be identified and adjusted for within multivariable statistical analyses. One of the advantages of prospective over retrospective studies is the ability to ensure data collection on important confounding factors. However, there are many unmeasurable or unknown confounding factors that cannot be collected and adjusted for. It is for these factors that randomization is crucial as it is the best way to balance these unknown or unmeasurable factors between groups. The method of randomization (usually a computer program) should be mentioned in the methods of any trial. Another vital aspect of randomization is allocation concealment. This refers to the concealment of the randomization process from the investigators so that it is unknown what group a patient will be randomized into. If not done properly, investigators can intentionally or unintentionally direct patients towards the group they feel is most suitable thus introducing selection bias into the process and losing much of the benefit of randomization. In the study by Löfgren et al. [7] the operation list and order of patients was determined the day before but randomization was not performed until the patient was brought into the operative suite. In this way, randomization was concealed from the surgeons. In addition, randomization was done by a computer program in blocks of 4 and 6, rather than randomizing single individuals which allows for more balance of factors.

Were Study Personnel "Blinded" to Treatment and Apart from the Experimental Intervention, Were the Groups Treated Equally?

Another major methodological concept is blinding. This is often confused with allocation concealment but they are distinct concepts. Blinding refers to ensuring that stakeholders in the trial do not know what treatment patients received as knowing this can influence the behavior of patients and investigators. While blinding of both patients and investigators is relatively straightforward in drug trials, it is often not possible in surgical trials as surgeons will often need to know the treatment the patient had. One way to minimize this issue in surgical trials is to have different clinicians provide the postoperative care to patients. In the study by Löfgren et al. [7], after randomization was done, the surgeons in the operative suite did know the type of mesh to be used within the procedure (blinded-patient). However, to minimize bias due to this, the two physicians performing the follow-up did not participate in the surgeries and were unaware of the study group assignments. Considering the study question, this was probably the strongest level of blinding possible.

Were All Patients Who Entered the Trial Accounted for and Was Follow-up Adequate?

Another major issue with trials of all types is patient attrition rate. Readers should be concerned if not all patients are accounted for at a trial's conclusion. If a large proportion of patients are unaccounted for at the end of a trial, the benefits of randomization may be lost. Moreover, bias can be introduced if the dropout is related to some aspect of the procedure itself. If the dropout was random, then the benefits of randomization should be maintained. Therefore, a full report of patient attrition is required. In addition, the follow-up should be rigorous, blinded and equal between groups to ensure that all adverse effects are accounted for. It should also be assessed similarly between groups and be long enough to ensure that the outcomes of interest can manifest themselves. In the Löfgren et al. [7] study, the follow-up was thoroughly conducted by two physicians who were blinded to the study group assignments. Overall, 4.4% of patients were lost to follow-up which was not different between groups. In addition, the time from surgery to follow-up was similar between groups. This is not unsurprising as there is little morbidity from a hernia repair and the follow-up period was relatively short.

Were Patients Analyzed According to the "Intention to Treat" Principle?

The intention-to-treat principle is also fundamental to ensuring causal inference of results. This principle states that patients should be analyzed in the groups they were originally allocated to, regardless of the treatment actually received. This is vital in surgical trials as patients of poor operative status sometimes may not receive surgery, despite being randomized for surgery. If these patients were to be analyzed in the nonsurgical group, they can bias the results by having healthier people in the surgical group. Sometimes, this principle can lead to issues of validity of conclusions if there are too many patients that did not receive the treatment but in most cases the strategy is sound. In addition, in surgical trials, if there are many patients not receiving the treatment it may provide a pragmatic answer as to the feasibility of the treatment.

In the Löfgren et al. [7] study, the intention to treat principle was followed for the final analysis. However, they make no mention of how the missing data was dealt with. It is likely, based on the small number of missing patients that the authors used a complete case analysis including data from only those patients who completed follow-up. This method of handling missing data is likely unbiased in this case due to the small numbers and did not likely substantially change the power for this study. Had patients dropped out due to measured or unmeasured confounders, the analysis will be biased. Furthermore, if too many patients were lost, even at random, the power of the study would be called into question.

Was the Study Large Enough to Detect a Difference?

Ensuring an adequate sample size is essential to answering any clinical question. A randomized trial should clearly describe an a priori sample size and what factors they used to determine the sample size. Generally, calculating a sample size requires the rate of type I error (usually 5%), rate of type II error (usually 20%, also known as 80% power), the allocation ratio between groups (1:1, 2:1, etc.), the expected effect and the variance of that effect. While the first three are fairly standard in the sample size calculation, the last few variables can be controlled by investigators. A larger a priori expected effect means a smaller sample size but if that effect is unreasonable then it could lead to an underpowered trial. Conversely, the effect size chosen should also be large enough to be clinically relevant. Power is the complement of the type II error rate for a trial, and can be described as the chance for a trial to produce a false negative result. Therefore, before a negative result can be truly established, the sample size and statistical power should be scrutinized and found to be adequate (see Chap. 29). In addition, the conclusions of other outcomes assessed, for which there was no sample size calculation, should not be assumed to be adequately powered. In the Löfgren et al. [7] study, the sample size was calculated at 150 patients within each group. This would give the study a power of 80% and a significance level of 5% to detect a five-percentage-point absolute difference in the rate of hernia recurrence at one year. Upon completion of the trial, this study failed to achieve the desired power level. The inability to reach power based on accrual issues should have been mentioned in the limitations so that it can be considered by the reader (see Chap. 29).

What Are the Results?

The key findings of the Löfgren et al. [7] study are found in Table 6.2.

What Outcomes Were Used and How Were They Measured?

Because of the wide variety of outcomes that can be assessed and the use of sophisticated statistical analyses, simply understanding what the results are can be a challenge for a surgeon. This section will provide a brief summary of how the most common outcomes are reported.

Binary Versus Continuous Outcomes

The vast majority of outcomes in the surgical literature are measured as either binary or continuous variables. Binary outcomes represent dichotomous occurrences where patients either have an outcome or they do not (e.g., death or anastomotic leak). Continuous outcomes represent data that are measured by real numbers such as weight or length of stay. The study by Löfgren et al. [7] had two primary outcomes, both binary, which were the hernia recurrence at 1 year and the overall complication rate at 2 weeks.

Univariate Testing: Univariable and Multivariable Analyses

There is considerable confusion in the literature as to the nomenclature for testing let alone the actual test themselves. Univariate testing refers to statistical tests with a single response variable per observation. This represents the vast majority of tests in the surgical literature where a single patient will have a single outcome associated with them. Multivariate analyses refer to when a single patient has multiple outcomes associated with them and are rarely used (i.e., a patient has several weight changes over the course of the study) [10]. Univariate testing can take the form of univariable or multivariable tests. Univariable tests occur when the outcome is tested against only a single predictor. Examples include the chi-square test for dichotomous data and a t-test for continuous data. For observational data, these usually represent preliminary tests and are used to give some exposition to the data rather than as actual conclusions. Alternatively, for randomized trials, these may represent the final analysis because randomization precludes the need for multivariable analysis.

Multivariable analyses use multiple predictors to explain the outcome of interest. The simplest examples are linear regression for continuous data and logistic regression for binary data. These studies demonstrate the effect of a single predictor of interest while holding all other predictors steady. These analyses, therefore, account for the effect of many different potential confounders which is not done in univariable analyses. In the study by Löfgren et al. [7], because of the fact that it is a randomized clinical trial, multivariable regression was not required. This is because the groups are expected to be balanced due to randomization. Therefore, the main analysis was done using a chi-square test or the Fisher exact test, where appropriate.

Multivariable Regression Results: Odds Ratios (OR) and Risk Ratios (RR)

Every surgeon has seen the results of a multivariable regression but correctly interpreting the results can be a bit more difficult. For linear regressions, the conclusions are represented by the effect on the outcome of interest by a one unit change in the predictor. For example, if an outcome was weight and the predictor was age, the results would be represented as the amount the weight has changed for each year in age. For dichotomous data analyzed by logistic regression, results are represented by odds ratios. Odds ratios are related to risk ratios but are less intuitive. Their predominant use stems from the fact that they are much easier to calculate within statistical models. Risk ratios (also known as relative risks or the incidence rate ratios) represent the ratio between the actual event rate between groups. For example, if the event happened 60% of the time in group A and 40% in group B then the risk ratio would be 1.5. Similarly, odds ratios are the proportion of the odds of occurrence between the two groups. It is not vital to truly understand the difference between odds and risks but it is important to know that odds ratios approximate risk ratios when outcomes are rare but *overestimate* risk when the outcomes are common (>10%). Relative risks are common in randomized trials where multivariable logistic regression analyses are not required due to randomization. Although not utilized in the study by Löfgren et al. [7], one could easily calculate the risk ratio of postoperative complications (refer to Table 6.3 for calculation). In the commercial mesh group, the rate of complication was 29.7% whereas the rate of complication in the low-cost mesh group was 30.8%, therefore, the relative risk of complications in the low-cost mesh group was 1.04, or 4% higher, not a statistically significant difference. Furthermore, a relative risk of 4% is unlikely to be clinically important even if statistically different. One could use the 95% confidence interval and an a priori selected clinically important difference benchmark (non-inferiority margin) to determine whether the change is a large one to persuade us to accept the low-cost mesh. This is the basis of non-inferiority trials (see Chap. 13). Table 6.3 explains the measures that are used to explain the magnitude and precision of the treatment effect of a surgical intervention. The Löfgren et al. [7] article is explained through these measures in Column 3.

How Large Was the Treatment Effect?

Importantly, the difference between absolute and relative measures needs to be understood by the surgeon contextualizing any results. Odds ratios and risk ratios represent a percentage change from the occurrence of an event. The absolute risk represents the change of the occurrence of an event on an absolute scale. From a clinical perspective, the latter is usually the much more important measure. For example, a study may report a predictor increases the event rate by 30% (risk ratio 1.30). This number seems large but if the event only occurs 1% of the time then the absolute risk only goes up to 1.3%. The same study could have reported a 0.3% increase in absolute risk—a much less provocative number. Conversely, a study could report a 5% relative increase (risk ratio 1.05) but if the event occurs 50% of the time then the absolute risk increase is 2.5%. Despite the clinical utility, absolute risks are usually only reported in randomized trials because they are much more difficult to model in regression analyses. Accordingly, surgeons must keep in mind the absolute risk of an event to contextualize the results of many trials. The study by Löfgren et al. [7] does report the absolute risk difference which is 1.1% and this was not seen as statistically significant. This, and calculations for the other results from the Löfgren et al. [7] study are shown in Table 6.2. The number needed to treat (NNT) of 91 (see column 3 Table 6.3) is an important measure which adds context to our interpretation of the data. It tells us that we have to treat 91 patients with the commercial mesh (instead of the low-cost mesh) to avoid one complication. Many surgeons may not see this as a huge benefit and may opt for the low-cost alternative.

Table 6.3 Terms used to show the magnitude and precision of the treatment effect

Term	Description	Example from Löfgren et al. [7]
Risk	The probability that an event would occur calculated as the number of events of interest divided by the total number within the group. Also, known as the relative risk	Risk in treatment group: 44/143 = 0.308 (30.8%) Risk in the control group: 44/148 = 0.297 (29.7%)
Risk ratio	The ratio of the risk between 2 different groups	Risk in treatment 0.308 versus control 0.297 RR: 30.8/29.7 = 1.04
Odds	A ratio of the probability that the event will happen to the probability that the event will not happen within the same group	Risk in the treatment group: 44/(143−44) = 0.44 Risk in the control group: 44/(148−44) = 0.42
Odds ratio	The ratio of odds between 2 different groups	Odds in treatment 0.44 versus in control 0.42 RR: 0.44/0.42 = 1.05
Absolute risk reduction	Absolute reduction in events in one group compared with the other	Complication in treatment 30.8% versus in control 29.7%. ARR: 30.8 −29.7 = 1.1%
Number needed to treat	The average number of patients who need to be treated to prevent one additional bad outcome. It is defined as the inverse of the absolute risk reduction	ARR from article:1.1% NNT = 1/ARR = 1/0.011 NNT = 91 patients
Relative risk reduction	Complement of relative risk, expressed as a percentage	Complication in treatment 30.8% versus in control 29.7%. RR (30.8−29.7)/ 30.8 = 3.6%
95% confidence interval	An interval of values that include the true value 95% of the time (calculated)	Various methods of calculation

How Precise was the Estimate of the Treatment Effect?

The last thing a surgeon should examine are the measures of statistical significance and precision. The significance is represented by *p* values. *p* values represent the probability of obtaining the results if the null hypothesis (i.e. the assumption that the predictor has no effect) were true. Generally, when this probability is less than 5% (<0.05) we consider the result statistically significant. It should be noted that this specific threshold is completely arbitrary and there is nothing magical between a *p*-value of 0.051 and 0.049. This threshold exists to limit the rate of Type I error (e.g. false positives) to 5%. Lastly, even if the *p*-value is below this threshold, statistical significance does not equate to clinical relevance. As a standard, most trials use a two-sided *p*-value of 0.05 as the threshold for statistical significance (see Chap. 27). In addition to *p* values, confidence intervals exist to better characterize the precision of the result. The 95% confidence interval is routinely used and can be interpreted as the interval in which the true effect lies 95% of the time if the same study with the same sample was repeated (see Chap. 28). Therefore, in studies with small sample sizes, the confidence interval can be quite large but with increasing sample size, the confidence interval becomes smaller. In the Löfgren et al. [7] study, the two-sided 95% confidence interval were calculated and for the main outcome of postoperative complication rate difference, this interval varied from −9.5 to 11.6%. One way to interpret this interval is by saying that if this same study was repeated multiple times, the true rate difference would lie within this interval 95% of the time.

Are the Results Applicable to My Patients?

External validity refers to the applicability of results to other groups of patients [11]. After the results are understood and the internal validity assessed, this aspect of any trial should be clearly investigated by the reader and the questions from Table 6.1 should be asked.

Were the Study Patients Similar to My Patients?

Comparing the patient population of a trial to the patient in front of you is essential to the application of evidence to surgical practice. Many trials have restricted criteria for enrollment and the results may not be directly applicable to the patient you are treating. In addition, they may only be enrolled from a specific patient group (e.g., veterans, men, uncomplicated surgical problems) which may not be the patient in front of you. Often, the patients we treat are older, have more comorbidities, and complex surgical problems than a trial would allow. These factors may mitigate the expected benefit of a treatment and thus the surgeon should know how the evidence relates to the patient in front of them before making any treatment decisions. The protocol for this study clearly outlines the inclusion and exclusion criteria. Specifically, it included patients 18 years of age or older with reducible, unilateral, primary inguinal hernias. It excluded females, recurrent hernias, femoral hernias, those on anticoagulation, those with current drug abuse and ASA 3 or above. In addition, these men were all from Uganda with a mean age of around 45 years old, mean BMI of 21 and ASA score of 1 for nearly 90% of the patients. These criteria give a clear picture of the type of patient these results can be applied to. Based on the mean BMI and ASA score of the patients within the study, this trial may not be as applicable in North America; however, it may be applicable to a low-income country. Considering the differences, it is important to carefully determine whether extrapolation to a different patient group is reasonable or whether this patient group has several things that may be too different to apply to your patients.

Were the Measured Outcomes Clinically Relevant?

Another area that surgeons should question before accepting a "superior treatment" is the choice of main outcomes considered in the study. The choice of main outcomes should be relevant to both the surgeon and the patient, and should be clinically meaningful. Certain biochemical markers may be relevant to surgeons but of no relevance to patients while postoperative pain and the return of function may be less important to surgeons but of great substance to patients. The main outcomes of the study include complication rate at 2 weeks and recurrence rate at 1 year. While a 1-year follow-up is relatively long, many recurrences occur after this and therefore the long-term durability of this treatment cannot be determined based on the results of this trial.

Are My Surgical Skills Similar to Those of the Study Surgeons?

Surgeons should also evaluate whether the treatment itself is feasible within their own practice. Trials on robotic surgery or expensive/difficult to obtain materials may have little relevance to a surgical practice, especially in low-resource settings. Moreover, certain surgical techniques may be beyond the technical proficiency of an individual surgeon and thus the treatment effect would largely be lost in the hands of that surgeon. If clearly published evidence does favor a certain treatment that is available but the surgeon does not perform it well then the surgeon is faced with three options: proceed with another operation that surgeon performs well while discussing all options for the patient, refer the patient to a colleague or seek additional training to master the new technique. Surgical proficiency creates a dilemma for surgical trials utilizing complex procedures and provides a major difference between surgical and medical trials. If the trial uses inexperienced surgeons it could bias the results away from the treatment, even if it does have a benefit in experienced hands. However, if the trial only utilized highly skilled surgeons the result may not be applicable to the larger surgical community. The trial by Löfgren et al. [7] utilized a relatively simple surgical procedure which is outlined in the protocol. Specifically, these were day surgeries under local anesthesia which used a Lichtenstein tension-free method. This method could likely be replicated by most general surgeons.

Resolution of the Clinical Scenario

A careful critique of this article demonstrates that the internal validity is quite high and therefore the results are likely valid to their goals. The resident who appraised this article likely felt that it was appropriate for her staff to use the low-cost mosquito net in this instance. It was comparable to the hernia mesh used in North America when used in these patients. However, it was clear that this conclusion may not be applicable to other groups at home in North America and the extrapolation of the results should be limited.

References

1. Garas G, Ibrahim A, Ashrafian H, Ahmed K, Patel V, Okabayashi K, et al. Evidence-based surgery: barriers, solutions, and the role of evidence synthesis. World J Surg. 2012;36(8):1723–31.
2. Baker A, Young K, Potter J, Madan I. A review of grading systems for evidence-based guidelines produced by medical specialties. Clin Med. 2010;10(4):358–63.
3. Kavanagh BP. The GRADE system for rating clinical guidelines. PLoS Med. 2009;6(9):e1000094.
4. Higgins J, Green S, editors. 8.2: "Bias" and "risk of bias." In: Cochrane handbook for systematic reviews of interventions version 510 [Internet]. The Cochrane Collaboration; 2011 [cited 14 June 2018]. Available from: www.handbook.cochrane.org.
5. Dickersin K, Scherer R, Lefebvre C. Identifying relevant studies for systematic reviews. BMJ. 1994;309:1286–91.
6. Balshem H, Helfand M, Schünemann HJ, Oxman AD, Kunz R, Brozek J, et al. GRADE guidelines: 3. Rating the quality of evidence. J Clin Epidemiol. 2011;64(4):401–6.
7. Löfgren J, Nordin P, Ibingira C, Matovu A, Galiwango E, Wladis A. A randomized trial of low-cost mesh in groin hernia repair. N Engl J Med. 2016;374:146–53.

8. Urschel JD, Goldsmith CH, Tandan VR, Miller JD. For the evidence-based surgery working group. Users' guide to evidence-based surgery: how to use an article evaluating surgical interventions. Can J Surg. 2001; 44(2):95–100.
9. Guyatt GH, Sackett DL, Cook DJ. Users' guides to the medical literature. II. How to use an article about therapy or prevention. A. Are the results of the study valid? Evidence-based medicine working group. JAMA. 1993;270:2598–601.
10. Hidalgo B, Goodman M. Multivariate or multivariable regression? Am J Public Health. 2013;103: 39–40.
11. Sedgwick P. External and internal validity in clinical trials. BMJ. 2012;344:e1004.

A Primer on Outcome Measures for Surgical Interventions

7

Joy MacDermid

Clinical Scenario

Patient: Mary is a 50-year-old woman who fell on ice in her driveway. Her X-ray revealed an undisplaced distal radius fracture (DRF). She was managed with a plaster cast in the Emergency Department, and arrangements were made for her to be seen in the fracture room within a week. She is experiencing a lot of pain. She is otherwise healthy. She is well educated, English is her first language and she enjoys reading and watching TV. What kind of outcome measures might I consider?

Information on Outcome Measures

An outcome measure is a standardized assessment of patient status. This includes patient-reported outcome measures (PRO) and clinician-based outcome measures (CBO).

We measure patient status for different reasons to:

- Evaluate change over time in individuals or groups,
- Differentiate pathology—diagnosis; or other clinically relevant subgroups within a population or
- To predict a future outcome (prognosis).

One of the most critical aspects of selecting an outcome measure is defining the concept (construct) that is to be measured [1]. The next step is matching the most salient constructs and measurement purposes to an appropriate outcome measure. Outcome measures can be used to assess broad or narrow constructs. Ideally, outcome measure developers have defined a clear conceptual framework or construct variables that guide the development process and support validation analyses (Table 7.1). Content validity is the extent to which a measure assesses the defined construct by presenting a sufficient set of salient items that adequately represent the content and measurement spectrum of the construct. Users of outcome measures should carefully consider the concordance between the construct they intend to measure, the expected impacts of the treatment plan, and the status of the individual patient. There is a wide variety of outcome measures available for many of the constructs assessed in clinical practice [2–10] (Table 7.2). Users should consider the scope of the construct,

J. MacDermid (✉)
Roth|McFarlane Hand and Upper Limb Centre, London, Canada
e-mail: jmacderm@uwo.ca

J. MacDermid
Western University, London, ON, Canada

J. MacDermid
School of Rehabilitation Science, McMaster University, Hamilton, ON, Canada

A. Thoma et al. (eds.), *Evidence-Based Surgery*,
https://doi.org/10.1007/978-3-030-05120-4_7

Table 7.1 Measurement parameters affecting outcome measurement construct and structure

Scope of construct	Items evaluated	Response scoring	Item perspectives	Respondent
Quality of life, e.g. *EQ-5D*	Consistent items—multiple items arranged in subscales that represent subdomains or related constructs, e.g. pain and disability	Numeric (e.g. 0–10)	Symptom/impairment intensity rating	Clinician—observation based
Health status, e.g. *SF-36*	Consistent items—multi-items from a single construct	Visual analog (e.g. 100 mm line)	Emotional or impact evaluation of a symptom/impairment	Clinician rating—subjective
Change in a construct/overall status, e.g. *Global rating of change*	Adaptive items	Likert	Actual performance of an activity or participation role	Instrumented
Utility, e.g. *Health utility index*, GRC	Single item	Categorical, e.g. Yes/no or dead/perfect health	Perceived capability to perform an activity or participation role	Patient rating
Pain e.g. *numeric pain rating or McGill pain questionnaire*,NRS, MPQ	Patient-generated items	Graphic indicators (e.g. faces)	Emotional evaluation of an aspect of activity or participation	Family member or caregiver rating
Specific symptom, e.g. *Sleep, fatigue*	–	Instrument output (e.g. force, motion)	Opinion/attitude evaluation	Independent observer
Symptoms and function global status, e.g. *The short musculoskeletal function assessment questionnaire* , SMFA	–	Time	Reporting of need for services, aids, social assistance or other supports	–
Function/disability status-regional or joint-specific	–	Qualitative	Comparative rating to a standard, e.g. normality, preferred health state	–
Symptoms/function-global e.g. *SMFA*				
Symptoms/function - region or joint specific e.g *DASH, PRWE or MHQ*				
Symptoms/function- condition-specific e.g *CTS-SSS, PRUNE*				
Symptoms/function- context specific e.g *WLQ*				
Function- Patient-specific e.g. *COPM, PSFS*				
Function/disability/disease specific, e.g. *DASH or PRWE or MHQ*	–	–	Importance rating	–
Function—context specific, *e.g. The work limitations questionnaire*	–	–	–	–
Satisfaction with outcome	–	–	–	–
Satisfaction with process/care	–	–	–	–

VAS visual analog scale, *NRS* numeric rating scale, *GRC* Global rating of change, *HUI* Health utility Index, *NRS* Numeric rating scale, *MPQ* McGill pain questionnaire, *SMFA* Short musculoskeletal function assessment, *DASH* Disability arm shoulder and hand, *PRWE* Patient-rated wrist evaluation, *MHQ* Michigan hand questionnaire, *CTS-SSS* Carpal tunnel syndrome- Symptom severity scale, *PRUNE* Patient-rated Ulnar Nerve Evaluation, *WLQ* Work limitations questionnaire, *COPM* Candian occupational performance measure, *PSFS* Patient-specific functional scale

Table 7.2 Sources of outcome measures

Outcome measure databases	
Name	Link
Patient-reported health instruments	http://phi.uhce.ox.ac.uk/
ePROVIDE™	https://eprovide.mapi-trust.org/
Rehabilitation outcome measure database	https://www.sralab.org/rehabilitation-measures
Orthopedic scores	http://www.orthoscores.com/
PROMIS® (patient-reported outcomes measurement information system)	http://www.healthmeasures.net/explore-measurement-systems/promis
NIH Toolbox®	http://www.healthmeasures.net/explore-measurement-systems/nih-toolbox

the nature of the items evaluated, how they are scored and the perspectives that the items are measuring as these all influence the nature and efficiency of the measurement.

Constructs measured can be quite broad, to be used generically across health conditions, such as health-related quality of life (HRQoL) or health status. HRQoL measures, like the EQ-5D [11–15] can take on a variety of formats that may appear like health status measures, like the SF-36 [16, 17] or SF-12 [18–20], since both sample important domains of life. The distinction between these is often subtle, but quality of life (QoL) measures infer evaluation of the extent to which a given health status meets the patient's needs or expectations. Utility measures provide an overall evaluation on the value of different health states, which, makes them ideally suited for economic analyses. Most generic outcome measures are multi-item scales that reflect different dimensions of QoL or health status. Single item global constructs can provide a brief overall assessment of change (e.g. the global rating of change), function, or how normal patients perceive themselves to be (e.g. the Single Assessment Numerical Evaluation [SANE]) [21]. Generic measures can be compared across different health conditions as a global outcome or to better understand what dimensions of health are impacted by a health condition or intervention. Disadvantages, particularly in upper extremity surgery, are that the generic measures often do not adequately sample upper extremity function and can be less responsive to detecting clinical change [22–24]. The more diffuse a concept/item is, the more likely that it will be understood and calibrated differently by different patients. For example, a single item, like the SANE [21], is appealing to clinicians as it provides a quick barometer of patient status. However, how patients define how 'normal' they are can be influenced by a variety of factors, which may not be related to the treatment provided. These global single item ratings are useful in combination with other scales, rather than as a sole indicator of outcome.

An outcome measure strategy often includes both observer/clinician-based outcomes (CBOs) and PRO. CBO measurements are important because they often are directly related to the treatment targets. The effects of surgery, fracture reduction and strengthening programs can only be assessed as being beneficial if they successfully change the underlying anatomy/impairments that are being targeted. Therefore, the measurement of these constructs is important to enhance our understanding of the treatment mechanisms. Ultimately, improving the patient's symptoms and functioning are often the primary goal of surgery, and these impacts are typically measured by PRO. PRO can contain consistent standardized items, adaptive items that are presented to patients, based on a computer algorithm or blank items where the patients can define the item to be rated. Advantages of the consistent format are that the clinician and patient can monitor responses to specific individual items, which can be useful when tracking functional goals. Further, the administration is feasible in either paper or electronic formats (not dependent on technology). A disadvantage of these standardized PRO is that they may not be appropriately targeted to some individuals. Further, patients often must answer items that are not relevant to them. Many standardized PRO focus on activities of daily life that might not adequately reflect important domains of life for people with high occupational or sport demands, which can result in ceiling or floor effects. Ceiling or floor effects occur when a patient score is already at the top or bottom of the scale and so no further worsening or improvement can be detected. Ceiling or floor effects for groups have been defined as when more than 15% of the population scores at the bottom or top [25], which should include the need for scores to be able to change a clinically important difference. Adaptive measures have the advantage of being efficient since the computer selects an item of appropriate difficulty based on a previous response. A disadvantage is that a different set of items is presented on each occasion and the change in specific functional tasks is not tracked. The items selected by the computer are not necessarily relevant to patients. Further, technology barriers may exclude some clinics or patient groups. The most patient-centred outcome measures are those where the patient selects the items. Patient-specific PRO, like the patient-specific functional scale (PSFS) [26] measures provide the highest level of responsiveness [27–29] since patients select items that are salient and problematic. Further, these items are often aligned with the patient's goals. A downside of patient-specific measures is that the scores cannot be compared between patients because the difficulty of the items is not calibrated.

Disease or symptom-specific PRO measures are indicated where the condition is sufficiently unique that important elements are not captured by generic instruments. For example, median (Symptom Severity Scale) [30] or the ulnar nerve (Patient-Rated Ulnar Nerve Evaluation [PRUNE])-[26] specific scales have been developed for neuropathies to capture the unique sensory and motor symptoms. Since pain is often a primary reason for patient consultation it can be measured with a variety of PROs. The most commonly used symptom outcome measure is a numeric pain rating scale, which can be administered verbally or by paper to measure pain intensity. However, multidimensional pain scales that assess other dimensions of pain, such as the McGill Pain Questionnaire [31], are gaining popularity. Regional measures of symptoms and function for example, the (Quick)DASH [32–34] MHQ [35–38] or PRWE [7, 39–42] are highly validated PROs that are useful in hand surgery practice and research. A 2014 practice survey found that the most used PROs in hand therapy clinical practice was the DASH and second most used was the PRWE, followed by the Quick-DASH, PSFS, the patient-rated elbow evaluation (PREE) and the upper limb functional index (ULFI) [43]. More recently, some larger centres are adopting computer adaptive testing such as the PROMIS system [44–46], which, like the DASH, MHQ and PRW(H)E possess strong measurement properties.

Choosing the Proper Outcome Measure

The ideal characteristics of an outcome instrument include:

- Interval level scaling properties
- Strong reliability, validity and responsiveness
- Validated for the proposed measurement purpose (responsiveness, diagnosis or prediction) and population
- Measures constructs relevant to your clinical population and planned interventions
- Low clinician burden: Time, scoring complexity and training
- Low respondent burden: time, cognitive and health literacy
- Relevant and acceptable to respondents
- Has clinical applicability: published comparative scores, decision-making benchmarks minimal detectable change (MDC) and clinically important difference (CID)
- Cross-cultural translations available for multiple groups
- Feasible Cost/availability
- Minimal expertise-required; or training easily accessed
- Common usage or recommended by international consensus panels

Multiple factors determine what is the best outcome measure for any given scenario; both measurement properties and feasibility issues are important. Outcome measures function for a given population, spectrum of the phenomenon and measurement purpose. Performance cannot be certain outside of those characteristics. For example, PROs that are validated for evaluating change (responsiveness), may not be ideal for discrimination or prediction. Therefore, it is important to have validation studies that apply both to the context and purpose of measurement.

How Can I Know if I Can Trust the Score?

Measurement threats are listed in Table 7.3. If the score provides consistent scores in stable patients (reliable) and is valid; it should consider capable of providing trustworthy scores. However, all scores are associated with some measurement error. The following guideposts are often considered when considering measurement error.

- Reliability is high (intraclass correlation coefficient (ICC) ≥ 0.90 for individual patients, or ≥ 0.75 for group's comparisons or evaluating trends with repeated measures [1]
- The amount of measurement error is low as indicated by a low standard error of measurement (SEM*); which is expressed in the original units of measurement

$$\text{SEM} = \text{Standard deviation}\left(\sqrt{1 - ICC}\right)$$

- Minimal detectable change (MDC) is considered; often set at a 90% confidence level

$$MDC90 = \text{SEM}_{\text{test-retest}}(z\text{-value})(\sqrt{2})$$

*The standard error of measurement (SEM) = 1, is associated with the 68% confidence interval. To obtain higher confidence levels, the SEM can be multiplied by z-values associated with different confidence levels (typically 90% = 1.65).

Table 7.3 Key measurement threats and respective solutions in outcome measures

Measurement threat	Impact	Solution
Ceiling or floor effects	No room to assess CID; Failure to measure change	Choose an appropriately targeted instrument; patient-specific scales
Reliability or validity established in different patient population	Measurement properties may not generalize; items may not be appropriately targeted	Conduct validation or choose a different instrument
Reliability less than excellent	Difficulty evaluating change	Multiple assessments; larger margins of error; large sample sizes in clinical studies
Lack of interval level scoring	Inaccurate measurement of change; compromise of statistical test assumptions	Rasch-based scoring [47]
Lack of factor structure/unidimensionality	Inaccurate attribution of constructs or areas of treatment impact	Use of separate subscales rather than total scores
English PRO	Exclusion of some people; biased assessments	Cross-cultural validation; surrogate completion (PRO)
(Health) literacy gaps between the measure and the patient's ability	Exclusion of segments of the population; nonadherence or invalid measurement	Assess literacy; Choose scales with low cognitive and literacy demands; surrogate completion
Intentional bias or effort failure	Invalid measurement	Assess respond patterns; Cross-reference PRO with objective measures

How Can I Interpret the Score in Clinical Practice?

- Evaluate the outcome trajectory over time
  - Compare the score to published benchmarks/trajectories
  - Compare the observed change to the clinically important difference (CID) specific to the patient population, intervention and context
- Evaluate if the score achieved is consistent with patient goals
- Use the score to differentiate subgroups or predict the future outcome

Numerous studies indicate that the best baseline predictor of a future score on a PRO is the baseline score on that PRO. When predicting the meaning of PRO, the initial baseline score, the expected trajectory, published clinical prediction rules and studies on outcome mediators should be considered. There has been substantial focus on defining CID for different PRO, and these can be useful benchmarks. However, these should be interpreted as loose benchmarks since they are often highly variable between studies with different patient populations or interventions [1]. Further since many PRO are ordinal scores, the CID can vary over the values of possible scores. Further, the CID for a group (research study) is different than for an individual. Because of differences in methods of computation between the CID and MDC, the MDC can equal or exceed the CID. Studies reporting scores for clinical subgroup scores can provide useful benchmarks; e.g. those who return to work versus those who do not.

What Cautions Should I Exercise?

Outcome measures may be invalid if not administered correctly, if not appropriately constructed or targeted, or if respondents are unwilling or unable to fully cooperate with the assessment. Outcome measures should be administered by an unbiased person or independent process to reduce bias in administration. Key measurement threats and solutions are listed in Table 7.3. Prognostic factors affect the baseline score and outcome trajectory, and these should be considered when comparing outcomes across individuals or groups. Potential prognostic factors include age, gender, disease severity, psychological status, comorbid health and socio-economic factors. Outcome measures indicate patient status and may be useful for signaling the need for further investigation but cannot diagnose a problem.

Conversely, while some people criticize PROs as being 'subjective', they have an important role in the assessment of patient status. They indicate outcomes that are important to patients, and the reason(s) for clinical intervention. In general, PROs used in hand surgery practice are as reliable, or more reliable, than impairment measures [39, 48, 49]; and are more associated with important outcomes like return to work [50]. Impairment measures like grip and range of motion (ROM) require patient cooperation, as do PROs. The objective outcome measures are those where the patient or evaluator input is not required (e.g. nerve conduction). These measures, while important for directing care, are not indicators of the patient's functional outcome. Therefore, a balanced measurement strategy that includes diagnostic/mechanism-based impairment measures, physical impairments like grip/motion and patient-based outcomes measured by PRO are typically needed as core measures in hand surgery.

Application of Above-Mentioned Concepts to Resolve the Clinical Scenario

In keeping with Mary's condition, imaging will be used to monitor fracture alignment. Constructs that are deemed relevant for assessing outcomes of Distal Radial Fracture (DRF) management include joint and hand function. Unlike some aspects of literature searching, no methodological filters have been developed specifically for clinical measurement studies. However, using a simple Boolean search strategy, we can combine the content constructs, measurement property terms and clinical populations in a search strategy to identify appropriate articles, e.g. (pain and disability) and (reliability or validity or responsiveness or Rasch or factor analysis) and (distal radius fractures). We can also consult outcome measure databases (Table 7.2) to identify potential candidates since often the measurement tools are not included with the clinical measurement studies evaluating their properties.

To assess joint function, we measure grip and range of motion; to assess hand function at the level of the person we will use a PRO.

The functional consequences of a distal radius fracture are well documented, and international panels have defined the core concepts as pain and disability [51, 52]. In this case we decide to use The patient-rated wrist evaluation [39, 53] because it is specific to this patient population, is highly reliable and valid [7], contains a separate pain score (salient given Mary's pain), is brief, has a low cognitive demand, has been translated into multiple languages [42, 54] and has been recommended as a core measure by international panels [51, 52]. The PRWE presents 15 items scored on a 0–10 numeric rating scale. The pain scale is scored out of 50 by summing the 5 pain items. The function score is comprised of 6 items on specific activities and 4 items on usual activities that are summed to provide a score out of 100. This score is divided by 2 to provide the second 50% of the total score. Thus, the total score equally waits for pain and disability on a scale ranging from 0 to 100, with 100 representing the maximum pain and disability.

Mary has a pain score of 40/50 on the PRWE pain subscale, and a total score of 70/100 on PRWE. Her pain is constant, a 4/10 at rest, a 9/10 at worst or when lifting heavy objects. Her function ratings include two low scores 'fastening buttons', indicating minimal problems with fine dexterity; and 'recreation' given that her main pastime is watching TV. Otherwise, the other functional items indicate high levels of difficulty in tasks that require motion or strength.

The SEM for the PRWE is 4–5 points [7]. The MDC_{90} is 9. This means that there is a 90% chance that Mary's true score is within 9 points of the measured score; so, given her measured score of 70, the true score is likely to fall between 65.5 and 74.5.

The CID for the PRWE is 11 [7, 54, 55]. To be confident that Mary score of 70 has changed an important amount, it would need to improve to 59 or less. We know that recovery is rapid in the first three months and slower thereafter [56], and should approach 12, by 1-year post-DRF [57, 58]. After reading some of the clinical measurement studies that investigate how the PRWE can be used to improve our prediction of Mary's future outcome, we find studies related to both return to work and chronic pain. One study demonstrated that patients with high baseline scores and who do not improve on successive evaluations are likely to have a delayed return to work [50]. We will watch Mary's scores carefully given that she has a high pain score to see whether improvement can be quickly obtained. Delayed improvement on the PRWE would suggest she might be at risk of a slow return to work. Another study investigated how baseline scores can be used to predict future chronic pain. A score of $\geq 35/50$ on the PRWE pain subscale of the PRWE has high sensitivity (85%) and specificity (79%), Area under the Curve = 89%, for predicting chronic pain at 1 year [59]. For more information on sensitivity and specificity, please see Chap. 21: Diagnostic Studies in Surgery. This study also reported that data as a relative risk. Thus, Mary is 8.4 times more likely to experience chronic pain at one year because her score exceeds that risk threshold of 35 out of 50.

Mary is provided the PRWE by administrative staff in the clinic to reduce social desirability bias. Translations are kept in reserve and used when needed for non-English speaking patients. Her forms are kept in her medical chart, and comparison data from published studies are kept on hand for comparison. The clinic develops a database to use for comparison data, quality assurance or research.

References

1. Frost MH, Reeve BB, Liepa AM, Stauffer JW, Hays RD, Group TMPOCM. What is sufficient evidence for the reliability and validity of patient-reported outcome measures? Value Heal. 2007 Nov;10(s2):S94–105.
2. Roy J-S, MacDermid JC, Amick BC, Shannon HS, McMurtry R, Roth JH, et al. Validity and responsiveness of presenteeism scales in chronic work-related upper-extremity disorders. Phys Ther. 2011;91(2):254–66.
3. Schmidt S, Ferrer M, González M, González N, Valderas JM, Alonso J et al. Evaluation of shoulder-specific patient-reported outcome measures: a systematic and standardized comparison of available evidence. J Shoulder Elb Surg. 2014;23(3).
4. Wasiak J, McMahon M, Danilla S, Spinks A, Cleland H, Gabbe B. Measuring common outcome measures and their concepts using the international classification of functioning, disability and health (ICF) in adults with burn injury: a systematic review. Burns. 2011;37(6):913–24.
5. Packham T, MacDermid JC, Henry J, Bain J. A systematic review of psychometric evaluations of outcome assessments for complex regional pain syndrome. Disabil Rehabil. 2012;34(13).
6. Coenen M, Kus S, Rudolf KDK-D, Müller G, Berno S, Dereskewitz C et al. Do patient-reported outcome measures capture functioning aspects and environmental factors important to individuals with injuries or disorders of the hand? J Hand Ther. 2013;26(4):332–42.
7. Mehta SP, MacDermid JC, Richardson J, MacIntyre NJ, Grewal R. A systematic review of the measurement properties of the patient-rated wrist evaluation. J Orthop Sport Phys Ther. 2015;45(4):289–98.
8. de Vries NM, Staal JB, van Ravensberg CD, Hobbelen JSM, Olde Rikkert MGM, Nijhuis-van der Sanden MWG. Outcome instruments to measure frailty: a systematic review, vol. 10, Ageing research reviews; 2011. p. 104–14.
9. Oltman R, Neises G, Scheible D, Mehrtens G, Grüneberg C. ICF components of corresponding outcome measures in flexor tendon rehabilitation—a systematic review. BMC Musculoskelet Disord. 2008;9(1):139.
10. Chung P, Yun SJH, Khan F. A comparison of participation outcome measures and the international classification of functioning, disability and health core sets for traumatic brain injury. J Rehabil Med. 2014;46(2):108–16.
11. Herdman M, Gudex C, Lloyd A, Janssen M, Kind P, Parkin D et al. Development and preliminary testing of the new five-level version of EQ-5D (EQ-5D-5L). Qual Life Res. 2011.
12. Rabin R, Oemar M, Oppe M, Janssen B, Herdman M. EQ-5D-5L user guide. Basic information on how to use the EQ-5D-5L instrument; 2015.
13. Van Hout B, Janssen MF, Feng YS, Kohlmann T, Busschbach J, Golicki D et al. Interim scoring for the EQ-5D-5L: mapping the EQ-5D-5L to EQ-5D-3L value sets. Value Heal. 2012.
14. Makai P, Brouwer WBF, Koopmanschap M, Stolk E, Nieboer AP, Melorose J et al. Can the EQ-5D detect meaningful change? A systematic review. Health Qual Life Outcomes. 2013.
15. van Reenen M, Oppe M. EQ-5D-3L user guide: basic information on how to use the EQ-5D-3L instrument. EuroQol Research Foundation; 2015.
16. Contopoulos-Ioannidis DG, Karvouni A, Kouri I, Ioannidis JPA. Reporting and interpretation of SF-36 outcomes in randomised trials: systematic review. BMJ. 2009.
17. Lins L, Carvalho FM. SF-36 total score as a single measure of health-related quality of life: Scoping review. SAGE Open Med. 2016.
18. Ware J, Kosinski M, Keller SD. A 12-item short-form health survey: construction of scales and preliminary tests of reliability and validity. Med Care. 1996;34(3):220–33.
19. Jenkinson C, Layte R, Jenkinson D, Lawrence K, Petersen S, Paice C, et al. A shorter form health survey: can the SF-12 replicate results from the SF-36 in longitudinal studies? J Public Health Med. 1997;19(2):179–86.
20. Farivar SS, Cunningham WE, Hays RD. Correlated physical and mental health summary scores for the SF-36 and SF-12 health survey, vol. 1. Health qual life outcomes; 2007.
21. Shelbourne KD, Barnes AF, Gray T. Correlation of a single assessment numeric evaluation (SANE) rating with modified cincinnati knee rating system and IKDC subjective total scores for patients after ACL reconstruction or knee arthroscopy. Am J Sports Med. 2012;40(11):2487–91.
22. MacDermid JC, Drosdowech D, Faber K. Responsiveness of self-report scales in patients recovering from rotator cuff surgery. J Shoulder Elb Surg. 2006;15(4):407–14.
23. Amadio PC, Silverstein MD, Ilstrup DM, Schleck CD, Jensen LM. Outcome after colles fracture: The relative responsiveness of three questionnaires and physical examination measures. J Hand Surg Am. 1996;21(5):781–7.
24. Angst F, Goldhahn J, Drerup S, Kolling C, Aeschlimann A, Simmen BR, et al. Responsiveness of five outcome measurement instruments in total elbow arthroplasty. Arthritis Care Res (Hoboken). 2012;64 (11):1749–55.
25. Terwee CB, Bot SDM, de Boer MR, van der Windt DAWM, Knol DL, Dekker J, et al. Quality criteria were proposed for measurement properties of health status questionnaires. J Clin Epidemiol. 2007;60(1):34–42.
26. Westaway MD, Stratford PW, Binkley JM. The patient-specific functional scale: validation of its use in persons with neck dysfunction. J Orthop Sports Phys Ther. 1998;27(5):331–8.

27. Abbott JH, Schmitt J. Minimum important differences for the patient-specific functional scale, 4 region-specific outcome measures, and the numeric pain rating scale. J Orthop Sport Phys Ther. 2014.
28. Gross DP, Battié MC, Asante AK. The patient-specific functional scale: validity in workers' compensation claimants. Arch Phys Med Rehabil. 2008.
29. Hefford C, Abbott JH, Arnold R, Baxter GD. The patient-specific functional scale: validity, reliability, and responsiveness in patients with upper extremity musculoskeletal problems. J Orthop Sport Phys Ther. 2012.
30. Levine DW, Simmons BP, Koris MJ, Daltroy LH, Hohl GG, Fossel AH, et al. A self-administered questionnaire for the assessment of severity of symptoms and functional status in carpal tunnel syndrome. J Bone Joint Surg Am. 1993.
31. Dworkin RH, Turk DC, Trudeau JJ, Benson C, Biondi DM, Katz NP, et al. Validation of the short-form McGill pain questionnaire-2 (SF-MPQ-2) in acute low back pain. J Pain. 2015;16(4):357–66.
32. Kennedy CA, Beaton DE, Smith P, Van Eerd D, Tang K, Inrig T, et al. Measurement properties of the QuickDASH (Disabilities of the arm, shoulder and hand) outcome measure and crosscultural adaptations of the QuickDASH: a systematic review, vol. 22, Quality of life research; 2013. p. 2509–47.
33. Beaton DE, Wright JG, Katz JN, Group UEC. Development of the QuickDASH: comparison of three item-reduction approaches. J Bone Jt Surg Am. 2005;87(5):1038–46.
34. Kennedy CA, Beaton DE. A user's survey of the clinical application and content validity of the DASH (disabilities of the arm, shoulder and hand) outcome measure. J Hand Ther. 2017;30(1):30–40.
35. Chung KC, Pillsbury MS, Walters MR, Hayward RA. Reliability and validity testing of the Michigan hand outcomes questionnaire. J Hand Surg Am. 1998.
36. Shauver MJ, Chung KC. The minimal clinically important difference of the Michigan hand outcomes questionnaire. J Hand Surg Am. 2009.
37. Chung KC, Hamill JB, Walters MR, Hayward RA. The Michigan hand outcomes questionnaire (MHQ): assessment of responsiveness to clinical change. Ann Plast Surg. 1999.
38. Kotsis SV, Lau FH, Chung KC. Responsiveness of the Michigan hand outcomes questionnaire and physical measurements in outcome studies of distal radius fracture treatment. J Hand Surg Am. 2007.
39. MacDermid JC, Turgeon T, Richards RS, Beadle M, Roth JH. Patient rating of wrist pain and disability: a reliable and valid measurement tool. J Orthop Trauma. 1998;12(8):577–86.
40. MacDermid JCJC, Tottenham V. Responsiveness of the disability of the arm, shoulder, and hand (DASH) and patient-rated wrist/hand evaluation (PRWHE) in evaluating change after hand therapy. J Hand Ther. 2004;17(1):18–23.
41. MacDermid JC, Richards RS, Donner A, Bellamy N, Roth JH. Responsiveness of the short form-36, disability of the arm, shoulder, and hand questionnaire, patient-rated wrist evaluation, and physical impairment measurements in evaluating recovery after a distal radius fracture. J Hand Surg Am. 2000;25(2):330–40.
42. Goldhahn J, Shisha T, MacDermid JC, Goldhahn S. Multilingual cross-cultural adaptation of the patient-rated wrist evaluation (PRWE) into Czech, French, Hungarian, Italian, Portuguese (Brazil), Russian and Ukrainian, vol. 133, Archives of orthopaedic and trauma surgery; 2013. p. 589–93.
43. Valdes K, MacDermid J, Algar L, Connors B, Cyr LM, Dickmann S, et al. Hand therapist use of patient report outcome (PRO) in practice: a survey study. J Hand Ther. 2014;27(4):299–307; quiz 308.
44. Döring AC, Nota SPFT, Hageman MGJS, Ring DC. Measurement of upper extremity disability using the patient-reported outcomes measurement information system. J Hand Surg Am. 2014.
45. Tyser AR, Beckmann J, Franklin JD, Cheng C, Hon SD, Wang A et al. Evaluation of the PROMIS physical function computer adaptive test in the upper extremity. J Hand Surg Am. 2014.
46. Hung M, Voss MW, Bounsanga J, Crum AB, Tyser AR. Examination of the PROMIS upper extremity item bank. J Hand Ther. 2017.
47. Tennant A, Conaghan PG. The Rasch measurement model in rheumatology: what is it and why use it? when should it be applied, and what should one look for in a Rasch paper? Arthritis Care Res. 2007;57 (8):1358–62.
48. Vincent JI, Macdermid JC, Michlovitz SL, Rafuse R, Wells-Rowsell C, Wong O, et al. The push-off test: development of a simple, reliable test of upper extremity weight-bearing capability. J Hand Ther. 2014;27(3):185–91.
49. MacDermid JC, Kramer JF, McFarlane RM, Roth JH. Inter-rater agreement and accuracy of clinical tests used in diagnosis of carpal tunnel syndrome. Work; 1997.
50. MacDermid JC, Roth JH, McMurtry R. Predictors of time lost from work following a distal radius fracture. J Occup Rehabil. 2007;17(1):47–62.
51. Goldhahn J, Beaton D, Ladd A, Macdermid J, Hoang-Kim A. Recommendation for measuring clinical outcome in distal radius fractures: a core set of domains for standardized reporting in clinical practice and research. Ugeskr Laeger. 2014;175 (23):1638–41.
52. Waljee JFJF, Ladd A, MacDermid JCJC, Rozental TDTD, Wolfe SWSW, Benson LS, et al. A unified approach to outcomes assessment for distal radius fractures. J Hand Surg Am. 2016;41(4):565–73.
53. MacDermid JC. Development of a scale for patient rating of wrist pain and disability. J Hand Ther. 1996;9(2):178–83.
54. Weinstock-Zlotnick G, Mehta SP. A structured literature synthesis of wrist outcome measures: an evidence-based approach to determine use among

common wrist diagnoses. J Hand Ther. 2016;29(2): 98–110.

55. Walenkamp MMJ, de Muinck Keizer RJ, Goslings JC, Vos LM, Rosenwasser MP, Schep NWL. The minimum clinically important difference of the patient-rated wrist evaluation score for patients with distal radius fractures. Clin Orthop Relat Res. 2015;473(10):3235–41.
56. MacDermid JC, Richards RS, Roth JH. Distal radius fracture: a prospective outcome study of 275 patients. J Hand Ther. 2001;14(2):154–69.
57. Lalone EA, Rajgopal V, Roth J, Grewal R, MacDermid JC. A cohort study of one-year functional and radiographic outcomes following intra-articular distal radius fractures. Hand (N Y). 2014;9(2):237–43.
58. Grewal R, MacDermid JC, Pope J, Chesworth BM. Baseline predictors of pain and disability one year following extra-articular distal radius fractures. Hand. 2007;2(3):104–11.
59. Mehta SP, MacDermid JC, Richardson J, MacIntyre NJ, Grewal R. Baseline pain intensity is a predictor of chronic pain in individuals with distal radius fracture. J Orthop Sport Phys Ther. 2015; 45(2):119–27.

Patient-Important Outcome Measures in Surgical Care

8

Katherine B. Santosa, Anne Klassen and Andrea L. Pusic

Scenario

A 65-year old otherwise healthy woman comes to your office for a consultation regarding post-mastectomy breast reconstruction after being diagnosed with invasive lobular carcinoma in her left breast. After discussing her options with her surgical oncologist, she decides to undergo a simple mastectomy of the left breast and is interested in learning about her options for unilateral breast reconstruction.

After examination and a review of her oncologic plan, you conclude that she would be a good candidate for either implant-based or autologous reconstruction. You discuss the two main types of reconstructive options as well as the expected risks, course and outcomes of surgery. She then states: 'I am not too concerned with my appearance—I'm 65 years old. But, I am wary about having a foreign body inside of my breast'. You note her personal preferences and give her the opportunity to consult with her family and she states: 'Doc, you're the expert. What do women like me tell you about having an implant or using their own tissue?' Realizing the importance of shared-decision-making in this process, and that you remain uncertain about the current literature assessing outcomes reported by patients regarding their experiences with implant-based versus autologous breast reconstruction, you decide to search the literature prior to the patient's next appointment.

Searching the Literature

The article that you are trying to find and would be most applicable to your patient would be a systematic review that compared the experiences as reported by patients who underwent post-mastectomy breast reconstruction with implant-based versus autologous techniques. Using the Medical Subject Headings (MeSH) Database from Medline PubMed's home page, you discover that the MeSH term for 'breast reconstruction' is 'mammaplasty', which was introduced into the database in 1992. Also, you find that the MeSH term for the concept 'patient outcome' is 'patient reported outcome measures', first introduced in 2017. Using these MeSH terms, you combine them and find 32 citations.

K. B. Santosa
Department of Surgery, University of Michigan, 1500 East Medical Center Drive, 2130 Taubman Center, Ann Arbor, MI 48109, USA
e-mail: ksantosa@med.umich.edu

A. Klassen
Department of Pediatrics, McMaster University, 1280 Main Street West, HSC-3N27, Hamilton, ON 8S 4K1, Canada
e-mail: aklass@mcmaster.ca

A. L. Pusic (✉)
Department of Surgery, Brigham Health, 75 Francis Street, Boston, MA 02115, USA
e-mail: apusic@bwh.harvard.edu

A. Thoma et al. (eds.), *Evidence-Based Surgery*,
https://doi.org/10.1007/978-3-030-05120-4_8

After reviewing the titles and abstracts for the studies that met your search strategy, you do not find a systematic review but do find a 2017 article in a high impact journal (Journal of Clinical Oncology) entitled, 'Patient-Reported Outcomes 1 Year After Immediate Breast Reconstruction: Results from the Mastectomy Reconstruction Outcomes Consortium', by Pusic and colleagues [1]. Although the abstract of the manuscript seems to meet your needs, you also keep in mind that one of the MeSH terms in your search, 'patient-reported outcome measures' was only introduced in 2017 so you find other relevant articles from the paper and from the remaining 31 citations.

In the Introduction of the paper by Pusic and colleagues [1], the authors state that few studies in the breast reconstruction literature have evaluated 'patient perceptions of outcomes' and of those that do, most have relied on generic measures or surveys with limited reliability or validity. Therefore, the goal of their study was to evaluate patient-reported outcomes (PROs) of women undergoing immediate post-mastectomy breast reconstruction with implant-based or autologous techniques at 1 year using a patient-reported outcome measure (PROM) termed the BREAST-Q [1]. After reviewing the manuscript, you are encouraged that it will help the shared decision-making process with your patient and review other articles to learn more about PROMs and their importance.

Introduction

What is a Patient-Reported Outcome?

Over time, there has been a realization of the importance of patient-centered care and evaluation of outcomes as reported by the patients themselves in surgical care [2]. The term 'patient-reported outcome (PRO)', as defined by the U.S. Food and Drug Administration (FDA) refers to 'any report of the status of a patient's health condition that comes directly from the patient, without interpretation of the patient's response by a clinician or anyone else' [3]. Broadly speaking, PROs encompass symptoms (e.g. post-operative pain or fatigue), health-related quality of life (HRQoL) , such as physical and psychosocial well-being, and satisfaction with care (e.g. satisfaction with preoperative information and postoperative follow-up provided by the care team).

HRQoL is a multidimensional concept that describes quality-of-life (QoL) as it pertains to health and disease and includes domains related to physical, mental, emotional and social functioning [4]. HRQoL is more encompassing than symptomology. Although symptoms describe the patient's condition or treatment effect, it usually mirrors a clinician-reported measure [5]. HRQoL on the other hand can be impaired by a patient's symptoms but also reflects disease or treatment characteristics that may not be captured by clinical symptomology alone.

In a variety of conditions and circumstances such as in our clinical scenario (QoL after breast reconstruction), it may be best to summarize outcomes and the importance of those outcomes with input from patients through PROs. Furthermore, despite advances in our ability to collect physical, physiological and biochemical data that can inform us about a patient's condition, there are certain data that cannot be obtained or adequately assessed without the patient's perspective [6]. It is the addition of the patients' perspective that emphasizes the importance of PROs in clinical research, patient care and quality improvement [6].

Other Important Concepts and Definitions

There are several key concepts and terms used when discussing and applying PROs; Table 8.1 summarizes these [3, 7]. Importantly, every PRO measure (PROM) has a conceptual framework, which, defines: (1) the concepts of interest or importance to patients; and (2) a description of the relationships between the questions asked and concepts being measured. From the conceptual framework, scales are developed to measure unidimensional concepts (or constructs).

Table 8.1 Common terminology used in the field of patient-reported outcomes

Instrument	A means to capture data, such as a questionnaire or scale, as well as all the information and documentation that supports its use. Generally, that includes: (1) clearly defined methods and instructions for administration or responding; (2) a standard format for data collection, and; (3) a well-documented method for scoring, analyzing and interpreting results for a given target population
Item	An individual question, statement or task (and the respective response options) completed by the patient to address a particular concept
Concept	The specific item that is to be measured by a PRO instrument. In clinical trials, a PRO instrument may be used to measure the effect of one intervention on one or more concepts. Concepts measured by a PRO represent aspects of how patients function or feel related to a health condition or its treatment
Domain	A sub-concept represented by a score on an instrument that measures a larger concept. Each concept is comprised of multiple domains; for example sleep function would be a concept, sleep disturbance and sleep-related impairment would be a domain
Health-related quality of life (HRQoL)	A multi-domain concept representing the patient's general perception of how an illness or treatment influences their physical, psychological and social aspects of life

Created using information from [3]

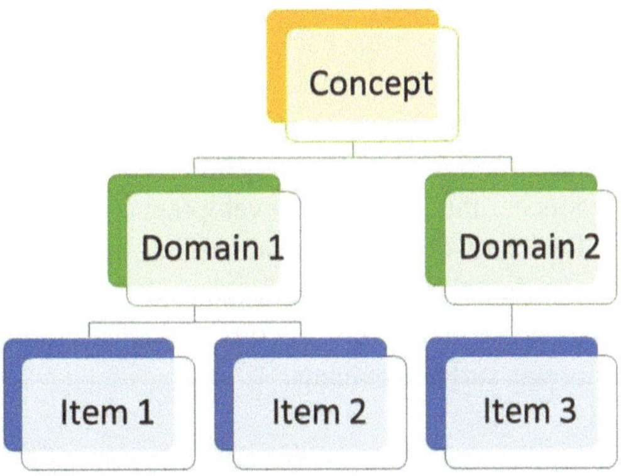

Fig. 8.1 General conceptual framework of any PRO instrument. Created using information from [3]

Each scale is composed of a series of 'items' or individual questions which are scored together to provide a measurement of the construct (Fig. 8.1).

In the initial development of any PROM, a conceptual framework is first defined. In the case of the BREAST-Q for example, Pusic and colleagues [8] defined six key themes based on patient interviews, research literature and expert opinion that formed the conceptual framework. In this PROM, there are two main concepts: (1) HRQoL; and (2) patient satisfaction in breast surgery. The three quality of life domains are: (1) physical well-being; (2) psychosocial well-being; and (3) sexual well-being [8]. Additionally, the three themes or domains that comprise the concept of satisfaction in breast surgery include: (1) satisfaction with breasts; (2) satisfaction with outcome; and (3) satisfaction with care [8]. Within each domain, there are a specific set of items that have been selected and evaluated and together map out a clinical hierarchy. Each item corresponds to a score in the domain.

How is a PROM Developed?

Developing a PROM is a very large undertaking. Guidelines for the development of a PROM have been described by governing bodies such as the Scientific Advisory Committee of the Medical Outcomes Trust [9], the International Society for Pharmacoeconomics and Outcomes Research [10, 11], and the FDA. The FDA has described the development in five steps (Fig. 8.2) below, these five steps are described in relation to the BREAST-Q:

1. *Hypothesize conceptual framework*: During the initial phase of the development of the BREAST-Q, a systematic review was performed and found a paucity in PROMs for the breast surgery population. Additionally, only

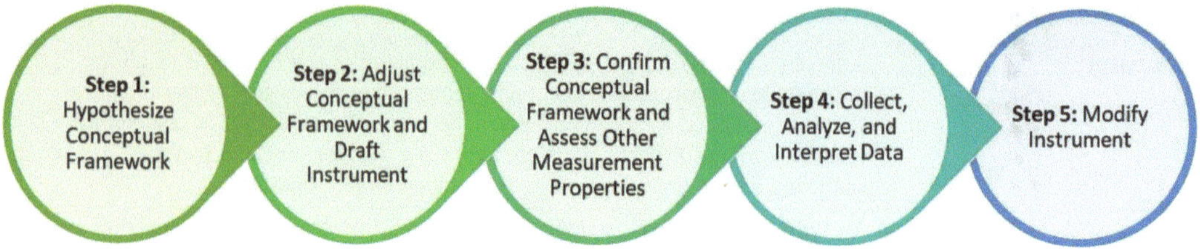

Fig. 8.2 Steps in the development of a PRO instrument as described by the FDA

one instrument was found to have properties that met internationally accepted criteria. The goal was to develop a conceptual framework of patient satisfaction and health-related quality of life in breast surgery. As such, qualitative interviews were conducted on breast reconstruction, reduction and augmentation patients. Together with expert opinion from plastic surgeons, oncologist breast surgeons, nurses, and psychologists, six key themes were identified and formed the conceptual framework. In addition to clinical expertise, mastery in other skill sets such as biostatistics, psychology, and measurement development are important to have in the development of a PROM.

2. *Adjust conceptual framework and draft instrument*: Using patient input, items and preliminary scales were generated. Items within each pool of patients (reconstruction, reduction and augmentation) were grouped into domains based on their conceptual meaning. Content validity was established during this step of development. Additionally, a recall period of two weeks was determined to be acceptable to patients, clinically relevant, and reflective of 'current status' of patients for all domains except sexual well-being.
3. *Confirm conceptual framework and assess other measurement properties*: Items were reduced such that half of the preliminary items were retained in the different modules. Rasch analysis [12], which will be discussed later in this chapter, allowed for the summing of items to form a total score for each scale within each of the modules. In a subsequent study, different aspects of validity and reliability of the instrument were performed.
4. *Collect, analyze, and interpret data*: In the first round of field testing of the BREAST-Q, questionnaires were sent to 2715 women with 1950 (72%) women returning the questionnaire for analysis. A subsequent study in 2012 was performed to test the instrument for other measures of validity and reliability with the inclusion of data from 817 women.
5. *Modify instrument*: Final cognitive debriefing interviews were performed with 30 patients (10 patients from each procedure group) to review the final draft of the questionnaire. During this step, the research team obtained the average completion times for patients. Since the initial development of the BREAST-Q, the questionnaire has been translated into 13 languages and has helped facilitate important outcomes studies among breast surgery patients.

Another example is the development of the CLEFT-Q, a PROM designed to assess outcomes for patients with cleft lip or palate. To develop the conceptual framework for this PROM, 138 heterogenous individuals across 6 countries, spanning different ages, genders, socioeconomic classes and cleft types participated in rigorous qualitative interviews. Data from the interviews were transcribed and contributed to the development of this PROM [13]. Successful completion of each step ensures that the PROM accomplishes three key things. First, it is imperative that the PROM evaluates the concept of interest. Next, the measure should integrate experiences important to the patient population of interest. Finally, the language utilized in the PROM should not only be easily understandable to the patient but should also allow the patient to respond without confusion. Asking irrelevant questions for a specific patient population or including questions that are poorly written could result in measurement error and bias [3].

After a literature search has been performed to identify existing PROMs and potential gaps in their utility in the subject area, qualitative research is performed. Careful qualitative research forms the basis of any new PROM. Data are derived from patient interviews or focus groups, which are audio recorded to facilitate transcription and analysis. Transcribed verbatim, patient interviews and focus group data are used to identify key concepts of interest and to form the conceptual framework. In addition, expert opinion from a heterogeneous group of individuals can also be utilized to refine a PROM [14]. During development of the BREAST-Q, for example a total of 48 patients were interviewed in a semi-structured fashion, generating a total of 2749 statements about patient satisfaction and HRQoL after breast surgery [8].

How Do You Evaluate a PROM?

Validity

Validity is a key property to consider in evaluating any PROM. Validity, or the ability of a PROM to measure what it is intended to measure, can be described by content validity, criterion validity, and construct validity [15]. *Content validity*, which has been referred to as 'the cornerstone of validity' [5, 15] describes 'the degree to which the content of a measurement is an adequate reflection of the construct measured' [15]. When assessing a PROM, it is important to ask: Is the questionnaire asking the important questions for the clinical question at hand? In other words, is this PROM appropriate for your patient or patient population? It is apparent to see why performing high-quality patient interviews and establishing content validity during the development of the PROM are so imperative. Content validity is arguably the most important aspect of validity and is largely established in the initial qualitative phase of PROM development [3, 16]. Establishment of content validity is, however, ongoing and refers not only to the measurement itself, but also to how it is used [7]. When deciding on which PROM to use, researchers should consider content validity, or the overall ability of the instrument to measure its stated concepts, and its ability to measure its stated concept in the patient population being studied.

Criterion validity is the process whereby a PROM is assessed against a true value or 'gold standard' [7, 15]. Importantly, often, criterion validity cannot be examined when there is no gold standard to which to compare the PROM. Criterion validity includes both concurrent validity and predictive validity. Concurrent validity compares scores from the PROM of interest with the gold standard administered at the same time, whereas predictive validity refers to the assessment of how well the measure predicts the gold standard in the future [7].

Another form of validity is *constructed validity*, which 'describes the relationship between PROM scores and factors that describe something that we can observe' [14]. Physical attributes such as a patient's height or weight are concrete measurements; however, measuring an abstract construct such as depression, for example, is more challenging and cannot be directly observed [7]. Instead, there are behaviors that are consequences of depression such as decreased energy, irritability, and changes in sleep that can be used to refer to abstract ideas that we construct in our minds to explain observed patterns or differences in behavior, attitudes, or feelings [7]. A main goal of any PROM is to measure these abstract concepts as there are no direct measurements to summarize such experiences. Construct validity, therefore, refers to the ability of a PROM to assess the abstract concept or construct it is trying to measure [14, 17, 18]. It is evaluated by hypothesizing how scores are associated with factors hypothesized to be associated with the constructs measured by the PROM [14, 18].

In 2010, the Consensus-based Standards of Health Status Management Instruments (COSMIN) study released a checklist to evaluate the methodological quality of studies measuring PROs [18, 19]. This consensus-based study included opinions of international experts in psychology, epidemiology, statistics and clinical medicine, and is used as a guide to evaluate validity and reliability of PROMs. The BREAST-Q was developed prior to the release of this consensus-based checklist [8]. Nonetheless, it meets the rigorous criteria for content, criterion and construct validity set forth by the COSMIN. In Phase I of development, data from qualitative interviews of 48 patients, expert opinion and literature review generated the items included in the instrument. Assessment of all items led to three pools of items from augmentation, reconstruction and reduction patients, which formed the domains of the conceptual framework for each type of surgery and was not just applied to all breast surgery patients. The research team then evaluated each of the item lists in each of the domains to retain the most appropriate items to form the best potential scale. In a subsequent study, the research team performed further validation tests of the BREAST-Q by analyzing questionnaires from 817 women [20]. With regards to criterion validity, BREAST-Q scales were compared to other 'gold standard' scales such as the Short Form 12/36, Breast Evaluation Questionnaire, Breast-Related Symptoms Questionnaire, Breast Reduction Assessment Severity Scale, European Organization for Research and Treatment of Cancer Scales, Body Image Scale, Body Image after Breast Cancer Questionnaire Body Stigma Scale [21–27]. Moderate correlations between BREAST-Q scores and other scales with related constructs and low correlations with dissimilar constructs were observed, confirming that this PROM meets criteria for criterion validity. The research team also determined the extent to which subscales of the BREAST-Q measured separate but related constructs by calculating inter-correlations to establish construct validity. Taken together, the BREAST-Q exceeds criteria for validity [28].

Reliability

In addition to validity, another important psychometric property to consider is reliability. Reliability assesses the precision of the measurements of the PROM and has been defined as 'the degree to which measurement is free from measurement error', [15] and is inversely related to measurement error. Reliability is typically referred to in terms of its reproducibility [15, 29]. Importantly, validity and reliability are not independent of each other—in other words, a PROM may be shown to be valid but not reliable, reliable but not valid, neither valid nor reliable, or both valid and reliable. However, validity can be limited by reliability in that inconsistent responses may affect the validity of the measurement [7].

There are two approaches to assessing the reliability of a PROM: (1) internal consistency reliability; and (2) repeatability reliability. Internal reliability is applied to multi-item scales and refers to the consistency of responses to the different items that form the scale. According to the Steering Committee of the COSMIN, Cronbach's alpha coefficient is the preferred statistic to measure internal consistency [20]. Cronbach's alpha coefficient is a statistic that is calculated from the pairwise correlations between items [7]. Values for Cronbach's alpha coefficient vary from 0 to 1, with >0.70 being a minimal requirement for internal consistency [7, 17]. Repeatability reliability on the other hand, can be applied to single-item or multi-item scale and evaluates the variances between repeated measurements on the same group of subjects. Repeatability reliability can be further divided into: (1) test–retest reliability; (2) interrater reliability; and (3) equivalent-forms reliability. Test–retest reliability is used when measurements are repeated on more than one occasion separated by a time interval that is sensible to how the PROM will be used. A minimum of a intra-class correlation coefficient (ICC) of 0.70 in studies with at least 50 patients is generally considered to meet criteria for acceptable test–retest reliability [13, 29]. Interrater reliability is used when measurements are made at the same time by different observers; and equivalent-forms reliability is used when measurements involve different variants of the same attribute on construct [7].

In addition to meeting the validity criteria set forth by COSMIN, the BREAST-Q also meets the reliability criteria. With regards to internal consistency, the uni-dimensionality of each scale of the BREAST-Q was checked and Cronbach's alpha coefficient was calculated for each scale separately. All domains within each module of the BREAST-Q (i.e. Augmentation, Reduction and Reconstruction) had Cronbach's alpha coefficients of >0.80. With regards to test–retest reliability, the intra-class correlation coefficient was calculated as >0.70 across all domains and modules after 462 patients retook the BREAST-Q after two weeks.

Classical Test Theory Versus Modern Psychometric Test Theory

There are two main techniques for the development and validation of PROMs: classical test theory (CTT) and item response theory (IRT) [30]. While CTT is the most commonly used, it has some drawbacks which IRT attempts to address [31]. In CTT for example, the psychometric properties only relate to a specific population and situation in which the questionnaire was developed and may only be valid for group-level-based research. Second, the assumption is that all items in a scale contribute equally to the final score. Third, it is difficult to equate scores that a person achieves on different tests [14]. In contrast, IRT focuses on individual items rather than an overall test score and assumes that individual items contribute differently to the final score [14]. One statistical method within the umbrella of IRT is Rasch Measurement Theory (RMT) [12], which was utilized in the development of the BREAST-Q [8]. Advantages of using Rasch measurement methods during the development and item reduction of the BREAST-Q scales have been described previously [8]. One important advantage of RMT over CTT, particularly for surgeons, is the ability to measure clinically meaningful change for individuals with RMT as questionnaires developed with CTT may only be applicable to group-based level research [8].

What Are the Different Types of PROMs?

Various types of PROMs exist that differ by content and the primary intended purpose of their use [19]. Instruments can be classified into different categories including: (1) disease/condition-specific; (2) generic; (3) dimension specific; (4) region/site-specific; (5) individualized; and (6) utility measures. Although they can be classified into different groups, they are not mutually exclusive, as some PROMs fit into more than one category. Here, we delve into the advantages and disadvantages between disease or condition-specific versus generic PROMs and briefly define the different types of instruments that exist.

Disease or condition-specific instruments measure the patient's perception of a specific disease or health problem. An important advantage of these types of instruments is that they are composed of relevant content that is important when used in a clinical trial or in clinical care of a specific patient group. It has been shown that disease-specific instruments are more likely to detect important changes that occur over time in the particular disease being studied [32, 33]. Because this type of PROM is more specific, it is also possible that a lower sample size may be needed to detect clinically important differences among a sample with the disease or condition of interest or differences following treatment or both [33, 34]. Additionally, patients may be more likely to complete questionnaires that ask about relevant concepts that are important to their condition or disease [32]. *Region or site-specific* PROMs, which can be considered a type of condition-specific measures, are particularly useful in surgery. These measurements were developed to assess problems in a specific part of the body. For example, the Shoulder Disability Questionnaire consists of 22-items to evaluate disability arising from the shoulder [35].

The major disadvantage of using a disease or condition-specific PROM is the inability to use the instrument on a generalized population without the disease or condition being measured. Therefore, it is not possible to compare the health status or well-being of the study sample to a general sample of well individuals. Moreover, disease or condition-specific measures may not capture health problems associated with a disease or its treatment that was not anticipated in the initial design of the instrument [32], further emphasizing the importance of establishing content validity during the development of the PROM.

Generic PROMs cover a broad spectrum of aspects of health status and can be applied to a wide group of patient groups. The SF-36 is an example of a generic PROM that has been widely used across many disciplines and patient groups [17]. Another common and more recently developed generic measurement is the Patient-Reported Outcomes Measurement Information System-29 (PROMIS-29). This generic, publicly available approach to measuring HRQoL was developed by the National Institutes of Health with the goal of comparing across different health conditions [36–40]. The main advantage of using generic measurements like the SF-36 or PROMIS-29 is the ability to use them across a broad spectrum of health problems and patient populations. Generic measurements are particularly useful if no condition-specific measures exist for a particular patient group [41]. Additionally, because they have been tested against healthy individuals, normative values exist for these different measurements, allowing for comparison to a baseline of healthy individuals [32].

An important disadvantage of using a generic PROM is that not all items may be relevant for the patient group or study question. Because generic measurements tend to have fewer relevant items to a particular condition or disease, they can be less sensitive in detecting differences with an intervention than using a condition-specific measurement [14]. For example, if we wanted to evaluate the impact of a new technique in breast reconstruction on sensation or natural-feeling aspect of the newly reconstructed breast, questions in generic measurement such as 'Are you able to walk a flight of stairs?' or 'How is your energy level?' are not as useful as a condition-specific measurement like the BREAST-Q that specifically asks about how satisfied the patient is with the feel of her breasts or appearance in clothing after reconstruction.

Depending on the research question, it may be appropriate to use a condition-specific, generic, or both in any given study. The advantages of any measurement tool should be weighed against the potential disadvantages of its use. In addition to condition-specific and generic measurements, other types of measures exist.

Dimension-specific measurements evaluate one specific aspect of health status [32]. For example, a common type of dimension-specific measurement is one that assesses different aspects of psychological function. The Beck Depression Inventory consists of 21 items addressing symptoms of depression [41]. Initially developed for use in patients with psychiatric illness, this dimension-specific measurement has been increasingly used to assess depression in patients with physical illnesses [42, 43].

Certain PRO platforms provide for a customizable measure specific to the treatment area or specific device. For example, the FACE-Q is a PROM designed to measure the satisfaction and quality of life for facial aesthetic procedures [44]. The instrument was developed with multiple modules of quality of life scales, appearance scales, adverse event checklist and patient experience of care scales. Modules can be chosen for a clinical study based on the specific treatment or general facial location where the device is used. For example, for a lip device, only modules relevant to the lip are utilized in the clinical study. Modules pertaining to other facial features (e.g. forehead) are removed for the specified clinical study. The customization limits the patient burden and assures all questionnaire items are relevant and appropriate for the patient cohort [45].

Individualized measures allow respondents to select issues, domains, or concerns that are of particular interest to them [32]. Without a predetermined list of questions selected by the investigator or researcher, individualized measurements encourage patients to identify the issues that are of personal concern or importance. The McMaster-Toronto Arthritis Patient Preference Disability Questionnaire (MACTAR) is an individualized PROM that asks patients to identify and subsequently prioritize five activities that are most affected by their arthritis [46]. Following an intervention, changes in the activities that patients identified are measured [46, 47].

Utility measures are typically considered a class of generic measurements, and have been derived from economics and decision-analysis [32]. Widely used in cost-effectiveness and decision-analysis studies, utility scores ascribe personal preferences of individuals regarding health states and provide evidence regarding the value of a particular intervention or treatment to society as a whole [32]. It is beyond the scope of this chapter to summarize and fully describe all the key aspects of utility measures; for more information please see Chap. 23.

Applying the Literature to Patients

How Do You Interpret Results?

Being able to assign qualitative meaning to a quantitative score from a PROM or interpretability, is of paramount importance. If a measurement tool shows validity and reliability but has not measured the issues that matter to patients it is not useful [14]. Calculating the minimal important difference (MID) or the minimal important change (MIC), standard error of measurement (SEM) is one approach to establishing interpretability of a PROM. Defined by Jaeschke and colleagues, MID refers to 'the smallest difference in score in the domain of interest which patients perceive as beneficial and which would mandate in the absence of troublesome side effects and excessive cost, a change in the patient's management' [48]. The MID or MIC should be defined to provide information regarding what changes in score would be considered to be clinically meaningful [14, 48].

Resolution of the Scenario

After reviewing the literature and finding the evidence from the study by Pusic and colleagues [1] to be the most directly relevant, you decide to share the main findings of the study with your patient. In summary, the primary goal of the study was to evaluate PROs after immediate implant-based versus autologous breast reconstruction. The main outcome of the study was PROs as measured by BREAST-Q and Patient-Reported Outcomes Measurement Information System (PROMIS) scores at 1 year after reconstruction.

After reading more about how the BREAST-Q was developed, you conclude that it is an appropriate condition-specific measure to assess PROs after breast reconstruction. In addition, the manuscript describes the scores from 7 domains of the PROMIS-29, a widely used generic PROM. The study found that patients who underwent autologous reconstruction were more satisfied with their breasts and had greater psychosocial and sexual well-being than those who underwent implant-based techniques. Despite these results favoring autologous reconstruction, there was a notable decrease physical well-being of the abdomen scores at 1 year compared to baseline. You find a similar article assessing similar outcomes, but among patients with longer follow-up [49].

You share these results and their implications with your patient. The patient is appreciative of the information and states that it has helped her come to an informed decision. Using a shared-decision-making approach, she utilizes the data from this study to opt for autologous reconstruction after mastectomy.

Appendix 1. Articles found in literature search

1. Cohen WA, Ballard TN, Hamill JB, Kim HM, Chen X, Klassen A, et al. Understanding and optimizing the patient experience in breast reconstruction. Ann Plast Surg. 2016;77(2):237–41.
2. Dayicioglu D, Tugertimur B, Zemina K, Dallarosa J, Killebrew S, Wilson A, et al. Vertical Mastectomy incision in implant breast reconstruction after skin sparing

mastectomy: advantages and outcomes. Ann Plast Surg. 2016;76(Suppl 4):S290–4.
3. de Blacam C, Healy C, Quinn L, Spillane C, Boyle T, Eadie PA, et al. Is satisfaction with surgeon a determining factor in patient reported outcomes in breast reconstruction? J Plast Reconstr Aesthet Surg. 2016;69 (9):1248–53.
4. Dean NR, Crittenden T. A five year experience of measuring clinical effectiveness in a breast reconstruction service using the BREAST-Q patient reported outcomes measure: a cohort study. J Plast Reconstr Aesthet Surg. 2016;69(11):1469–77.
5. Hart AM, Pinell-White X, Losken A. The psychosexual impact of postmastectomy breast reconstruction. Ann Plast Surg. 2016;77(5):517–22.
6. Huber KM, Zemina KL, Tugertimur B, Killebrew SR, Wilson AR, DallaRosa JV, et al. Outcomes of breast reconstruction after mastectomy using tissue expander and implant reconstruction. Ann Plast Surg. 2016;76(Suppl 4):S316–9.
7. Ng SK, Hare RM, Kuang RJ, Smith KM, Brown BJ, Hunter-Smith DJ. Breast reconstruction post mastectomy: patient satisfaction and decision making. Ann Plast Surg. 2016;76(6):640–4.
8. Razdan SN, Patel V, Jewell S, McCarthy CM. Quality of life among patients after bilateral prophylactic mastectomy: a systematic review of patient-reported outcomes. Qual Life Res. 2016;25(6):1409–21.
9. van Verschuer VM, Mureau MA, Gopie JP, Vos EL, Verhoef C, Menke-Pluijmers MB, et al. Patient satisfaction and nipple-areola sensitivity after bilateral prophylactic mastectomy and immediate implant breast reconstruction in a high breast cancer risk population: nipple-sparing mastectomy versus skin-sparing mastectomy. Ann Plast Surg. 2016;77(2):145–52.
10. Aguiar IC, Veiga DF, Marques TF, Novo NF, Sabino Neto M, Ferreira LM. Patient-reported outcomes measured by BREAST-Q after implant-based breast reconstruction: a cross-sectional controlled study in Brazilian patients. Breast (Edinburgh, Scotland). 2017;31:22–5.
11. Bennett KG, Qi J, Kim HM, Hamill JB, Wilkins EG, Mehrara BJ, et al. Association of fat grafting with patient-reported outcomes in postmastectomy breast reconstruction. JAMA Surg. 2017;152(10): 944–50.
12. Berlin NL, Momoh AO, Qi J, Hamill JB, Kim HM, Pusic AL, et al. Racial and ethnic variations in one-year clinical and patient-reported outcomes following breast reconstruction. Am J Surg. 2017;214 (2):312–7.
13. Cogliandro A, Barone M, Cassotta G, Tenna S, Cagli B, Persichetti P. Patient satisfaction and clinical outcomes following 414 breast reductions: application of BREAST-Q. Aesthetic Plast Surg. 2017;41 (2):245–9.
14. Cooke AL, Diaz-Abele J, Hayakawa T, Buchel E, Dalke K, Lambert P. Radiation therapy versus no radiation therapy to the neo-breast following skin-sparing mastectomy and immediate autologous free flap reconstruction for breast cancer: patient-reported and surgical outcomes at 1 year-a mastectomy reconstruction outcomes consortium (MROC) substudy. Int J Radiat Oncol Biol Phys. 2017;99(1):165–72.
15. Di Micco R, O'Connell RL, Barry PA, Roche N, MacNeill FA, Rusby JE. Standard wide local excision or bilateral reduction mammoplasty in large-breasted women with small tumours: surgical and patient-reported outcomes. Eur J Surg Oncol. 2017;43(4):636–41.
16. Fuzesi S, Cano SJ, Klassen AF, Atisha D, Pusic AL. Validation of the electronic version of the BREAST-Q in the army of women study. Breast (Edinburgh, Scotland). 2017;33:44–9.
17. Jeevan R, Browne JP, Gulliver-Clarke C, Pereira J, Caddy CM, van der Meulen JHP, et al. Surgical determinants of patient-reported outcomes following postmastectomy reconstruction in women with breast

cancer. Plast Reconstr Surg. 2017;139 (5):1036e–45e.
18. Kelsall JE, McCulley SJ, Brock L, Akerlund MTE, Macmillan RD. Comparing oncoplastic breast conserving surgery with mastectomy and immediate breast reconstruction: case-matched patient reported outcomes. J Plast Reconstr Aesthet Surg. 2017;70(10):1377–85.
19. Khavanin N, Clemens MW, Pusic AL, Fine NA, Hamill JB, Kim HM, et al. Shaped versus round implants in breast reconstruction: a multi-institutional comparison of surgical and patient-reported outcomes. Plast Reconstr Surg. 2017;139(5):1063–70.
20. Kuykendall LV, Tugertimur B, Agoris C, Bijan S, Kumar A, Dayicioglu D. Unilateral Versus Bilateral Breast Reconstruction: Is Less Really More? Ann Plast Surg. 2017;78 (6S Suppl 5):S275–s8.
21. McCarthy CM, Hamill JB, Kim HM, Qi J, Wilkins E, Pusic AL. Impact of bilateral prophylactic mastectomy and immediate reconstruction on health-related quality of life in women at high risk for breast carcinoma: results of the mastectomy reconstruction outcomes consortium study. Ann Surg Oncol. 2017;24(9):2502–8.
22. Mundy LR, Homa K, Klassen AF, Pusic AL, Kerrigan CL. Breast cancer and reconstruction: normative data for interpreting the BREAST-Q. Plast Reconstr Surg. 2017;139(5):1046e–55e.
23. Mundy LR, Homa K, Klassen AF, Pusic AL, Kerrigan CL. Normative data for interpreting the BREAST-Q: augmentation. Plast Reconstr Surg. 2017;139(4):846–53.
24. Pusic AL, Matros E, Fine N, Buchel E, Gordillo GM, Hamill JB, et al. Patient-reported outcomes 1 year after immediate breast reconstruction: results of the mastectomy reconstruction outcomes consortium study. J Clin Oncol. 2017;35 (22):2499–506.
25. Qureshi AA, Odom EB, Parikh RP, Myckatyn TM, Tenenbaum MM. Patient-reported outcomes of aesthetics and satisfaction in immediate breast reconstruction after nipple-sparing mastectomy with implants and fat grafting. Aesthet Surg J. 2017;37 (9):999–1008.
26. Srinivasa DR, Garvey PB, Qi J, Hamill JB, Kim HM, Pusic AL, et al. Direct-to-implant versus two-stage tissue expander/implant reconstruction: 2-Year risks and patient-reported outcomes from a prospective, multicenter study. Plast Reconstr Surg. 2017;140(5):869–77.
27. Erdmann-Sager J, Wilkins EG, Pusic AL, Qi J, Hamill JB, Kim HM, et al. Complications and patient-reported outcomes after abdominally based breast reconstruction: results of the mastectomy reconstruction outcomes consortium study. Plast Reconstr Surg. 2018;141(2):271–81.
28. Lagendijk M, van Egdom LSE, Richel C, van Leeuwen N, Verhoef C, Lingsma HF, et al. Patient reported outcome measures in breast cancer patients. Eur J Surg Oncol. 2018;44(7):963–8.
29. Mylvaganam S, Conroy EJ, Williamson PR, Barnes NLP, Cutress RI, Gardiner MD, et al. Adherence to best practice consensus guidelines for implant-based breast reconstruction: results from the iBRA national practice questionnaire survey. Eur J Surg Oncol. 2018;44(5):708–16.
30. Steele KH, Macmillan RD, Ball GR, Akerlund M, McCulley SJ. Multicentre study of patient-reported and clinical outcomes following immediate and delayed Autologous breast reconstruction and radiotherapy (ABRAR study). J Plast Reconstr Aesthet Surg. 2018;71(2):185–93.
31. Vrouwe SQ, Somogyi RB, Snell L, McMillan C, Vesprini D, Lipa JE. Patient-reported outcomes following breast conservation therapy and barriers to referral for partial breast reconstruction. Plast Reconstr Surg. 2018;141(1):1–9.
32. Yoon AP, Qi J, Brown DL, Kim HM, Hamill JB, Erdmann-Sager J, et al. Outcomes of immediate versus delayed breast reconstruction: results of a multicenter prospective study. Breast (Edinburgh, Scotland). 2018;37:72–9.

References

1. Pusic AL, Matros E, Fine N, Buchel E, Gordillo GM, Gamill JB, et al. Patient-reported outcomes 1 year after immediate breast reconstruction: results of the mastectomy reconstruction outcomes consortium study. J Clin Oncol. 2017;35(22):2499–506.
2. Cano SJ, Hobart JC. Watch out, watch out, the FDA are about. Dev Med Child Neurol. 2008;50(6):408–9.
3. US Department of Health and Human Services. Guidance for Industry: Patient-Reported Outcome Measures: Use in Medical Product Development to Support Labeling Claims. [Internet]. 2009 [cited 2018 May 5]. Available from https://www.fda.gov/downloads/drugs/guidances/ucm193282.pdf.
4. Office of Disease Prevention and Health Promotion (ODPJP). Healthy People 2020: Foundation Health Measure Report Health-Related Quality of Life and Well-Being. [Internet]. 2010 [cited 2018 June 3]. Available from https://www.healthypeople.gov/sites/default/files/HRQoLWBFullReport.pdf.
5. Deshpande PR, Rajan S, Sudeepthi BL, Abdul Nazir CP. Patient-reported outcomes: a new era in clinical research. Perspect Clin Res. 2011;2(4):137–44.
6. Kerr C, Nixon A, Wild D. Assessing and demonstrating data saturation in qualitative inquiry supporting patient-reported outcomes research. Expert Rev Pharmacoecon Outcomes Res. 2010;10(3):269–81.
7. Cappelleri JC, Zou KH, Bushmakin AG, Alvir JMJ, Alemayehu D, Symonds T. Patient-Reported outcomes: measurement, implementation and interpretation. Boca Raton, FL: CRC Press; 2014.
8. Pusic AL, Klassen AF, Scott AM, Klok JA, Cordeiro PG, Cano SJ. Development of a new patient-reported outcome measure for breast surgery: the BREAST-Q. PRS. 2009;124(2):345–53.
9. Lohr KN. Assessing health status and quality-of-life instruments: attributes and review criteria. Qual Life Res. 2002;11(3):193–205.
10. Walton MK, Powers JH 3rd, Hobart J, Patrick D, Marquis P, Vamvakas S, et al. Clinical outcome assessments: conceptual foundation-report of the ISPOR clinical outcomes assessment—emerging good practices for outcomes research task force. Value Health. 2015;18(6):741–52.
11. Patrick DL, Burke LB, Gwaltney CJ, Leidy NK, Martin ML, Molsen E, et al. Content validity-establishing and reporting the evidence in newly developed patient-reported outcomes (PRO) instruments for medical product evaluation: ISPOR PRO good research practices task force report: part 1–eliciting concepts for a new PRO instrument. Value Health. 2011;14(8):967–77.
12. Smith EV, Conrad KM, Change K, Piazza J. An introduction to Rasch measurement for scale development and persona assessment. J Nurse Meas. 2002;10(3):189–206.
13. Wong Riff KWY, Tsangaris E, Goodacre TEE, Forrest CR, Lawson J, Pusic AL, et al. What matters to patients with cleft lip and/or palate: an international qualitative study informing the development of the CLEFT-Q. Cleft Palate Craniofac J. 2018;55(3):442–50.
14. Dobbs TD, Hughes S, Mowbray N, Hutchings HA, Whitaker IS. How to decide which patient-reported outcome measure to use? A practical guide for plastic surgeons. J Plast Reconstr Aesthetic Surg. 2018;71(7):957–66.
15. Mokkink LB, Terwee CB, Patrick DL, Alonso J, Stratform PW, Knol DL, et al. The COSMIN study reached international consensus on taxonomy, terminology, and definitions of measurement properties for health-related patient-reported outcomes. J Clin Epidemiol. 2010;63(7):737–45.
16. Patrick DL, Burke LB, Gwaltney CJ, Leidy NK, Martin ML, Molsen E, et al. Content validity–establishing and reporting the evidence in newly developed patient-reported outcomes (PRO) instruments for medical product evaluation: ISPOR PRO Good Research Practices Task Force report: part 2–assessing respondent understanding. Value Health. 2011;14(8):978–88.
17. Streiner DL, Norman GR, Cairney J. Health measurement scales: a practical guide to their development and use. New York: Oxford University Press; 2015.
18. Mokkink LB, Terwee CB, Knol DL, Stratford PW, Alonso J, Patrick DL, et al. The COSMIN checklist for evaluating the methodological quality of studies on measurement properties: a clarification of its content. BMC Med Res Methodol. 2010;10(1):22.
19. Mokkink LB, Terwee CB, Patrick DL, Alonso J, Stratford, Knol DL, et al. The COSMIN checklist for assessing the methodological quality of studies on measurement properties of health status measurement instruments: an international Delphi study. Qual Life Res. 2010;19(4):539–49.
20. Cano SJ, Klassen AF, Scott AM, Cordeiro PG, Pusic AL. The BREAST-Q: further validation in independent clinical samples. Plast Reconstr Surg. 2012;129(2):293–302.
21. Ware JEJ, Kosinski MA, Keller SD. SF-36 physical and mental health summary scales: a user's manual. Boston, Mass: The Health Institute, New England Medical Center; 1994.
22. Kerrigan C, Collins E, Striplin D, et al. The health burden of breast hypertrophy. Plast Reconstr Surg. 2001;108:1591–9.
23. Aaronson N, Ahmedzai S, Bergman B, et al. The European organization for research and treatment of cancer QLQC30: a quality-of-life instrument for use in international clinical trials in oncology. J Natl Cancer Inst. 1993;85:365–76.
24. Anderson R, Cunningham B, Tafesse E, Lenderking W. Validation of the breast evaluation questionnaire for use with breast surgery patients. Plast Reconstr Surg. 2006;118:597–602.

25. Sigurdson L, Kirkland S, Mykhaloyskiy E. Validation of a questionnaire for measuring morbidity in breast hypertrophy. Plast Reconstr Surg. 2007;120:1108–14.
26. Hopwood P, Fletcher I, Lee A, Al Ghazal S. A body image scale for use with cancer patients. Eur J Cancer. 2001;37:189–97.
27. Baxter N, Goodwin P, McLeod R, Dion R, Devins G, Bombardier C. Reliability and validity of the body image after breast cancer questionnaire. Breast J. 2006;12: 221–32.
28. Bohrnstedt GW. Measurement. In: Rossi PH, Wright JD, Anderson AB, editors. Handbook of survey research. New York: Academic Press; 1983. p. 69–121.
29. Giraudeau B, Mary JY. Planning a reproducibility study: how many subjects and how many replicates per subject for an expected width of the 95 per cent confidence interval of the intraclass correlation coefficient. Stat Med. 2001;20:3205–14.
30. Crocker LAJ. Introduction to classical and modern test theory. Rinehart and Winston: Holt; 1986.
31. DeVellis RF. Classical test theory. Med Care. 2006;44(11):S50–9.
32. Fitzpatrick R, Davey C, Buxton MJ, Jones DR. Evaluating patient-based outcome measures for use in clinical trials. Health Technol Assess. 1998;2(14): i–iv, 1–74.
33. Deyo RA, Patrick DL. Barriers to the use of health status measures in clinical investigation, patient care, and policy research. Med Care. 1989;27(3 Suppl): S254–68.
34. Deyo RA, Patrick DL. The significance of treatment effects: the clinical perspective. Med care. 1995;33(4 Suppl):As286–291.
35. Croft P, Pope D, Zonca M, O'Neill T, Silman A. Measurement of shoulder related disability: results of a validation study. Ann Rheum Dis. 1994;53(8):525–8.
36. Jensen RE, Potosky AL, Reeve BB, Hahn E, Cella D, Fries J, et al. Validation of the PROMIS physical function measures in a diverse US population-based cohort of cancer patients. Qual Life Res. 2015;24 (10):2333–44.
37. Hahn EA, Beaumont JL, Pilkonis PA, Garcia SF, Magasi S, DeWalt DA, et al. The PROMIS satisfaction with social participation measures demonstrated responsiveness in diverse clinical populations. J Clin Epidemiol. 2016;73:135–41.
38. Teresi JA, Jones RN. Methodological issues in examining measurement equivalence in patient reported outcomes measures: methods overview to the two-part series, "measurement equivalence of the patient reported outcomes measurement information system((R)) (PROMIS((R))) Short Forms". Psychol Test Assess Model. 2016;58(1):37–78.
39. Craig BM, Reeve BB, Brown PM, Cella D, Hays RD, Lipscomb J, et al. US Valuation of health outcomes measured using the PROMIS-29. Value Health. 2014;17(8):846–53.
40. Visser MC, Fletcher AE, Parr G, Simpson A, Bulpitt CJ. A comparison of three quality of life instruments in subjects with angina pectoris: the Sickness Impact Profile, the Nottingham Health Profile, and the quality of well being scale. J Clin Epidemiol. 1994;47(2):157–63.
41. Beck AT, Ward CH, Mendelson M, Mock J, Erbaugh J. An inventory for measuring depression. Arch Gen Psychiatry. 1961;4:561–71.
42. Grabowska-Fudala B, Jaracz K, Gorna K, Miechowicz I, Wojtasz I, Jaracz J, et al. Depressive symptoms in stroke patients treated and non-treated with intravenous thrombolytic therapy: a 1-year follow-up study. J Neurol. 2018. [Epub ahead of print] https://doi.org/10.1007/s00415-018-8938.
43. Daniel M, Agewall S, Berglund F, Caidahl K, Collste O, Ekenbäck C, et al. Prevalence of anxiety and depression symptoms in patients with myocardial infarction with non-obstructive coronary arteries. AM J Med. 2018. [Epub ahead of print] https://doi.org/10.1016/j.amjmed.2018.04.040.
44. Klassen AF, Cano SJ, Scott A, Snell L, Pusic AL. Measuring patient-reported outcomes in facial aesthetic patients: development of the FACE-Q. Facial Plast Surg. 2010;26(4):303–9.
45. Administration USFaD. Value and Use of Patient-Reported Outcomes (PROs) in Assessing Effects of Medical Devices. [Internet]. 2017. [cited 2018 July 14]. Available from https://www.fda.gov/downloads/AboutFDA/CentersOffices/OfficeofMedicalProductsandTobacco/CDRH/CDRHVisionandMission/UCM588576.pdf.
46. Tugwell P, Bombardier C, Buchanan WW, Goldsmith CH, Grace E, Hanna B. The MACTAR patient preference disability questionnaire–an individualized functional priority approach for assessing improvement in physical disability in clinical trials in rheumatoid arthritis. J Rheumatol. 1987;14(3):446–51.
47. Brodin N, Grooten WJA, Strat S, Lofberg E, Alexanderson H. The McMaster Toronto arthritis patient preference questionnaire (MACTAR): a methodological study of reliability and minimal detectable change after a 6 week-period of acupuncture treatment in patients with rheumatoid arthritis. BMC Res Notes. 2017;10(1):687.
48. Jaeschke R, Singer J, Guyatt GH. Measurement of health status: ascertaining the minimal clinically important difference. Control Clin Trials. 1989;10 (4):407–15.
49. Santosa KB, Qi J, Kim HM, Hamill JB, Wilkins EG, Pusic AL. Long-term patient-reported outcomes in postmastectomy breast reconstruction. JAMA Surg. 2018. [Epub ahead of print] https://doi.org/10.1001/jamasurg.2018.1677.

9 Surrogate Endpoints

Seper Ekhtiari, Ryan P. Coughlin, Nicole Simunovic and Olufemi R. Ayeni

Clinical Scenario

You are an orthopedic surgeon who has recently started your practice. You are seeing a new patient in the clinic. She is an otherwise healthy active 41-year-old female (body mass index [BMI] of 25 kg/m^2) with an acute symptomatic meniscal tear who is considering arthroscopic surgery to manage this injury. The procedure would be performed under regional anesthesia. Her only medication is an oral contraceptive pill (OCP). She does not smoke. She explains that she has heard that oral contraceptives increase her risk of a "blood clot in the lung which can kill". As well, her next-door neighbor recently developed a "blood clot" following anterior cruciate ligament reconstruction. The patient wants to know if she should be taking any medications before and after the surgery to prevent "dying from a blood clot". She has no family history of venous thromboembolism.

You know that lower limb surgery is a risk factor for venous thromboembolic (VTE) events [1]. As well, if this patient's tear is amenable to repair, you may want to restrict her weight bearing which is also a risk factor for VTE. On the other hand, she is young and active and will likely be able to ambulate shortly after the operation. Her history of OCP use also concerns you because it increases her baseline risk of a VTE [2]. You tell the patient that you would like to find some evidence to help you make an informed decision regarding whether anticoagulation is appropriate. You know that there is a considerable amount of research that has been done on deep vein thrombosis (DVT) following knee surgery but you wonder if this evidence will help you address the patient's concern about pulmonary embolism and death particularly given the fact that she has an added risk factor (the OCP). You decide to do some further research and get back to the patient.

Introduction

Surrogate endpoints, sometimes referred to as "biomarkers" (although these terms are not strictly interchangeable) or "surrogate outcome measures", can be defined as "an endpoint that is used in clinical trials as a substitute for a direct measure of how a patient feels, functions, or survives [3]." These outcomes do not directly measure "patient important outcomes", but rather

S. Ekhtiari · R. P. Coughlin · N. Simunovic
O. R. Ayeni (✉)
Department of Surgery, Division of Orthopaedic Surgery, McMaster University, Hamilton, ON, Canada
e-mail: femiayeni@gmail.com

O. R. Ayeni
Department of Health Research Methods, Evidence, and Impact, McMaster University, Hamilton, ON, Canada

A. Thoma et al. (eds.), *Evidence-Based Surgery*,
https://doi.org/10.1007/978-3-030-05120-4_9

act as a substitute for the true outcome of interest. For example, measuring joint range-of-motion following orthopedic surgery and using it as an endpoint to estimate function and recovery is such a surrogate outcome.

Surrogate endpoints offer multiple advantages, hence their popularity in the literature. They do, however, have some important limitations that must be recognized and understood before using them. The "LDL cholesterol mortality paradox" is a finding of large well-designed trials that high-intensity statin drugs (compared to low- or moderate-intensity statins) result in a statistically significant reduction in serum low-density lipid (LDL) values, but do not affect overall mortality [4]. In this case, LDL is used as a surrogate endpoint for the severity of atherosclerosis and the likelihood of eventual cardiac events. The cholesterol mortality paradox example displays many of the advantages of surrogate endpoints, as well as a major disadvantage. Some of the most important advantages of surrogate endpoints include the following [5, 6]:

1. **They are easier and cheaper to measure than "true" endpoints**: Measuring blood pressure is simple, cheap and routinely performed. Detecting a stroke requires thorough clinical evaluation and detailed cross-sectional imaging. Thus, using blood pressure as a surrogate endpoint for risk of stroke is much cheaper and easier than focusing on stroke itself as an endpoint.
2. **They can often be measured more objectively and precisely than patient-important endpoints**: For a postoperative patient, particularly in the elderly and those with a history of cardiac disease, myocardial injury is always a concern. Measuring serum troponin levels as a surrogate endpoint for the presence and extent of cardiac injury is more precise and objective than a clinical history and physical exam [7].
3. **They are often present earlier than the clinical manifestation of the outcome, thus making them useful particularly in early stages of pharmacological trials**: Surrogate endpoints are often used as a "proof-of-concept" in the development and evaluation of pharmaceuticals and surgical techniques alike. For example, we know that hemoglobin A1c (HbA1c) is an important marker of sugar control in diabetic patients, and thus a predictor of long-term disease outcomes [8]. It is much more practical to measure HbA1c to assess the potential benefit of a new antihyperglycemic medication than to wait for the long-term micro- and macrovascular sequela of diabetes to declare themselves.
4. **They reduce the sample size required to observe an effect**: In the randomized controlled trial (RCT) discussed later in this chapter [9], all postoperative patients routinely underwent Doppler ultrasonography. Thus, even patients who were completely asymptomatic but had a positive ultrasound would be considered as DVT events. Clearly, this means that patients with "subclinical" DVTs that in routine practice would have been inconsequential and gone unnoticed were now being identified. This increases the event rate, thus decreasing the total sample size that is needed for the study to be sufficiently powered.

Overall, the surrogate endpoints are indispensable in both research and clinical settings. Their ease of use, relative inexpensiveness, objectivity, and early presentation make them ideal in both contexts if used appropriately.

That being said, there are certainly drawbacks to the use of surrogate endpoints. Some of these limitations include misleading conclusions, misrepresentation of the effect size of an intervention, and challenges in evaluating the safety of an intervention.

One potential pitfall is that the surrogate endpoint produces results that are misleading—meaning they make the risk–benefit balance appear opposite to its "true" direction. This is a rare but not unprecedented scenario. Generally, this brings into question the validity of the surrogate endpoint, and the relationship between the surrogate and true endpoints should be reassessed. Anti-arrhythmic medications provide a good case study for this phenomenon. Cardiac arrhythmias are dangerous conditions which can cause severe complications including heart failure and death [10]. It would seem to make sense then, that a medication that stops or reverses an arrhythmia would be beneficial to the patient's health and longevity. Interestingly, a recent meta-analysis of randomized controlled trials found an increase in noncardiac mortality and all-cause mortality with anti-arrhythmic medication; the risk of cardiac death was not different in patients on these medications [11]. Thus, what may have seemed like quite a suitable endpoint (the reversal of an arrhythmia), turned out in fact to show a net harm in patient outcomes.

More commonly, surrogate endpoints correctly identify the direction of the treatment effect, but over- or underestimate the magnitude of the effect. As mentioned earlier, one of the advantages of surrogate endpoints is that they allow for a trial to be conducted with a smaller sample size than would be necessary otherwise. The potential downside of this is that they may overestimate the effect size [12]. An interesting example of this pitfall has been demonstrated in ophthalmological trials for treatment of glaucoma. Clearly, glaucoma is a disease of increased intraocular pressure [13]. Thus, it makes sense that reducing intraocular pressure (IOP), whether medically or through a procedure, will lead to better functional outcomes. Interestingly, however, there are medications that provide quite clinically important structural improvements (i.e., lower IOP), but relatively smaller functional gains [14]. Using a hypothetical example, gains in knee range-of-motion beyond a certain limit may not provide any further functional benefit—does 150° of knee flexion provide any additional benefit beyond 140°? Thus, using range-of-motion as a surrogate endpoint for the function may overestimate the effect of the intervention.

Finally, surrogate endpoints are often unable to accurately quantify the overall safety of an intervention in terms of patient-important complications, such as death or major adverse clinical events. The detection of differences in these outcomes requires large RCTs that are specifically designed and powered to detect such events.

Balancing these advantages and disadvantages is important when performing or evaluating RCTs that employ surrogate endpoints. With the advancement of laboratory medicine and technology, the number of surrogate endpoints available to clinicians and researchers has increased [15]. Thus, it can be tempting to "treat the numbers" in an effort to help patients. Caution should be exercised, however; normalizing or improving laboratory or structural measurements does not always yield clinical improvement [4]. For a surrogate endpoint to be valid, it has to meet two major, important criteria:

1. **Is there strong documented/published evidence that connects the surrogate outcome to the patient-important outcome under consideration?** Troponin is a protein expressed in both skeletal and cardiac muscle, with specific subtypes only being expressed in the myocardium and nowhere else. Myocardial necrosis causes the release of troponins into the bloodstream, where they can be easily measured [16]. In addition, angiographic studies have confirmed that troponin concentration is directly related to the presence and extent of a coronary artery clot [16]. Therefore, we can be assured that the co-occurrence of myocardial injury and troponin elevation is not simply by chance either— there is no confounding effect here (more on this later). Thus, the use of serum troponin as a surrogate for myocardial injury meets the first criterion for a valid surrogate endpoint.
2. **Is there strong clinical data available to correlate improvement in the surrogate endpoint with improvement in the patient-important outcome of interest?** Myocardial injury after noncardiac surgery (MINS) refers to a phenomenon where serum troponin levels elevate after noncardiac surgery, in the absence of other classic findings

of myocardial injury [17]. In a large, international, multicentre RCT, postoperative rise in troponin was been found to independently predict 30-day mortality. In other words, if we can find ways to reduce the likelihood of postoperative troponin rise, then we can reduce the likelihood of postoperative death within 30 days. Thus, troponin rise after noncardiac surgery satisfies the second criterion as well because it is directly related to a very important patient outcome: death.

Beware! Confounders

A strong correlation between a surrogate endpoint and a patient-important outcome is not enough to satisfy the first criterion of a "plausible, causal relationship" between the two. A patient's risk of myocardial infarction (MI) is higher in the acute postoperative period following a total joint arthroplasty compared to the preoperative period. After about 6 months, however, the risk of MI returns to baseline [18]. Similarly, pain scores peak in the early postoperative period and begin to gradually improve from there, reaching a new steady baseline somewhere between 3 and 6 months postoperatively [19]. Thus, if plotted together on a graph, MI risk (y-axis) and pain scores (x-axis) may be correlated. Of course, joint pain has no causal relationship to cardiac injury, and using pain scores as a surrogate endpoint for cardiac risk would not meet our first criterion. In this case, there is a ***confounder***—a third variable that independently affects two unrelated variables, causing them to be correlated despite a complete lack of a causal relationship (see Fig. 9.1). The confounding variable, in this case, is the surgery itself—undergoing the joint replacement has independently and simultaneously increased the risk of MI *and* caused the patient to experience joint pain. While this particular example may seem rather obvious, many real-life examples are often more nebulous, and mistaking or misrepresenting correlation as causation is not an uncommon error in the academic world [20].

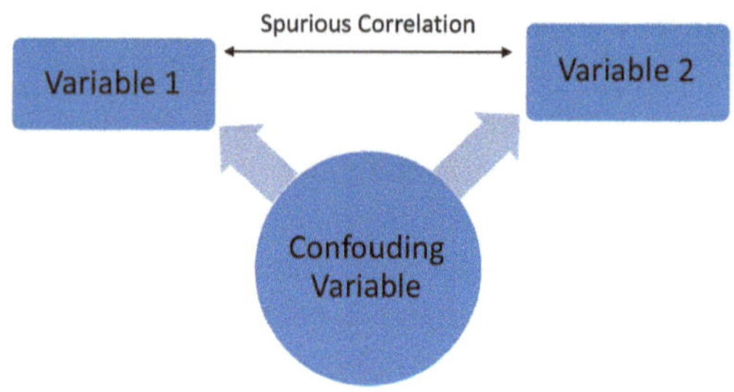

Fig. 9.1 Demonstration of the concept of a confounding variable

Literature Search

You use PubMed, a search engine to access online reference databases, to conduct a search strategy to find the evidence for VTE events following arthroscopic knee surgery. You know there has been a fair bit of research on the subject, so you restrict your search to Level 1 Evidence only (i.e., RCTs) . Your search terms include "knee", "arthroscop*" (to encompass terms such as arthroscopic and arthroscopy), "venous thromboembolism", "deep vein thrombosis", and "pulmonary embolism". You combine "venous thromboembolism", "deep vein thrombosis", and "pulmonary embolism" using the "OR" operator, and then combine this trio with "knee" and "arthroscop*" using the "AND" Boolean operator. The search has no date limitations and was performed on April 14, 2018. This search produced 13 results.

After screening the abstracts, you identify 7 of the 13 articles that directly compared prophylactic anticoagulation regimens in patients undergoing knee arthroscopy. The remaining 6 studies were either on related topics or did not directly analyze VTE events. Of the remaining 7 articles, 5 have sample sizes of fewer than 250 randomized patients. The remaining 2 studies both appear to be of high quality, with over 1000 randomized patients and 3-month follow-up. Ultimately, you choose the study by Camporese et al. because it also compares differing durations of anticoagulant therapy [9]. In this study, the authors enrolled 1761 consecutive patients undergoing knee arthroscopy and randomized them to (a) graduated compression stockings

Table 9.1 Key findings from the article by Camporese et al. [9]

	7 day GCS	7 day LMWH	14 day LMWH [95% CI]	*p*-value
N	660	657	444	–
Age (year)	42.3 (14.4)	41.9 (15.1)	42.5 (16.7)	–
Male:Female	1.66:1	1.62:1	1.60:1	–
Use of hormonal compounds, *n*(%)	154 (23.3)	194 (29.5)	114 (25.7)	–
Primary efficacy end point, *n*(%) – Death – Symptomatic PE – Asymptomatic proximal DVT – Symptomatic proximal DVT – Symptomatic distal DVT	21 (3.2) 0 2 (0.3) 7 (1.1) 1 (0.2) 11 (1.7)	6 (0.9) 0 2 (0.3) 2 (0.03) 0 2 (0.3)	4 (0.9[0.4–2.3]) 0 2 (0.5 [0.1–1.6]) 0 1 (0.2 [0.0–1.3]) 1 (0.2 [0.0–1.3])	0.005
Secondary efficacy end point, *n*(%) – Asymptomatic distal DVT	31 (4.7) 10 (1.5)	12 (1.8) 6 (0.9)	11 (2.5 [1.4–4.4]) 7 (1.6 [0.8–3.2])	0.005
Primary safety end point, *n*(%) – Major bleeding event – Clinically relevant bleeding	2 (0.3) 1 (0.2) 1 (0.2	6 (0.9) 2 (0.3) 4 (0.6)	2 (0.5 [0.1–1.6]) 1 (0.2 [0.0–1.3]) 1 (0.2 [0.0–1.3])	–
Secondary safety end point, *n*(%) – Minor bleeding event	22 (3.3) 20 (3.0)	29 (4.4) 23 (3.5)	18 (4.1 [2.6–6.3]) 16 (3.6 [2.2–5.8])	–

(GCS), (b) low-molecular-weight heparin (LMWH) for 7 days, or (c) LMWH for 14 days. All patients had bilateral ultrasonography performed at follow-up (or earlier if necessary). Patients suspected of having sustained a pulmonary embolism (PE) also underwent a ventilation–perfusion scan. The primary endpoint in the article was a 3-month composite outcome measure consisting of asymptomatic DVT, symptomatic venous thromboembolism (VTE), and all-cause mortality [9]. Table 9.1 summarizes demographics and key efficacy and safety results from this study.

Are the Results Valid?

Let us evaluate whether or not our surrogate endpoint is valid. The patient has stated that she is worried about "dying from a blood clot in her lung"; thus, PE-related mortality is your true end goal. You wonder if DVT is a valid surrogate endpoint in this case. Clearly, DVT as a surrogate endpoint for PE meets the first criterion: there is a causal relationship between DVT and PE, and a PE can certainly be fatal. This causal relationship makes sense—a thrombus formed in the veins of the leg (or arm for that matter) has the potential to embolize, travel back via the venous system to the heart, pass through the right-sided chambers, and eventually end up in the lungs, where it can cause a blockage in the pulmonary vasculature (i.e., a PE). Thus, we can be confident that the strong relationship between these two events is causal and unlikely to be confounded. The second criterion is also satisfied in this case: there is good evidence to show that treating DVT and PE with anticoagulant therapy results in significant reductions in morbidity and mortality [21]. Thus, DVT is a valid surrogate endpoint to use for risk of mortality from a PE.

What Are the Results?

You now review the results of the Camporese et al. [9] study, confident that DVT is a valid surrogate endpoint to look at. You turn your attention to the results section of the article. Interestingly, you notice that the authors report that among 877 patients with DVT symptoms (i.e., "suspected DVT"), only 16 had a confirmed

DVT on ultrasound (1.8%) [9]. As well, the total number of patients with asymptomatic DVT ($N = 32$) is twice the number of patients with a symptomatic DVT ($N = 16$) [9]. After lamenting the seemingly limited utility of symptoms in guiding the diagnosis of DVT, you turn your attention to the data comparing the three groups. You note that there were zero deaths across the three groups. In addition, there was an identical number of PEs across the three groups, though the percentages are slightly different. Given that the primary endpoint was a composite outcome, these individual outcomes are not directly compared. You note that the authors report a p-value of 0.005 for their primary endpoint, with the LMWH groups having fewer events than the GCS group. Finally, you look at the safety data: the study reports that the rate of major and minor bleeding events across the three groups was similar, though no direct statistical comparison was performed.

Are the Results Applicable to My Patients?

You are satisfied that using DVT as a surrogate endpoint for PE-related mortality is valid. You are somewhat concerned about the fact that the study reported composite endpoints, and that these included many cases of asymptomatic DVT. Nonetheless, you turn your attention to the demographics of the study to decide whether the results are applicable to your practice in general, and this patient in particular. You notice that the study had a ratio of approximate 1.6:1, males versus females enrolled, and that the patient groups had a mean age of about 42 years. Based on your knee arthroscopy patient population, this seems like a close representation. Given that your patient is female, however, the sex distribution does make you somewhat cautious. Fortunately, the authors do specifically mention that close to 10% of the patients were using a "hormonal compound", such as the OCP. Unfortunately, however, these patients' results were not separately reported or analyzed. Interestingly, the study includes a range of arthroscopic procedures, including longer and more complex surgeries such as ligament reconstruction. You note that the study was conducted in Italy, and thus, the patient group may have had different risk factors and lifestyle patterns than your Canadian patient group. Finally, you wonder about the applicability of LMWH—this study is nearly a decade old, and there have been a number of newer, more effective anticoagulant medications developed since then. Overall, you decide that the patient groups are relatively similar to your practice and patient, but you do have some reservations about the generalizability of the results.

Resolution of Clinical Scenario

Having considered the study, you come to the following conclusions:

- The study was well-designed and well-conducted.
- The sample size was large enough (as the authors performed a prospective sample size calculation and met their target [9]) and generalizable to your patients. Demographic data similar to your patient included: age, BMI, smoking status and family history of venous thromboembolism. Furthermore, the included patients had arthroscopic knee surgery (38–44% meniscectomies) performed under regional anesthesia.
- The sample included patients on hormonal therapies, though their outcomes were not separately analyzed or reported.
- The rate of the composite outcome, which included asymptomatic DVTs, was lower in the 7-day LMWH group compared to the GCS group.
- The rate of adverse events was similar for LMWH compared to nonmedical treatment, though a direct statistical comparison was not performed.

Overall, you decide that you have a number of concerns about the study which make it difficult to use this paper to help counsel your patient. Ultimately, you decide that she is likely quite low risk, with OCP use being her only risk factor. As well, the composite outcome makes it difficult to assess how much real clinical benefit LMWH confers.

Your hunch is that LMWH is likely not necessary after knee arthroscopy, particularly for low risk patients. Thus, you decide to dig a little bit deeper into the literature and find two very helpful articles: A recent meta-analysis of RCTs found that anticoagulant therapy did significantly decrease the risk of DVT, but not of symptomatic VTE or PE [22]. The other is a large case-control study which found that the use of OCP in women over 46 years old had an odds ratio of 46.6 for DVT [23]. In the end, you decide that while a PE, particularly a fatal one seems quite unlikely, anticoagulation for the prevention of DVT may be a reasonable choice in this case. You plan to bring this information back to the patient and decide on a course of action together with her.

Conclusion

Surrogate endpoints are outcome measures that can be measured directly, objectively, and often inexpensively. They are meant to serve as a more practical substitute for true, patient-important outcomes. When applied correctly, surrogate endpoints are indispensable to conducting well-designed clinical trials. To ensure a surrogate endpoint is valid, it must meet two main criteria: (1) have a direct causal relationship to the true outcome and (2) have been shown with strong evidence to be correlated with change in the true outcome. It is always important to consider confounding variables, and try to ensure that they are not producing misleading results. The downside of surrogate endpoints is that they may mislead us on the direction and magnitude of the risk-benefit analysis, and that they are not well-suited to assess the safety of an intervention. When appraising any study, remember to ask: (1) is the study valid? (2) What are the results? and (3) Can I apply the results to my practice?

References

1. Barker RC, Marval P. Venous thromboembolism: risks and prevention. Contin Educ Anaesthesia, Crit Care Pain. 2011;11(1):18–23. https://doi.org/10.1093/bjaceaccp/mkq044.
2. Trenor CC 3rd, Chung RJ, Michelson AD, Neufeld EJ, Gordon CM, Laufer MR, et al. Hormonal contraception and thrombotic risk: a multidisciplinary approach. Pediatrics. 2011;127(2):347–57. https://doi.org/10.1542/peds.2010-2221.
3. Robb MA, McInnes PM, Califf RM. Biomarkers and surrogate endpoints: developing common terminology and definitions. JAMA—J Am Med Assoc. 2016;315(11):1107–8. https://doi.org/10.1001/jama.2016.2240.
4. Nunes JPL. Statins and the cholesterol mortality paradox. Scott Med J. 2017;62(1):19–23. https://doi.org/10.1177/0036933016681913.
5. Aronson JK. Biomarkers and surrogate endpoints. Br J Clin Pharmacol. 2005;59(5):491–4. https://doi.org/10.1111/j.1365-2125.2005.02435.x.
6. Bucher H, Cook D, Holbrook A, Guyatt G. Surrogate Outcomes. In: Guyatt G, Rennie D, Meade MO, Cook DJ, editors. Users' guides to the medical literature: a manual for evidence-based clinical practice, 3rd ed. USA: McGraw-Hill Education; 2015, p. 271–84. (evidence; 2015).
7. Hallén J. Troponin for the estimation of infarct size: what have we learned? Cardiology. 2012;121(3):204–12. https://doi.org/10.1159/000337113.
8. Sherwani SI, Khan HA, Ekhzaimy A, Masood A, Sakharkar MK. Significance of HbA1c test in diagnosis and prognosis of diabetic patients. Biomark Insights. 2016;11:95–104. https://doi.org/10.4137/Bmi.s38440.
9. Camporese G, Bernardi E, Prandoni P, Noventa F, Verlato F, Simioni P, et al. Low-molecular-weight heparin versus compression stockings for thromboprophylaxis after knee arthroscopy: a randomized trial. Ann Intern Med. 2008;149(2):73–82. https://doi.org/10.7326/0003-4819-149-2-200807150-00003.
10. Fu DG. Cardiac arrhythmias: diagnosis, symptoms, and treatments. Cell Biochem Biophys. 2015;73(2):291–6. https://doi.org/10.1007/s12013-015-0626-4.
11. Pandya B, Spagnola J, Sheikh A, Karam B, Reddy Anuggu V, Khan A, et al. Anti-arrhythmic medications increase non-cardiac mortality—a meta-analysis of randomized control trials. J Arrhythmia. 2016;32(3):204–11. https://doi.org/10.1016/j.joa.2016.02.006.
12. Lantz B. The large sample size fallacy. Scand J Caring Sci. 2013;27(2):487–92. https://doi.org/10.1111/j.1471-6712.2012.01052.x.

13. Weinreb RN, Aung T, Medeiros FA. The Pathophysiology and treatment of glaucoma. JAMA. 2014; 311(18):1901. https://doi.org/10.1001/jama.2014.3192.
14. Medeiros FA. Biomarkers and surrogate endpoints: lessons learned from glaucoma. Investig Ophthalmol Vis Sci. 2017;58(6):BIO20–BIO26. https://doi.org/10.1167/iovs.17-21987.
15. Yudkin FJS, Lipska Robert KJ, Montori VM. The idolatry of the surrogate. BMJ. 2012;344(7839). https://doi.org/10.1136/bmj.d7995.
16. Korff S, Katus HA, Giannitsis E. Differential diagnosis of elevated troponins. Heart. 2006;92(7):987–93. https://doi.org/10.1136/hrt.2005.071282.
17. Botto F, Alonso-Coello P, Chan MT, Villar JC, Xavier D, Srinathan S, et al. Myocardial injury after noncardiac surgery: a large, international, prospective cohort study establishing diagnostic criteria, characteristics, predictors, and 30-day outcomes. Anesthesiology. 2014;120(3):564–78. https://doi.org/10.1097/ALN.0000000000000113.
18. Lu N, Misra D, Neogi T, Choi HK, Zhang Y. Total joint arthroplasty and the risk of myocardial infarction—a general population, Propensity score-matched cohort study. Arthritis Rheumatol. 2015: n/a–n/a. https://doi.org/10.1002/art.39246.
19. Wylde V, Rooker J, Halliday L, Blom A. Acute postoperative pain at rest after hip and knee arthroplasty: severity, sensory qualities and impact on sleep. Orthop Traumatol Surg Res. 2011;97(2):139–44. https://doi.org/10.1016/j.otsr.2010.12.003.
20. Coleman AB, Lam DP, Soowal LN. Correlation, necessity, and sufficiency: common errors in the scientific reasoning of undergraduate students for interpreting experiments. Biochem Mol Biol Educ. 2015;43(5):305–15. https://doi.org/10.1002/bmb.20879.
21. Kelly J, Hunt BJ. Do anticoagulants improve survival in patients presenting with venous thromboembolism? J Intern Med. 2003;254(6):527–39. https://doi.org/10.1111/j.1365-2796.2003.01206.x.
22. Zheng G, Tang Q, Shang P, Pan XY, Liu HX. No effectiveness of anticoagulants for thromboprophylaxis after non-major knee arthroscopy: a systemic review and meta-analysis of randomized controlled trials. J Thromb Thrombolysis. 2018;45(4):562–70. https://doi.org/10.1007/s11239-018-1638-x.
23. van Adrichem RA, Nelissen RGHH, Schipper IB, Rosendaal FR, Cannegieter SC. Risk of venous thrombosis after arthroscopy of the knee: results from a large population-based case-control study. J Thromb Haemost. 2015;13(8):1441–8. https://doi.org/10.1111/jth.12996.

How to Assess an Article that Deals with Health-Related Quality of Life

10

Achilles Thoma, Jenny Santos, Margherita Cadeddu, Eric K. Duku and Charles H. Goldsmith

Introduction

Traditionally, the results of surgery have been measured by clinical outcomes such as prolonged survival and reduced morbidity. Death or survival rates are critical outcomes that are usually difficult to dispute, unless a patient is comatose in a vegetative state in an intensive care unit or on a neurosurgical ward. Surgeons and patients, however, can interpret the morbidity outcomes differently. A hernia repair may be considered a success from the general surgeon's point of view but not so from the patient's point of view if the scar is painful due to skin scar neuromata or entrapment of deeper sensory nerves during the repair. Similarly, a successful digit replant may be considered a success from a hand surgeon's point of view if the digit is viable but not from the patient's point of view if there is stiffness of the whole hand making it difficult to work, potentially leading to loss of employment.

Since around 1990, the outcomes research movement has shifted the declaration of a "successful surgical outcome" from surgeon to patient. In other words, the evaluation of outcomes in surgery have begun to take into account the patient's experiences, preferences, and values. This is, in essence, one of the tenets of what Evidence-Based Surgery is all about. With the exception of some high-risk surgical subspecialties, such as cardiac surgery and oncological surgery, most of the surgical procedures we perform as surgeons are aimed at reducing morbidity or improving Quality of Life (QoL) . The broader term QoL can be defined as "an individual's perception of their position in life in the context of the culture and values systems in which they live and in relation to their goals,

A. Thoma (✉) · J. Santos
Department of Surgery, Division of Plastic Surgery, McMaster University, Hamilton, ON, Canada
e-mail: athoma@mcmaster.ca

J. Santos
e-mail: santoj8@mcmaster.ca

M. Cadeddu
Department of Surgery, Division of General Surgery, McMaster University, Hamilton, ON, Canada
e-mail: mocadeddu@yahoo.com

E. K. Duku
Offord Centre for Child Studies, Department of Psychiatry and Behavioral Neurosciences, McMaster University, Hamilton, ON, Canada
e-mail: duku@mcmaster.ca

A. Thoma · C. H. Goldsmith
Department of Health Research Methods, Evidence and Impact, McMaster University, Hamilton, ON, Canada
e-mail: cgoldsmi@sfu.ca

C. H. Goldsmith
Faculty of Health Sciences, Simon Fraser University, Burnaby, BC, Canada

C. H. Goldsmith
Department of Occupational Science and Occupational Therapy, Faculty of Medicine, The University of British Columbia, Vancouver, BC, Canada

A. Thoma et al. (eds.), *Evidence-Based Surgery*,
https://doi.org/10.1007/978-3-030-05120-4_10

expectations, standards, and concerns" [1]. A subcategory of QoL, Health-Related Quality of Life (HRQL), is a multi-dimensional concept that includes domains of physical, mental, emotional, and social functioning [2]. Since around 1990, there has been an increasing trend to evaluate the outcomes of health care interventions using sophisticated HRQL scales (instruments, measures) [3, 4]. The same has been espoused for surgical interventions [5].

With time, we see more and more articles in surgical literature where the results of novel interventions are reported with HRQL scales rather than the traditional physiologic outcomes. Decisions to adopt or reject novel interventions are based on such reports. It is therefore important for surgeons to be familiar with the appraisal of such articles that measure HRQL before they incorporate interventions into their practice and recommend them to their patients.

Clinical Scenario

At the last surgical oncology rounds, a surgical fellow asked his supervisor why she closed the temporary ileostomy of a 68-year-old male patient after rectal cancer resection at 12 days in contrast to her colleagues who tend to close it at 3 months after the creation of the temporary stoma. The senior surgeon responded that in her opinion, the early closure improved the patient's QoL and was associated with fewer complications. She challenged the surgical fellow to look at the literature evidence and let her know if she should change her practice.

Literature Search

The ideal article addressing this surgical question would be a meta-analysis of randomized controlled trials (RCTs) comparing early versus late closure of the temporary ileostomy after rectal cancer resection. In the absence of such a study design, one should look for a large single RCT that addresses the same question. Using the skills outlined by Banfield et al. in Chap. 5 and the Waltho et al. Users Guide to the Surgical Literature [6], we searched the literature after creating a clinical research question based on the PICOT format (see Chap. 4 on the clinical research question):

- **P**opulation: Patients who underwent rectal cancer resection.
- **I**ntervention: Early temporary ileostomy closure.
- **C**omparative Intervention: Late temporary ileostomy closure.
- **O**utcome: HRQL, complications.
- **T**ime Horizon: 12 months.

From the components of the PICOT format above, the research question is: "In patients who undergo rectal cancer resection, does early temporary ileostomy closure lead to improved HRQL and fewer complications after 12 months"?

Using a filtered database, COCHRANE, we performed a search using the key words rectal cancer, surgical resection, RCT and Health-Related Quality of Life. We did not identify any articles that were relevant to our research question. We, therefore, proceeded to use an unfiltered database, PubMed, and performed a search using the same keywords and identified 11 articles. After reviewing the titles and abstracts, only a few seemed relevant. Articles were eliminated if they did not address our question. This included studies that did not look at HRQL as the primary outcome, studies that were not comparing surgical procedures, as well as studies that were not designed as a randomized controlled trial (RCT).

One of the remaining articles by Park et al. (2018), which looked at the quality of life in a randomized trial of early closure of temporary ileostomy after rectal resection for cancer (the EASY trial), seems the most relevant [7]. In addition to the study being based on a prior RCT study, the interventions were surgical, HRQL was used as the main outcome and it was quite recent [8]. Therefore, this is the one appraised in the present chapter. The appraisal of an article with HRQL as an outcome follows the same format as other chapters in this book (see Box 1).

Box 1. Guidelines for the appraisal of an article in the surgical literature that purports to be reporting on Health-Related Quality of Life

A. **Are the results valid?**

Primary guides

i. Have the surgical investigators measured aspects of patients' lives that surgical patients consider important?
ii. Have important aspects of HRQL been omitted?
iii. Are the HRQL instruments chosen valid, reliable and responsive?

Secondary guides

i. Were HRQL assessments appropriately timed to evaluate the effects of the surgical intervention?
ii. If there were trade-offs between quantity and quality of life, did the investigators use an economic analysis?

B. **What were the results?**

i. What was the magnitude of the effect on HRQL?

C. **Will the results help me in caring for my patients in my practice?**

i. Will the information from this study help me inform my patients?

Primary Guides

Have the Investigators Measured Aspects of Patients' Lives that Patients Consider Important?

As mentioned in the introduction, traditionally, surgeons decide if an intervention is successful based on the restoration of some anatomical defect, reverting laboratory data to normal range, successful resection of malignant disease based on imaging or some laboratory marker or just simply by asking patients how they feel. The problem here is that we are not certain if we have considered all aspects of health that patients consider important. If one looks at the WHO definition of HRQL, one can see it is multi-dimensional [1]. One way to address this problem is to administer HRQL questionnaires to patients before and at various times after the surgical intervention and see if there has been a change.

The development of HRQL questionnaires is an arduous process that may take years to develop. Such an instrument requires the combined effort of methodologists, psychologists, biostatisticians, patients, and other experts. According to the U.S. Food and Drug Administration (FDA), there are four measurable outcomes; Patient-reported outcomes (PROs), clinician-reported outcomes, observer-reported outcomes, and performance outcomes [9].

Streiner et al. [10] provide an excellent source on how to design health-measurement scales. As mentioned above, it takes a lot of effort to develop a new HRQL scale. Surgeons do not have to develop such scales unless one does not exist for a particularly common condition. McDowell provides most of the known QOL questionnaires and surgeons are encouraged to use this helpful resource [11]. The nomenclature of these HRQL instruments has evolved to Patient-Reported Outcomes (PROs), a term that is used more frequently now [12]. Guidelines have been developed since 2010 for the development of a new patient-reported (PRO) instrument. For PROs or HRQL instruments to be valid, they need to have proper psychometric properties. By this, we mean that the PROs reliably attach a numerical value to patients' feelings so they can be assessed. If they are not constructed by the correct methods they are invalid and unreliable. Some commonly used valid HRQL instruments can be found in Table 10.1. Although generic PROs provide some important information about both health status and health utility, they are not always the most appropriate choice, if chosen as the sole HRQL instrument [13]. If the quality of life is

Table 10.1 Commonly used disease-specific and generic HRQL instruments

Instrument	Abbreviation	Condition
Michigan Hand Questionnaire	MHQ	Any condition of the upper extremities
European Organization for Research and Treatment of Cancer Quality-of-life Questionnaire Core 30	EORTC QLQ-C30	Cancer (more specific ones exist for different cancers)
Western Ontario and McMaster University Osteoarthritis Index	WOMAC	Osteoarthritis
Gastrointestinal Quality of Life Index	GIQLI	Gastrointestinal conditions
Short Form-36	SF-36	Generic: Health Status
EuroQol 5-Dimension	EQ-5D	Generic: Health Utility
Health Utility Index	HUI	Generic: Health Utility

greatly affected by a specific disease, such as in cancer patients, a disease-specific instrument should be used [13].

In appraising the Park et al. article, we need to assess whether the authors have measured aspects of patients' lives that the patients would consider important [7]. A temporary iliostomy may reduce the risk of pelvic sepsis after anastomotic dehiscence following rectal cancer resection. An iliostomy, however, carries with it certain risks such skin irritation, parastomal infection, leakage outside the appliance bag, parastomal hernia, stomal stenosis, stoma prolapse, and high-volume output that can lead to acute kidney injury. Certainly, all of the above can affect the quality of life of a patient who undergoes this procedure. The theoretical advantage of late closure after the procedure is the potential to ensure healing of the rectal colon anastomosis, avoiding dehiscence and pelvic sepsis, and allowing adjuvant chemotherapy to be undertaken with minimal delay. The disadvantages, on the other hand, are the potential complications related to the ileostomy site mentioned above. Measuring the HRQL in a comparative intervention, which in this case is the timing of the closure of the ileostomy, seems appropriate.

In terms of the HRQL assessment itself, Park and colleagues administered the Short Form Health Survey (SF-36) and two EORTC questionnaires, QLQ-C30 and QLQ-CR29. The SF-36 is a generic questionnaire and both the EORTC questionnaires are ones that relate directly to cancer and colorectal cancer patients.

As mentioned, conditions such as cancer can greatly impact one's quality of life and would require a disease-specific HRQL instrument. The investigators took this into account, ensuring they chose the correct HRQL measures to assess health status. However, they do not measure health utility, an important component of HRQL, with instruments such as the EQ-5D or the HUI-3. A utility instrument is useful since we can calculate quality-adjusted life years (QALYs), an important component of cost-effectiveness analysis.

Although there are only a select few instruments highlighted here, one should review what the objectives of the study are, the condition they are planning to focus on and whether there are any disease-specific measures for HRQL before moving forward.

Have Important Aspects of HRQL Been Omitted?

Depending on the condition assessed, it is important that clinical investigators remain unbiased in assessing HRQL. In other words, their assessment should be comprehensive. Inclusion of some HRQL issues and exclusion of others will bias the final results. A generic HRQL may not capture the specific differences of ileostomy reversal at early versus late time periods. On the other hand, a cancer-specific or preferably "ileostomy related PRO", if one exists should be able to discriminate between early and late reversal periods. It is for these reasons that in surgical trials we should administer three types of questionnaires, as suggested by Guyatt et al., to ensure that we are taking into account all aspects of the patients' health and quality of life [14]. As mentioned, Park and colleagues did not include a utility measure. They included only the generic (SF-36) and subscales (QLQ-C30, QLQ-CR29) of a condition-specific scale the EORTC. Investigators did, however, assess all domains of the SF-36 and QLQ-C30/CR29, ensuring a comprehensive assessment using the instruments they did include.

Death is always a possibility with any surgical procedure. Although death is rare in the closure of an ileostomy, it is important to assess if there is difference in the mortality rate among the comparative interventions. Park et al. reported one death in each group and in each case, it was attributed to cancer rather than the ileostomy closure timing [7]. If patients were of an employable age, reporting on their ability to return to work would be an important issue for the patients. If carrying an ileostomy bag for a prolonged period of time interfered with a patient's job then this would also be an important issue to consider.

Are the HRQL Instruments Chosen Valid, Reliable and Responsive?

For an HRQL instrument to be chosen, it must meet three important preconditions; validity, reliability, and responsiveness to change. This ensures that it is measuring HRQL (the outcome) in a way that provides consistent, valid results. In short, the validity of an instrument describes to what degree it measures what it was developed to measure.

Reliability is assessed by conducting tests of repeatability or reproducibility of the measure under consideration. It can be classified as either having high interobserver (between different observers) reliability, high intra-observer (within the same observers) reliability, or both. These measures provide information about whether the measure being used has a tendency to change depending on who is conducting the test or when it is being conducted. Ideally, we are after the least variable inter- and intra-observer scores. This would mean that regardless of assessor and time period, the measure under consideration is providing reliable information on which to base conclusions.

Test–retest reliability is measured by comparing scores from the same individual and then calculating a correlation between the different results. Park et al. did not assess test–retest reliability. This is important because it illustrates whether results are truly reliable based on whether the calculated correlation is strong. It is important to keep in mind that a reliable test is not always a valid one, but a valid test is always reliable so it is necessary to evaluate both these qualities of an assessment tool.

Last, responsiveness has two major aspects: internal and external. Internal responsiveness entails the ability of a measure to capture the change in a participant's outcome over a prespecified timeframe. In the case of Park et al., that would be 12 months. External responsiveness reflects the extent to which change in a measure relates to a corresponding change in a reference measure of clinical or health status [15, 16]. Responsiveness, therefore, tells us whether or not an assessment tool will be able to detect a change in the outcome (HRQL) over time (12 months).

Park and colleagues use the SF-36, which has validity and reliability that has been supported in clinical research [17, 18]. The responsiveness of the SF-36 has also been documented in relation to various common clinical conditions [19]. The other measures used by the investigators, the EORTC QLQ-C30 [20] and QLQ-CR29 [21], also have evidence of being valid and reliable in colorectal cancer patients. We conclude that the measures used for the measurement of HRQL by Park et al. meet the guidelines of validity, reliability, and responsiveness to change.

Secondary Guides

Were HRQL Assessments Appropriately Timed to Evaluate the Effects of the Surgical Intervention?

Although patients were enrolled and randomized after rectal resection but before ileostomy reversal, there was no preoperative assessment, which is not ideal. If there is no baseline information participants to include in the model, it is difficult to determine the actual overall impact of either intervention other than the information ascertained from comparing them.

Park et al. administered both questionnaires at the 3, 6, and 12-months post treatment. The timing of these assessments is critical since if you perform them too soon, or too close together, you may not measure a meaningful change, if any. If you measure the HRQL for example, at 1 week after the surgery, the patients may still be recovering from the actual surgery and no meaningful information will be obtained. Additionally, if the follow-up time is not long enough, there may not be the opportunity to observe any complications posttreatment.

The response shift, which is the patients' adaptation to their illness with time, may alter the HRQL questionnaire scores. As the Park et al. study was a randomized controlled trial, we would not; however, expect that this would be an issue, as the response shift should apply to both groups.

If There Were Trade-Offs Between Quantity and Quality of Life, Did the Investigators Perform a Economic Analysis?

The quantity versus quality of life is an important consideration because as mentioned earlier, the focus of surgical interventions in the past was prolonging life. Over the last decades, it has begun to become clear that more years or months of life does not necessarily translate to a "good" few years or months. Some patients may be willing to forgo longevity if this is associated with pain.

An economic evaluation may also be important from the perspective of the patient, third-party payers, and society. To do so, one needs to calculate the costs and effectiveness of the two comparative approaches and calculate an incremental cost-utility ratio (ICUR). This is explained in Chap. 23 of this book.

Park et al. did not conduct an economic analysis. In their case, they could have conducted a cost-effectiveness analysis using quality-adjusted life years (QALY) as an outcome to measure the quality of life for these rectal cancer patients and the ilesotomy closure timing. Specifically, QALYs represent the gains from reduced mortality and morbidity in a single measure [15]. To do so, they would have needed to choose the most appropriate health utility measure in addition to the ones they used to measure HRQL (SF-36, EORTC QLQ-C30, and QLQ-CR29).

A possibility could have been the use of the EQ-5D-5L. This is a utility measure with 25 items to assess general health status and health-related quality of life. From this instrument, one can calculate QALYs. There are five dimensions including; mobility, self-care, usual activities, pain/discomfort, and anxiety/depression. A health utility of 1.00 represents best possible health and a health utility of 0 or negative represents death or health worse than death [22]. There are utility scales of course such as the HUI, which is more powerful scale that can discriminate between close to million different health states [23].

What Were the Results?

What Was the Magnitude of the Effect on HRQL?

Investigators report the similarities or differences between scores obtained from the questionnaires, rather than whether one treatment over the other resulted in better outcomes. However, these similarities or differences need to be reported and interpreted in a meaningful way, so conclusions about HRQL of the patients following the treatments under evaluation can be made.

Park et al. found that SF-36 dimension scores were similar between the treatment groups, with no differences in the physical and mental component scores. They did find some significant differences in various other dimension scores including; role physical (3 months), bodily pain (12 months), and mental health (12 months). At 12 months, 52–85% of the patients scored higher than the late closure group, with physical functioning scoring the highest among the dimensions (Table 10.2). In terms of the other measures, EORTC QLQ-C30 and QLQ-CR29, scores were comparable between early and late closure groups. Emotional functioning was lower in the early closure group at 3 and 6 months, but similar to the late closure group at 12 months. No statistically significant differences were seen at 12 months in the dimensions of the QLQ-CR29 questionnaire (Table 10.4). Significant results are indicated in bold.

The difference in medians observed in relation to the MCIDs for these dimension scores fall in the 5–10-point interval making them clinically important even though not statistically important.

The original RCT (the EASY trial) outlines the sample size calculation (60 per group) and stated 80% power to detect a 62.5% reduction in annual mean number of complications [8]. Park et al. concluded that no significant differences were observed in HRQL within 12 months after

Table 10.2 SF-36® scores at 3, 6, and 12 months after rectal resection

Dimensions	3 months		6 months		12 months	
	Median (*Q*1–*Q*3)	*p*	Median (*Q*1–*Q*3)	*p*	Median (*Q*1–*Q*3)	*p*
Physical Functioning						
Early	90 (75–95)	0.646	90 (81.7-100)	0.630	95 (70–100)	0.322
Late	90 (80–95)		90 (80-95)		95 (90–100)	
Role Physical						
Early	75 (50–96.9)	**0.025**	81.3 (50–100)	0.140	81.3 (56.3–100)	0.718
Late	62.5 (43.8–75)		75 (50–93.8)		87.5 (75–100)	
Bodily Pain						
Early	80 (52–100)	0.858	74 (62–100)	0.264	79 (51–100)	**0.035**
Late	74 (62–100)		84 (63–100)		100 (74–100)	
General Health						
Early	71.6 (52–88.5)	0.139	77 (56–87)	0.820	74.5 (45–92)	0.279
Late	77 (67–87)		77 (65–87)		82 (72–87)	
Vitality						
Early	62.5 (43.8–81.3)	0.441	68.8 (50–81.3)	0.796	68.8 (50–81.3)	0.196
Late	68.8 (56.3–81.3)		68.8 (56.3–81.3)		75 (62.5–87.5)	
Social Functioning						
Early	75 (62.5–100)	0.468	87.5 (66.7–100)	0.976	87.5 (62.5–100)	0.415
Late	87.5 (75–100)		87.5 (75–100)		100 (75–100)	
Role Emotional						
Early	83.3 (58.3–100)	0.345	87.5 (66.7–100)	0.923	95.8 (66.7–100)	0.697
Late	83.3 (75–100)		83.3 (75–100)		95.8 (75–100)	
Mental Health						
Early	80 (55–90)	0.217	80 (60–90)	0.291	80 (60–90)	**0.020**
Late	85 (65–90)		85 (70–95)		85 (75–95)	
Mental Component Score						
Early	52.5 (40.7–58.6)	0.588	54.4 (42.8–58.6)	0.939	54.1 (42.6–58.5)	0.105
Late	53 (44.8–57.8)		54.6 (46.9–57.5)		56.6 (52.9–59.2)	
Physical Component Score						
Early	51.8 (40.9–58.2)	0.823	53.3 (43.3–57.1)	0.900	54.1 (44.5–59)	0.281
Late	51.2 (46.9–54.8)		52.2 (45.8–57.9)		56.8 (51–59.4)	

rectal resection for cancer when early and late closure of temporary ileostomy was compared. This was based on 5–10-point difference as a little change and 10–20-point difference as a moderate change [7]. We can conclude that the results are valid as investigators had an adequate sample size.

The values presented in these tables seem to be quite high, with many intervals for the dimension scores including a 100 (perfect state). Park et al. state that dimension scores were calculated based on guidelines given by the developers of these measures, and these results suggest the distributions of data are skewed.

The lack of statistically significant findings may also be due to the fact that the authors included many dimension scores in the model rather than choosing categories (such as mental component score and physical component score). These are a few of the many things to consider when using questionnaires like these ones.

For those of you who are statistically inclined, you will notice a few things about Tables 10.2, 10.3 and 10.4. First, the original

Table 10.3 EORTC QLQ-C30 scores at 3, 6, and 12 months after rectal resection

Dimensions	3 months		6 months		12 months	
	Median (*Q*1–*Q*3)	*p*	Median (*Q*1–*Q*3)	*p*	Median (*Q*1–*Q*3)	*p*
Global Quality of Life Early Late	 75 (50–83.3) 66.7 (58.3–83.3)	 0.941	 66.7 (50–83.3) 66.7 (66.7–83.3)	 0.961	 83.3 (50–91.7) 83.3 (66.7–91.7)	 0.889
Physical Functioning Early Late	 93.3 (73.3–100) 93.3 (73.3–100)	 0.634	 93.3 (80–100) 93.3 (80–100)	 0.433	 93.3 (73.3–100) 100 (80–100)	 0.137
Role Functioning Early Late	 83.3 (66.7–100) 66.7 (50–100)	 **0.066**	 100 (66.7–100) 83.3 (66.7–100)	 0.503	 100 (66.7–100) 100 (66.7–100)	 0.793
Emotional Functioning Early Late	 83.3 (66.7–100) 91.7 (83.3–100)	 **0.023**	 83.3 (66.7–100) 91.7 (75–100)	 **0.031**	 91.7 (66.7–100) 91.7 (83.3–100)	 0.409
Cognitive Functioning Early Late	 100 (83.3–100) 100 (83.3–100)	 0.447	 83.3 (83.3–100) 100 (83.3–100)	 0.131	 100 (66.7–100) 100 (83.3–100)	 0.652
Social Functioning Early Late	 83.3 (66.7–100) 83.3 (66.7–100)	 0.583	 83.3 (66.7–100) 83.3 (66.7–100)	 0.882	 83.3 (66.7–100) 100 (66.7–100)	 0.142

Table 10.4 EORTC QLQ-CR29 scores for functional scales at 3, 6, and 12 months after rectal resection

Dimensions	3 months		6 months		12 months	
	Median (*Q*1–*Q*3)	*p*	Median (*Q*1–*Q*3)	*p*	Median (*Q*1–*Q*3)	*p*
Urinary Frequency Early Late	 16.7 (0–33.3) 16.7 (0–50)	 0.323	 16.7 (0–50) 16.7 (8.3–41.7)	 0.353	 16.7 (0–33.3) 33.3 (0–50)	 0.268
Stool Frequency Early Late	 33.3 (16.7–50) 0 (0–16.7)	 **<0.001**	 33.3 (16.7–50) 16.7 (0–66.7)	 0.068	 33.3 (16.7–50) 33.3 (16.7–50)	 0.611
Body Image Early Late	 88.9 (66.7–100) 77.8 (66.7–100)	 0.715	 88.9 (77.8–100) 88.9 (66.7–100)	 0.364	 94.4 (77.8–100) 100 (88.9–100)	 0.502

tables presented by the authors use the abbreviation of "i.q.r." rather than "IQR" and the values presented were not the IQR. An IQR is a single number, which represents the ***difference*** between the lower (Q_1) and upper (Q_3) quartiles. Therefore, Park et al. presented the dimension scores varying from the lower quartile to the upper quartile. This was changed in Tables 10.2, 10.3, and 10.4 to indicate this.

Second, the authors interchanged mean and median values in their results section and then presented median values for their tables. This causes some confusion as to whether the authors examined the differences in dimension scores based on the median values reported, as mean values were not reported. This needs to be clarified and stated explicitly for the reader. In the field of colorectal cancer patients and health-related quality of life, mean values for measures such as the SF-36 and EORTC QLQ-C30 are often reported, rather than the median. However, as authors reported median and wanted to show the IQR, we can assume that there were outliers as reporting these statistics is common when outliers are present in the data.

As previously mentioned, patient-reported outcomes (PROs) have become increasingly utilized in clinical research. The questionnaires used in Park et al. (SF-36, EORTC QLQ-C30, and EORTC QLQ-CR29) are a great way to measure PROs. Interpreting the scores of these questionnaires properly is immensely important, as this is the information that is used to base the decision of whether a novel treatment will be used over the current gold-standard treatment. A way to interpret scores or responses is by using a minimal clinical important difference (MCID) that has been supported in previous literature for the surveys in question. The MCID has been defined as "the smallest difference in score in the domain of interest in which patients perceive as beneficial" [24].

Clinicians use the MCID to define the level of change an intervention creates to determine whether that change is a clinically important change in the population [24]. Park et al. reported they used the suggestion from a Swedish study that a difference of 5–10 points be considered a "little change" and a difference of 10–20 points a "moderate change" [7]. These standards were chosen as the study took place in Sweden and Denmark. When they compared their SF-36® scores with Swedish reference data, a general improvement was seen during the 12-month follow-up interval.

Will the Results Help Me in Caring for My Patients?

Will the Information from This Study Help Me Inform My Patients?

Surgeons know from their experience that patients who undergo similar surgical interventions can respond differently. To determine whether our patients will be helped by the results of the Park et al. study we would like to know if the patients in the Park et al. study are similar to our patient. We, therefore, look at the table that describes the demographic characteristics of their study group. We look to see if the Park et al. study patients were similar in age to our patient and any other prognostic factors. Our patient is 68 years in age and the mean patient age in the Park et al. study was 67 years, which is similar to ours. If we believe that their patient group (Scandinavian) is different from ours (North American), we may be skeptical of the generalizability of their findings. If we agree that there are no major differences in these two populations, we should accept their findings. As we do not have any evidence of major differences, we should accept their findings.

Resolution of the Scenario

The results from the Park et al. [7] study indicate that there is no difference in the HRQL of patients whether they undergo early or late closure of the ileostomy, even though the early closure was associated with fewer complications. This clinical advantage had no effect on the patients' HRQL. The surgical fellow informs the senior surgeon that in fact what she doing is just fine!

References

1. World Health Organization. WHOQOL: Measuring Quality of Life. [Internet]. Geneva; 2018 [cited 2018 Jan 10]. Available from: http://www.who.int/healthinfo/survey/whoqol-qualityoflife/en/.
2. Office of Disease Prevention and Health Promotion. Health-Related Quality of Life and Well-Being. [Internet]. Washington, DC; 2010 [cited 2018 Jan 10]. Available from: https://www.healthypeople.gov/2020/about/foundation-health-measures/Health-Related-Quality-of-Life-and-Well-Being.
3. Kirshner B, Guyatt G. A methodological framework for assessing health indices. J Chronic Dis. 1985;38:27–36.
4. Wood-Dauphinee S. Quality of life assessment: recent trends in surgery. Can J Surg. 1996;39: 368–72.
5. Wood-Dauphinee S. Assessing quality of life in clinical research: from where have we come and where are we going? J Clin Epidemiol. 1999;52: 355–63.
6. Waltho D, Kaur MN, Haynes RB, Farrokhyar F, Thoma A. Users' guide to the surgical literature: hot to perform a high-quality literature search. Can J Surg. 2015;58(5):349–58.
7. Park AK, Danielsen E, Angenete D, Bock AC, Marinez E, Haglind JE, et al. Quality of life in a randomized trial of early closure of temporary ileostomy after rectal resection for cancer (EASY trial). Wiley Online Libr. 2018;105:244–51.
8. Danielsen AK, Park J, Jansen JE, Bock D, Skullman S, Wedin A, et al. Early closure of a temporary ileostomy in patients with rectal cancer: a Multicenter randomized controlled trial. Ann Surg. 2017;265 (2):284–90.
9. US Food and Drug Administration. Clinical Outcome Assessment Qualification Program. [Internet]. Silver Spring, Maryland; 2018 [cited 2018 Jan 10]. Available from: https://www.fda.gov/Drugs/DevelopmentApprovalProcess/DrugDevelopmentToolsQualificationProgram/ucm284077.html.
10. Streiner DL, Norman RG, Cairney J. Health measurement scales: a practical guide to their development and use. 5th ed. Oxford: Oxford University Press; 2014.
11. McDowell I. Measuring health: a guide to rating scales and questionnaires. 3rd ed. Oxford: Oxford University Press; 2006.
12. Deshpande PR, Rajan S, Sudeepthi Nazir CPA. Patient-reported outcomes: a new era in clinical research. Perspect Clin Res. 2011;2(4):137–44.
13. Litwin MS. Health-related quality of life. In: Penson DF, Wei JT, editors. Chapter 13: Clinical research for surgeons. Totowa, NJ: Humma Press; 1998.
14. Guyatt GH, Naylor CD, Juniper E. Users' guides to the medical literature XII. How to use articles about health-related quality of life. JAMA. 1997; 277: 1232–7.
15. Thoma A, Cornacchi SD, Lovrics PJ, Goldsmith CH. Users' guide to the surgical literature: how to assess an article on health-related quality of life. Can J Surg. 2008;51(3):215–24.
16. Husted JA, Cook RJ, Farewell VT, Gladman DD. Methods for assessing responsiveness: a critical review and recommendations. J Clin Epidemiol. 2000;53:459–68.
17. Stansfeld SA, Roberts R, Foot SP. Assessing the validity of the SF-36 general health survey. Qual Life Res. 1997;6(3):217–24.
18. Jenkinson C, Wright L, Coulter A. Criterion validity and reliability of the SF-36 in a population sample. Qual Life Res. 1994;3:7–12.
19. Garratt AM, Ruta DA, Abdalla MI, Russell IT. SF 36 health survey questionnaire: II. Responsiveness to changes in health status in four common clinical conditions. Qual Health Care. 1994;3(4):186–92.
20. Ganesh V, Agarwal A, Popovic M, Bottomley A, McDonald R, Vuong S, et al. Comparison of the FACT-C, EORTC QLQ-CR38, and QLQ-CR29 quality of life questionnaires for patients with colorectal cancer: a literature review. Support Care Cancer. 2016;24(8):3661–8.
21. EORTC. EORTC QLQ-C30. [Internet]. Brussels; 2017 [cited 2018 Jan 5]. Available from: http://groups.eortc.be/qol/eortc-qlq-c30.
22. EuroQoL Group. EQ-5D-5L. [Internet]. Rotterdam; 2009 [cited 2018 Jan 5]. Available from: https://euroqol.org/eq-5d-instruments/eq-5d-5l-about/.
23. Horsman J, Furlong W, Feeny D, Torrance G. The health utilities index (HUI): concepts, measurement properties and applications. Health Qual Life Outcomes. 2003;1(54):1–13.
24. Jaeschke R, Singer J, Guyatt GH. Measurement of health status: ascertaining the minimal clinically important difference. Control Clin Trials. 1989;10: 407–15.

Randomized Controlled Trial Comparing Surgical Interventions

11

Max Solow, Raman Mundi, Vickas Khanna and Mohit Bhandari

Introduction

Despite years of training and schooling, clinicians routinely encounter difficult clinical scenarios that go beyond the scope of their everyday practice. To answer such questions, physicians often rely on high quality, research evidence—or in other terms, evidence-based practice. With high-quality research being integral to the practice of evidence-based medicine, it is to no surprise that the National Institutes of Health, in the United States, invests nearly $37.7 billion annually toward funding medical research projects [1].

Historically, physicians made therapeutic decisions based on anecdotal reports and personal experience. More recently, guidelines have been endorsed to eliminate variability among patient care and to highlight the importance of evidence from clinical research [2, 3]. These guidelines typically emphasize randomized controlled trials (RCTs) as the optimal study design for eliminating bias and capturing the truest estimates of treatment effect. Yet, not all RCTs are equal in terms of validity. Simply stating that a study was randomized does not ensure it is a high-quality study. The purpose of this chapter is to introduce strategies for clinicians to use while evaluating the evidence, with a particular focus on RCTs comparing surgical interventions. Arguably, conducting an RCT in a surgical setting poses some unique challenges, such as with blinding and the surgical learning curve that if not properly accounted for can lead to potential confounders. We will illustrate how physicians may apply these strategies and identify potential confounders with the help of a clinical scenario.

Scenario

A healthy 74-year-old woman comes into your clinic complaining of pain and a palpable mass on the lateral aspect of her right thigh. A year prior to her presentation, she had undergone open reduction and internal fixation with a sliding hip screw for a femoral neck fracture of her right femur due to a fall. On the anteroposterior radiograph, nonunion, deformed femoral neck, and implant migration are appreciated. You conclude that her implant has failed and she would likely benefit from a revision surgery. You discuss with her the nature of her problem, as well as the risks and benefits of further surgery. Your patient agrees to the procedure but asks you

M. Solow
St. George's University School of Medicine, St. George's, West Indies, Grenada

R. Mundi · V. Khanna · M. Bhandari (✉)
Department of Surgery, Division of Orthopaedic Surgery, McMaster University, Hamilton, ON, Canada
e-mail: bhandam@mcmaster.ca

R. Mundi
e-mail: Raman.mundi@medportal.ca

A. Thoma et al. (eds.), *Evidence-Based Surgery*,
https://doi.org/10.1007/978-3-030-05120-4_11

"If I had my initial fracture fixed with a different implant, would it still have failed?" Unsure initially of how to answer this question, you decide to review the literature and assure her that at her next clinical appointment, you will provide her with the best possible answer.

Literature Search

You begin your literature search by creating a well-defined research question that encompasses several aspects of the clinical scenario. Using the PICO(T) format [4], which incorporates information about the patient population (P), the intervention (I), comparative interventions (C), the outcome (O), and time period (T), you generate the following research question: In femoral neck fracture patients, does fixation with a sliding hip screw lead to higher revision rates compared with other methods of fixation? Using Medline, the National Library of Medicine's PubMed database [5], you enter "femoral neck fracture" AND "reoperation" in the search field. You limit your search to English articles, published in the last 3 years, clinical trials, and human subjects. The search yields five articles [6–10]. Three of the articles do not compare fixation methods [7, 8, 10] and one article compares hemiarthroplasty to internal fixation [6]. The article, "Fracture fixation in the operative management of hip fractures (FAITH): an international, multicentre randomized controlled trial" compares two methods of femoral neck fracture fixation and seems to address your clinical question.

Summary of the Appraised Article

The FAITH trial [9] was conducted to compare the sliding hip screw to cancellous screw fixation for patients with low-energy femoral neck fractures. The study was an international, multicentre, and randomized controlled trial, which included 1108 patients across 81 clinical centers from 8 countries. Following randomization, 557 patients were assigned to receive a sliding hip screw and 551 patients to receive cancellous screws. The primary outcome of this study was the need for reoperation within 24 months. Other important outcomes included mortality, fracture healing, complications, and health-related quality of life scores. The mean length of follow-up was 633 days (standard deviation [SD] 208 days).

Reoperations within 24 months, mortality, fracture healing, implant failures, nonunions, infections, medically related adverse advents, and health-related quality of life scores did not differ in either treatment arm. However, more cases of avascular necrosis were observed in the sliding hip screw group than in the cancellous screws group (50 patients [9%] vs. 28 patients [5%]; HR 1.91, 1.06–3.44; $p = 0.0319$). Likewise, prespecified subgroup analyses showed that sliding hip screws are favored in patients with displaced fractures, fractures at the base of the femoral neck, and in patients who currently smoke.

Evaluating a Randomized Controlled Trial

When reading a research article, it is always important to critique whether or not the study was carried out in a manner that would produce reliable results. Notably, three questions should be asked: Are the results valid? What are the results? And are the results applicable to my practice (see Box 1) [11]?

Box 1. Important points to consider when evaluating a surgical RCT

Are the results valid?

- Was the learning curve taken into consideration?
- How was randomization and allocation concealment performed?
- Who was blinded?
- Were the patient groups similar to one another?
- How were patients' data analyzed?

- Were treatments standardized and all patients accounted for?

What are the results?

- What impact did the treatment have?
- How precise were the results?

Are the results applicable to my practice?

- Do the results apply to my patient population?
- How clinically relevant are the results?
- How do these results impact me?

This list was modified from [11].

Are the Results Valid?

Learning Curve and Expertise-Based Randomized Controlled Trials

Compared with drug trials, surgical RCTs require special considerations. To begin with, a study comparing a "novel" intervention may need to factor in the surgical learning curve. A learning curve refers to the fact that a surgeon's proficiency, efficiency, and expectant outcomes of a procedure will improve with experience [12, 13]. Simply speaking, the more cases a surgeon has completed, the better they will become with the technical aspects of the procedure. Likewise, as experience increases, surgeons will have a better understanding of the necessary adjunctive medications, the appropriate patient selection, and the necessary pre- and postoperative care regimens to optimize outcomes. If an RCT does not consider (or mention) a learning curve, the results may be biased in favor of the traditional, or more common, intervention. One solution to this challenge is the "expertise based RCT", in which study patients are randomized directly to a surgeon, rather than the intervention. The surgeon, in turn, only delivers the intervention in which they are an expert [14]. Yet, these too are not without fault as determining expertise, achieving adequate recruitment, and the context-specific nature of such studies prove challenging [15, 16].

In the FAITH trial [9], surgeons had done at least 25 hip fracture fixation procedures during their career, with at least 5 fracture fixation procedures having been completed in the year prior to participation. With this in mind, we can assume that participating surgeons had sufficient expertise in performing either intervention.

Patient Randomization and Allocation Concealment

Randomization is a technique that assigns patients to either the treatment or control arm of the study in a manner that is entirely by chance and without taking into consideration patient or researcher preference [17]. The randomization schedule can often be created by computer-generated sequences. The purpose of randomization is to produce groups that are similar to one another in terms of both known and unknown characteristics that may influence the study outcome. Without randomization, researcher, patient, and physician bias may influence experimental outcomes and alter study results.

Similarly, allocation concealment aims to limit selection bias by concealing which treatment arm each prospective study patient will be assigned to [17]. In essence, it is a method to protect the integrity of the randomization sequence. An example of allocation concealment is the use of a central call-in center or computer program, which will reveal the treatment arm a patient has been randomized to only after enrolment. As such, physicians cannot predict which treatment the patient will receive prior to enrolment and randomization. Despite proper randomization, failure to adequately control allocation concealment may introduce bias and influence study results. For example, if investigators opened unsealed assignment envelopes and channeled participants with a better prognosis to the experimental group, this would lead to larger treatment effects [18].

In the FAITH trial [9], randomization and allocation concealment were performed with a centralised computer system, which provides a methodologically robust approach for randomization and allocation concealment.

Were Patients, Surgeons, and Researchers Aware of Group Assignment (Blinding)?

Within RCTs, blinding refers to the precautions taken to prevent the patient, surgeon, or researchers from knowing a participant's group assignment [19]. The importance of blinding is that it minimizes bias in intervention implementation, outcomes assessment, results analysis, and patient dropout. Take for example the placebo effect, a scenario where a patient's belief about their treatment influences their outcomes [20]. In a meta-analysis comparing osteoarthritis patients receiving a placebo to an untreated control group, patients in the placebo group experienced significantly more pain and stiffness relief than the control group [21]. If patients are aware of their group allocation they may alter their answers on quality assessments and subconsciously put forth more of an effort in their rehabilitation, exaggerating the experimental treatment effect. Similarly, surgeons may favor one intervention over another and may unintentionally be more precise during its implementation, ultimately overestimating study results [22, 23]. Unfortunately, the very nature of surgery makes it nearly impossible for surgeons to remain blinded during intervention implementation. Finally, the research personnel in charge of assessing the outcomes, if not blinded, may alter study results. If, for example, the researchers rounded outcomes from the treatment arm of the study upwards compared to the control group, or if preferential treatment were given to either group during rehabilitation or assessment, study results could be distorted [24, 25].

In the FAITH trial [9], both the surgeons and the patients were not blinded, while the data analysts were. Because both treatment strategies were similar from a patient experience perspective, unblinded patients likely would not have biased the study results. Furthermore, the primary outcome of reoperation was unlikely to be substantially altered by the lack of blinding of patients. Unfortunately, as there is no real solution to surgeon blinding, it is difficult to comment on whether or not differential care was provided to either care group. However, as this study was large and incorporated multiple surgeons from various countries, it may be fair to assume that any differences during procedure implementation would have been balanced between the two groups.

Were the Patients in Each Group Similar?

At the onset of the trial, it is imperative that the experimental and control groups be relatively homogenous. In other words, the more alike the two groups are to one another prior to trial commencement the less likely other factors can influence study results and the easier it will be to detect the true effects of the therapeutic intervention. Most commonly, studies present patient baseline demographic information and known prognostic variables—often presented in a table. In the FAITH trial [9], patients were included if they were 50 years or older and sustained a low-energy femoral neck fracture that required operative fixation and baseline patient characteristics were presented (Table 11.1).

Prior to randomization, it is important to consider whether or not any other variables exist that could influence treatment responsiveness. Stratification, another measure to ensure group balance, divides study participants into homogenous subgroups from which they are then randomized into the different arms of the trial [26]. Consider a study comparing two different treatment modalities for first-time traumatic anterior shoulder dislocations. Since patient age correlates very strongly with the rate of repeated dislocation, it would be critical to stratify patients in each trial group based on age [27]. Otherwise, the group with a larger proportion of younger patients may underestimate the treatment effect. Likewise, it is important to consider the variability among individual surgeons and clinical sites as these can influence outcomes [28]. In the FAITH trial [9], patients were stratified by clinical site, however, the authors did not report whether this had an impact on outcomes.

Table 11.1 Patient baseline characteristics [9]

		SHS	CS
Age	(Years)	72.2 (12.0)	72.0 (12.3)
Sex	Male	212/535 (40%)	210/535 (39%)
	Female	323/535 (60%)	325/535 (61%)
Ethnic origin	Native	1/533 (<1%)	3/535 (1%)
	South Asian	65/533 (12%)	65/535 (12%)
	East Asian	6/533 (1%)	4/535 (1%)
	Black	22/533 (4%)	18/535 (3%)
	Hispanic	3/533 (1%)	1/535 (<1%)
	White	436/533 (82%)	444/535 (83%)
Smoking history	Never smoked	268/533 (50%)	276/532 (52%)
	Current smoker	101/533 (19%)	100/532 (19%)
	Former smoker	164/533 (31%)	156/532 (29%)
Current drugs	None	170/535 (32%)	179/534 (34%)
	NSAIDS	86/535 (16%)	64/534 (12%)
	General cardiac	167/535 (31%)	167/534 (31%)
	Opioid analgesics	43/535 (8%)	56/534 (10%)
	Pulmonary drugs	58/535 (11%)	69/534 (13%)
	Anti-hypertension drugs	244/535 (46%)	252/534 (47%)
	Osteoporosis drugs	67/535 (13%)	73/534 (14%)
BMI	Underweight (BMI 18.5)	37/530 (7%)	33/528 (6%)
	Normal weight (18.5–24.9)	276/530 (52%)	300/528 (57%)
	Overweight (25–29.9)	159/530 (30%)	148/528 (28%)
	Obese (30–39.9)	58/530 (11%)	47/528 (9%)
Fractured hip	Left	280/535 (52%)	281/535 (53%)
	Right	255/535 (48%)	254/535 (47%)
Mechanism of injury	Fall	515/533 (97%)	521/534 (98%)
	Spontaneous	13/533 (2%)	6/534 (1%)
	Other low-energy trauma	5/533 (1%)	7/534 (1%)
History of surgery to affected hip	Yes	3/535 (1%)	0/535 (0%)
	No	532/535 (99%)	535/535 (100%)
Additional injuries	Yes	67/535 (13%)	72/535 (13%)
	No	468/535 (87%)	463/535 (87%)

SHS = sliding hip screw; CS = cancellous screws; NSAIDS = non-steroidal anti-inflammatory drugs; BMI = body-mass index

Intention-to-Treat Analysis

Once the trial has begun, it is important to consider how the analysis was carried out. Consider the hypothetical example of an RCT comparing the rates of surgical site infection in 200 patients who underwent total knee arthroplasty. In this study, 100 patients are assigned to receive intraoperative local vancomycin powder to their wound plus preoperative ancef (experimental group), while the remaining 100 only receive the preoperative ancef for prophylaxis (control group). The surgeon then decides that 10 patients

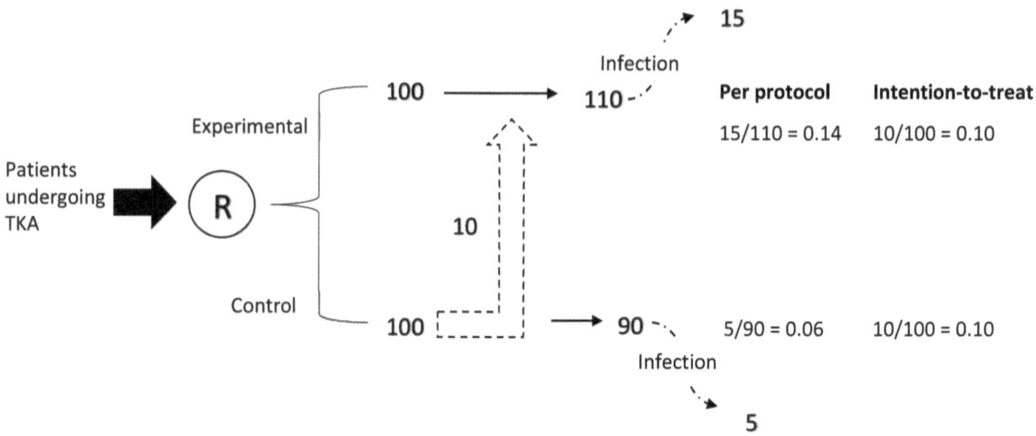

Fig. 11.1 Bias introduced when using a per-protocol analysis versus an intention-to-treat analysis. Per-protocol analysis includes all those patients who received vancomycin, irrespective of their initial assignment. With this analysis, the event rate in the experimental group is more than double that of the control group. The intention-to-treat analysis analyzes patients in their original groups irrespective of the treatment they actually received. Under this model, we see that the event rates are equal. R = randomization; TKA = total knee arthroplasty

in the ancef-only group would benefit from the local vancomycin powder due to intraoperative complications. If 10 of the 100 patients in the initial experimental group develop an infection, plus 5 of the 10 patients that switched group's perioperatively go on to develop an infection, then the event rate would be 14%; however, the rate in the control group would be 6% (Fig. 11.1). These values represent a spurious reduction in infection rates for the control group. Intention-to-treat analysis eliminates this potential bias by analyzing patients in an RCT according to the treatment arm they were originally assigned to, irrespective of the treatment they actually received [29, 30]. In our example, if patients were analyzed with an intention-to-treat model the event rates would be 10/100 for both groups. Incorporating this method of analysis into a study eliminates any bias that may arise from participant attrition or crossover. In the FAITH trial [9], the authors state that an intention-to-treat analysis was employed.

Treatment Standardization

Standardization of interventions is important in surgical trials to ensure treatment effects are not biased due to differential care between groups outside of the main surgical intervention (i.e., preoperative antibiotics, perioperative care, postoperative thromboprophylaxis, postoperative weight-bearing status, and rehabilitation). For example, differences in postoperative care could introduce bias if one group were given extra physiotherapy sessions. Standardization tries to address any bias that may be introduced in studies with multiple components by attempting to keep things as consistent as possible [31]. In the FAITH trial [9], patient positioning, fracture reduction, and surgical exposure were left to the surgeons' discretion. However, surgeons were given specific criteria for acceptability of post-fixation radiographic fracture alignment. The authors also provide supplemental materials in the appendix regarding procedural and rehabilitative standardization. Therefore, it is safe to assume that the necessary steps were taken to address any potential variability.

Sample Size Calculation and Follow-Up

A predetermined sample size calculation is integral to the conduct of an RCT (see Chap. 29). A study with too few participants may fail to reach its objective by lacking capacity to answer the primary study question due to being statistically underpowered. Conversely, a study should not simply recruit an excessive number of patients as this would overpower the study and may result in findings of statistical significance that are not actually clinically important [32]. As such, RCTs should have a sample size calculation based upon a determined minimally clinically important difference and desired study power [32]. Sample size calculations provide a study with adequate power to detect the minimally clinically important differences for outcomes used in the calculation. However, subgroup analysis is not included in this calculation.

Another caveat in any study is participant attrition. Patients that are lost to follow-up threaten the validity of the study since we do not know their outcomes, whether or not they died, or if demographic differences exist between them and the study group [33]. While there is not any hard and fast cutoff value at which attrition related bias becomes apparent, it is generally accepted that 5% loss to follow-up is of little worry, a loss of 20% should raise concern, and a loss between 5 and 20% may still produce bias but to a lesser degree [34]. To maintain the predetermined study power and avoid skewing study results, it is important to consider the anticipated loss to follow-up when calculating a trials minimum sample size in the planning phase of the study [35] (see Chap. 29 for further explanation). In the FAITH trial [9], the original sample size calculation found that enrolment of 1500 patients would give the trial a study power of 81.5%. However, upon reanalysis of completed follow-up data from the first 589 patients, it was found that a sample size of 1100 patients would provide 95.7% power to detect a relative risk reduction of 35%. The authors were able to recruit 1108 patients. The authors validate their study by providing details of sample size calculations and patient exclusion rationale in the appendix.

What Are the Results?

What Was the Impact from the Treatment?

Now that the study has been conducted, we want to know what the results mean and their clinical importance and statistical significance. Some common terminology used to report data are relative risk (RR), relative risk reduction (RRR), absolute risk reduction (ARR), and the number needed to treat (NNT) (Box 2). The RR describes the probability of an event occurring in one group of people versus another [36, 37] (see Chap. 6 for further explanation). In our study, the RR would tell us the probability of reoperation within 24 months in patients receiving a sliding hip screw (experimental) versus patients receiving cancellous screws (control). The RRR measures how much risk is reduced in the experimental group versus the control group [38]. Consider a hypothetical situation comparing stroke rates in hypertensive patients receiving an intensive treatment regimen (experimental) versus the standard of care (control). If 10% of the control group experienced a stroke, compared to 5% of patients in the treatment group, it can be said that the intensive treatment regimen resulted in a relative risk reduction of 50% (Table 11.2). The ARR describes the absolute difference in event rates between the control and treatment groups [38]. Using our hypothetical situation, the ARR for strokes would be 5%. The NNT refers to the number of patients that would need to be treated in order to prevent one additional adverse event from occurring and can be thought of as the inverse of the ARR [39, 40]. Referring to our hypothetical example once more, for every 20 patients treated with the intensive treatment regimen, 1 stroke would be prevented. In the FAITH trial [9], the authors report that reoperations of any kind within 24 months were roughly equal in the sliding hip screw group versus the cancellous screw group and there was no minimally clinically important difference or statistical significance (20% vs. 22%, $p = 0.18$); however, implant removal took place significantly less frequently in the sliding hip screw group than in the cancellous screws group although the findings were not clinically significant (5% vs. 9%, $p = 0.0009$). The authors also report that there were no statistically or clinically significant differences between the two groups in terms of mortality, fracture healing, complications, and health-related quality of life scores.

Table 11.2 Sample calculations from the hypothetical hypertensive drug trial

	Experimental group	Control group
Total number of patients	124	130
Number of strokes	6	13
Event rates	$x = 6/124 = 0.05$ (5%)	$y = 13/130 = 0.10$ (10%)
Relative risk: $x/y = 0.05/0.10 = 0.50$ (50%)		
Relative risk reduction: $(x - y)/y = (0.05 - 0.10)/0.10 = 0.50$ (50%)		
Absolute risk reduction: $x - y = 0.05 - 0.10 = 0.05$ (5%)		
Number needed to treat: $1/(x - y) = 1/(0.05 - 0.10) = 20$		

Patients in the control group were 50% more likely to experience a stroke (RR). Similarly, the experimental intervention reduced the risk of stroke by 50% (RRR). Likewise, for every 100 patients treated with the experimental intervention, there would be 5 fewer strokes (ARR). Furthermore, in order to prevent one stroke, 20 patients would need to be treated with the experimental intervention (NNT).

Box 2. Equations for common statistic terminology

Relative Risk (RR)
$RR = \frac{x}{y}$

Relative Risk Reduction (RRR)
$RRR = \frac{(x-y)}{y}$

Absolute Risk Reduction (ARR)
$AAR = x - y$

Number Needed to Treat (NNT)
$NNT = \frac{1}{AAR}$

x—# of events in experimental group/total # of patients in experimental group.

y—# of events in control group/total # of patients in control group.

How Precise Were the Results?

It is impossible to know the "true" reduction to reoperation rates within 24 months caused by the use of a sliding hip screw because of variables unbeknownst to researchers that may impact the study. The best we can do is come up with a close estimate, known as the point estimate, of the true value that would lie within that ballpark. To communicate the point estimate, researchers provide a variety of values, known as the confidence interval (CI), that specifies a probability within which one can be confident the true value lies [41, 42]. By convention, a 95% CI is generally used, meaning we can be 95% certain that the "true" value lies within the interval (see Chap. 28 for more information).

In the FAITH trial [9], results are reported using hazard ratios (HR), the chance of an event occurring in the treatment arm divided by the chance of the event occurring in the control arm [43], CIs, and *p* values. They report an HR of 0.83 with a 95% CI of 0.63–1.09 and a *p*-value of 0.18. This means that the patients who received a sliding hip screw are less likely to require a reoperation and that the true value for this rate lies between 0.63 and 1.09. However, the difference in event rates between the two groups is not statistically or clinically significant.

What Now?

Generalizability

Before we decide to implement a particular intervention, we need to assess how relevant the information is to our patient population. In our clinical scenario, our patient is a 74-year-old woman who sustained a femoral neck fracture due to a fall. In the FAITH trial [9], they enrolled patients who were 50 years or older with a low-energy femoral neck fracture requiring operative fixation. Looking at the table of patient baseline characteristics, we also see that the mean age of patients was 72.1 years and that 61% of the study participants were female, therefore these findings could apply to our patient.

Clinical Relevance

It is important to consider whether or not the outcomes that the researchers examined are clinically relevant. For example, a study comparing two treatment modalities for rotator cuff tears that looked at "return to sport time" would be clinically useful for a 20-year-old pitcher, but less relevant for a 74-year-old patient. In the FAITH trial [9], the outcomes assessed included reoperation within 24 months, mortality, fracture healing, complications, and health-related quality of life scores. All of these outcome measures would be relevant to both physicians and patients alike, as they are clinically important with important implications on the ultimate outcome. For instance, revision surgeries tend to be more technically complex, impose added expenses to the health care system, and expose patients to further risks and potential perioperative morbidity [44].

What Does This Mean for Me as a Healthcare Provider?

Now that we have assessed the evidence provided to us, how do we use it? For medical doctors, this may be straightforward because if a study shows that drug A is more efficacious than drug B, they can simply begin prescribing drug B. However, implementing new evidence poses potential challenges for surgeons. If a study shows that a particular intervention produces superior outcomes, how do they go about implementing it? Surgeons need to objectively critique their expertise and proficiency with a procedure and earnestly consider if they would be happy with the level of care provided. It would be unethical for a surgeon to perform a procedure they are not familiar with as patients would potentially experience a higher complication rate [45–47]. If a surgeon is not comfortable performing the procedure they can: (1) refer the patient to a colleague, (2) seek additional training, or (3) perform a different procedure after considering the evidence for it. Any of these options would be sufficient and the decision ultimately lies with each surgeon.

Resolving Our Clinical Scenario

After thoughtfully examining the information provided to us from the FAITH trial [9], it is fair to conclude that either a sliding hip screw or cancellous screws would be acceptable treatments for low-energy femoral neck fractures in terms of the primary endpoints assessed (reoperation within 24 months, death, complications, and quality of life). Although our patient in the clinical scenario experienced an implant failure within a year, and will likely require reoperation, we can be confident in answering her that her failure likely was not due to the choice of implant.

References

1. National Insititue of Health (NIH). What we do: budget [Internet]. 2018 Apr 11. [cited 2018 Aug 9]. Available from: https://www.nih.gov/about-nih/what-we-do/budget#note.
2. Graham R, Mancer M, Wolman Miller D, Greenfield S, Steinberg E, editors. Clinical practice guidelines we can trust. Washington, DC: The National Academies Press; 2011. p. 290.
3. Guyatt G, Cairns J, Churchill D, Cook D, Haynes B, Hirsh J, et al. Evidence-based medicine. A new approach to teaching the practice of medicine. JAMA. 1992;268(17):2420–5.
4. Richardson WS, Wilson MC, Nishikawa J, Hayward RS. The well-built clinical question: a key to evidence-based decisions. ACP J Club. 1995;123(3):A12–3.
5. Motschall E, Falck-Ytter Y. Searching the MEDLINE literature database through PubMed: a short guide. Onkologie. 2005;28(10):517–22.
6. Lu Q, Tang G, Zhao X, Guo S, Cai B, Li Q. Hemiarthroplasty versus internal fixation in super-aged patients with undisplaced femoral neck fractures: a 5-year follow-up of randomized controlled trial. Arch Orthop Trauma Surg. 2017;137(1):27–35.
7. Bhandari M, Jin L, See K, Burge R, Gilchrist N, Witvrouw R, Krohn KD, Warner MR, Ahmad QI, Mitlak B. Does teriparatide improve femoral neck fracture healing: results from a randomized placebo-controlled trial. Clin Orthop Relat Res. 2016;474(5):1234–44.
8. Sprague S, Slobogean GP, Bogoch E, Petrisor B, Garibaldi A, O'Hara N, Bhandari M, FAITH Investigators. Vitamin D use and health outcomes after surgery for hip fracture. Orthopedics. 2017;40(5):e868–75.
9. Fixation using Alternative Implants for the Treatment of Hip fractures (FAITH) Investigators. Fracture fixation in the operative management of hip fractures (FAITH): an international, multicentre, randomised controlled trial. Lancet. 2017;389(10078):1519–27.
10. Watts CD, Houdek MT, Sems SA, Cross WW, Pagnano MW. Tranexamic acid safely reduced blood

loss in hemi- and total hip arthroplasty for acute femoral neck fracture: a randomized clinical trial. J Orthop Trauma. 2017;31(7):345–51.
11. Guyatt G, Rennie D, Meade MO, Cook DJ. User's guides to the medical literature: essentials of evidence-based clinical practice. 2nd ed. Hamilton, ON: McGraw-Hill Professional; 2008. p. 380.
12. Hopper AN, Jamison MH, Lewis WG. Learning curves in surgical practice. Postgrad Med J. 2007;83 (986):777–9.
13. Maruthappu M, Duclos A, Lipsitz SR, Orgill D, Carty MJ. Surgical learning curves and operative efficiency: a cross-specialty observational study. BMJ Open. 2015;5(3):e006679.
14. Devereaux PJ, Bhandari M, Clarke M, Montori VM, Cook DJ, Yusuf S, et al. Need for expertise based randomised controlled trials. BMJ. 2005;330 (7482):88.
15. Cook JA. The challenges faced in the design, conduct and analysis of surgical randomised controlled trials. Trials. 2009;10:9.
16. Cook JA, Elders A, Boachie C, Bassinga T, Fraser C, Altman DG, et al. A systematic review of the use of an expertise-based randomised controlled trial design. Trials. 2015;16:241.
17. Kim J, Shin W. How to do random allocation (randomization). Clin Orthop Surg. 2014;6(1):103–9.
18. Schulz KF. Subverting randomization in controlled trials. JAMA. 1995;274(18):1456–8.
19. Boutron I, Estellat C, Guittet L, Dechartres A, Sackett DL, Hróbjartsson A, et al. Methods of blinding in reports of randomized controlled trials assessing pharmacologic treatments: a systematic review. PLoS Med. 2006;3(10):e425.
20. Kaptchuk TJ. Powerful placebo: the dark side of the randomised controlled trial. Lancet. 1998;351 (9117):1722–5.
21. Zhang W, Robertson J, Jones AC, Dieppe PA, Doherty M. The placebo effect and its determinants in osteoarthritis: meta-analysis of randomised controlled trials. Ann Rheum Dis. 2008;67(12):1716–23.
22. van der Linden W. Pitfalls in randomized surgical trials. Surgery. 1980;87(3):258–62.
23. Prescott RJ, Counsell CE, Gillespie WJ, Grant AM, Russell IT, Kiauka S, et al. Factors that limit the quality, number and progress of randomised controlled trials. Health Technol Assess. 1999;3(20):1–143.
24. Karanicolas PJ, Farrokhyar F, Bhandari M. Practical tips for surgical research: blinding: who, what, when, why, how? Can J Surg. 2010;53(5):345–8.
25. Miller LE, Stewart ME. The blind leading the blind: use and misuse of blinding in randomized controlled trials. Contemp Clin Trials. 2011;32(2):240–3.
26. Randelli P, Arrigoni P, Lubowitz JH, Cabitza P, Denti M. Randomization procedures in orthopaedic trials. Arthroscopy. 2008;24(7):834–8.
27. Kirkley A, Werstine R, Ratjek A, Griffin S. Prospective randomized clinical trial comparing the effectiveness of immediate arthroscopic stabilization versus immobilization and rehabilitation in first traumatic anterior dislocations of the shoulder: long-term evaluation. Arthroscopy. 2005;21(1): 55–63.
28. Farrokhyar F, Bajammal S, Kahnamoui K, Bhandari M. Practical tips for surgical research. Ensuring balanced groups in surgical trials. Can J Surg. 2010;53(6):418–23.
29. Herman A, Botser IB, Tenenbaum S, Chechick A. Intention-to-treat analysis and accounting for missing data in orthopaedic randomized clinical trials. J Bone Joint Surg Am. 2009;91(9):2137–43.
30. Montori VM, Guyatt GH. Intention-to-treat principle. CMAJ. 2001;165(10):1339–41.
31. Blencowe NS, Cook JA, Pinkney T, Rogers C, Reeves BC, Blazeby JM. Delivering successful randomized controlled trials in surgery: methods to optimize collaboration and study design. Clin Trials. 2017;14(2):211–8.
32. Zhong B. How to calculate sample size in randomized controlled trial? J Thorac Dis. 2009;1(1):51–4.
33. Dumville JC, Torgerson DJ, Hewitt CE. Reporting attrition in randomised controlled trials. BMJ. 2006;332(7547):969–71.
34. Fergusson D, Aaron SD, Guyatt G, Hébert P. Post-randomisation exclusions: the intention to treat principle and excluding patients from analysis. BMJ. 2002;325(7365):652–4.
35. Maggard MA, O'Connell JB, Liu JH, Etzioni DA, Ko CY. Sample size calculations in surgery: are they done correctly? Surgery. 2003;134(2):275–9.
36. Yelland LN, Salter AB, Ryan P. Relative risk estimation in randomized controlled trials: a comparison of methods for independent observations. Int J Biostat. 2011;7(1):1–31.
37. Sistrom CL, Garvan CW. Proportions, odds, and risk. Radiology. 2004;230(1):12–9.
38. Irwig L, Irwig J, Trevena L, Sweet M. Smart health choices: making sense of health advice. London: Hammersmith Press; 2008. p. 1–242.
39. Haas M, Schneider M, Vavrek D. Illustrating risk difference and number needed to treat from a randomized controlled trial of spinal manipulation for cervicogenic headache. Chiropr Osteopat. 2010;18:9.
40. Bender R. Calculating confidence intervals for the number needed to treat. Control Clin Trials. 2001;22 (2):102–10.
41. Flechner L, Tseng TY. Understanding results: P-values, confidence intervals, and number need to treat. Indian J Urol. 2011;27(4):532–5.
42. Sedgwick P. Randomised controlled trials: inferring significance of treatment effects based on confidence intervals. BMJ. 2014;349:g5196.
43. Trinquart L, Jacot J, Conner SC, Porcher R. Comparison of treatment effects measured by the hazard ratio and by the ratio of restricted mean survival times in oncology randomized controlled trials. J Clin Oncol. 2016;34(15):1813–9.
44. Bhandari M, Jon Smith, Larry E. Miller, Jon E. Block. Clinical and economic burden of revision

knee arthroplasty. Clin Med Insights Arthritis Musculoskelet Disord. 2012;(5):89–94.
45. Hammond JW, Queale WS, Kim TK, McFarland EG. Surgeon experience and clinical and economic outcomes for shoulder arthroplasty. J Bone Joint Surg Am. 2003;85–A(12):2318–24.
46. Jain N, Pietrobon R, Hocker S, Guller U, Shankar A, Higgins LD. The relationship between surgeon and hospital volume and outcomes for shoulder arthroplasty. J Bone Joint Surg Am. 2004;86–A(3):496–505.
47. Hervey SL, Purves HR, Guller U, Toth AP, Vail TP, Pietrobon R. Provider volume of total knee arthroplasties and patient outcomes in the HCUP-nationwide inpatient sample. J Bone Joint Surg Am. 2003;85–A(9):1775–83.

How to Assess a Pilot Trial in Surgery

12

Guowei Li, Gillian A. Lancaster and Lehana Thabane

Clinical Scenario

A hip fracture leads to much pain, bleeding, immobility and subsequent complications. Early surgery may reduce morbidity and mortality due to hip fractures. However, most patients with a hip fracture have to wait a long time to receive surgery mainly because of delayed medical clearance and operation room access. Therefore, you hope to run a multicenter randomized controlled trial (RCT) to assess whether accelerated care (i.e. accelerated medical clearance plus surgical access) would cause better outcomes compared with standard care (i.e. regular medical clearance plus surgery). But before you begin, you are uncertain about whether it is feasible to perform such a large clinical trial. You are concerned that you may not be able to recruit a sufficient number of willing patients and whether they will be able to complete the follow-up assessments. Therefore, you decide to review the literature first to see if any pilot study assessed the feasibility of the subsequent large trial.

G. Li · L. Thabane (✉)
Department of Health Research Methods, Evidence, and Impact, McMaster University, St. Joseph's Healthcare Hamilton, Hamilton, Canada
e-mail: thabanl@mcmaster.ca

G. A. Lancaster
Institute of Primary Care and Health Sciences, Keele University, Keele, UK

A. Thoma et al. (eds.), *Evidence-Based Surgery*,
https://doi.org/10.1007/978-3-030-05120-4_12

Definition of Pilot Trials

For a long time, there has been no consensus on the differences in definition of *pilot* and *feasibility* studies: some consider the terms pilot and feasibility as being synonymous, while others argue that these two terms have related but different meanings [1]. Multiple terms such as *pilot study, feasibility trial, pilot work, pilot trial and feasibility investigation,* have been used without clear distinction among them [2]. However, in 2016, as part of the process of developing the CONSORT extension to pilot trials [3, 4], Eldridge et al. introduced a conceptual framework and published definitions of what constitutes a feasibility study and a pilot study. A feasibility study is viewed as an overarching concept of uncertainty about aspects of a future study within which three distinct types of study are identified: randomized pilot studies in which part or all of the aspects of the future study are carried out on a smaller scale to see if it can be done; non-randomized studies which are similar but exclude randomization of participants; and other types of feasibility studies where some element of the future study is being addressed (e.g. intervention development or acceptability) but no part of the future trial is being conducted [4, 5]. Within this framework, the authors define a feasibility study as a study asking '*whether something can be done, should we proceed with it, and if so, how*' and a pilot study as '*a study in which a future RCT or part of it, is conducted on a smaller scale*' [4]. Essentially, Eldridge et al. appropriately note that '*the corollary of these definitions is that all pilot studies (including trials) are feasibility studies but not all feasibility studies are pilot studies*' [4].

Importance or Necessity of Conducting a Pilot Trial

Dependent upon the feasibility objective(s), reasons for conducting a pilot trial include procedural, resource- or management-related, scientific and methodological rationales. We refer readers to Table 2 in Thabane et al. paper regarding the importance of doing a pilot trial with specific examples [6]. In brief, a pilot study can help (1) assess whether the procedures (such as recruitment rates, adherence levels, and inclusion/exclusion criteria, among others) in a large-scale study can be feasible; (2) evaluate and identify the issues related to resources and management including budgets, time/personnel, data collection/storage, capacity in participating centres, etc.; (3) explore the scientific concerns such as preliminary safety evaluations, intervals/dosages of interventions, biological activity and estimating variation of treatment effect sizes, among others; and (4) investigate methodological issues, which includes assisting with sample size estimation for large-scale studies, study design modifications, statistical plan adjustment, to mention a few. For instance, the PROSPECT (Probiotics: Prevention of Severe Pneumonia and Endotracheal Colonization Trial) pilot study aimed to determine the feasibility of conducting a main trial of probiotics to prevent VAP (ventilator-associated pneumonia) in mechanically ventilated patients in the intensive care unit (ICU) [7]. The feasibility objectives included timely recruitment, protocol adherence levels, minimal contamination and an estimated VAP rate of $\geq 10\%$ [8]. Results from the pilot study showed all four objectives were met in 24 participating centres within a study duration of 10 months, indicating the feasibility of a further large-scale RCT to assess the effect of probiotics on VAP in patients in ICU [9].

Current Practice in Pilot Trials in the Literature

Even though given their notable importance and wide application in clinical areas, pilot studies have received little attention or suboptimal scrutiny in the scientific community. For example, publications of pilot studies rarely mention whether such studies are conducted to inform a subsequent large study; and journals adopt substantially varying editorial policies concerning publication of pilot studies. Lancaster et al. surveyed 7 journals (4 general medical journals: *BMJ [British Medical Journal], Lancet, JAMA [Journal of the American Medical Association*, and *NJEM [New England Journal of Medicine]*; and 3 subject-specific journals: *BJC [British Journal of Cancer], BJOG [British Journal of Obstetrics and Gynaecology]* and *BJS [British Journal of Surgery]*) [10]. They found 90 pilot studies published in these journals for the years 2000 and 2001. However, 4 (out of 90) pilot studies specifically stated that the pilot trial was in preparation for a main RCT. They also contacted the 7 journal editors and found that 4 (out of 7) journals had no publication policy for pilot studies, and 1 journal indicated the journal did not publish pilot studies. Arain et al. repeated this work to assess whether practice and editorial policy of pilot studies had changed over the years. They reviewed the years 2007 and 2008 [11] and found little change in practice compared with Lancaster et al. study [10]. Another editorial from the cardiovascular medicine journal *Circulation* reported that 41 pilot studies had been published since 2004 [12]. After peer review, most of the authors were requested to explicitly define their trials as pilots to alert the audience to the preliminary nature of the findings including small sample size and lack of generalizability. All the aforementioned findings indicate the suboptimal nature of the current practices of pilot studies in the literature.

The IDEAL (Idea, Development, Exploration, Assessment, and Long-term Follow-up) framework was set up to provide guidance and recommendations for an integrated evaluation system for surgical studies [13]. The adoption of the IDEAL framework has been slow but is gaining increased momentum in the surgical literature [14]. The IDEAL framework is currently being updated and is expected to explicitly incorporate pilot studies in the future under the 'exploration' category. It is hoped that the inclusion of pilot trials will address some of the inappropriate practices regarding the conduct and interpretation of small studies in surgery. For example, in surgical trials comparing two techniques, authors often conclude inappropriately that absence of evidence (i.e. p-value > 0.05 based on the data) is equivalent to evidence of absence (i.e. in fact, no difference between the two techniques) [14]. This incorrect interpretation may mislead researchers to thinking that further properly designed studies are not needed to detect the differences between interventions.

Key Considerations for Designing a Pilot Trial

Before conducting a pilot study, some key elements should be carefully considered. Several key considerations we emphasize here include study rationale, objective(s), feasibility and patient-centred outcome(s) , sample size justification, appropriate methods of analysis and criteria of success.

Study Rationale

It is important to show readers why a pilot trial is needed before a future main RCT is conducted, given the current scientific background and available evidence. The rationale for a pilot study is generally to explore areas of uncertainty that need to be addressed before the large-scale trial can be planned [4] because according to the principles of the Helsinki declaration, it is unethical to expose participants unnecessarily to the unknown risks of research [15]. An example can be found in Dingemans et al. study that aimed to assess the feasibility of a new portable single-use negative pressure wound therapy (NPWT) device in patients undergoing major foot ankle surgery: '… *However, as only one prospective study on prophylactic negative pressure wound therapy in patients undergoing major lower extremity fracture surgery is available, evidence on its beneficial effect is limited and it is uncertain whether the extra expenses of the NPWT device are justified. Additionally, lately portable, single-use devices have been developed, which allow early discharge without the need for specialized home care. It is however unknown whether the good results observed with regular NPWT devices are equalled by these newly developed devices*' [16].

Objective(s) and Outcomes(s)

The primary objective(s) of a pilot study should concern the feasibility of performing a subsequent main study. To address the feasibility objective(s), pre-specified outcome measurements should be carefully chosen. In general, outcomes of pilot studies may include recruitment rates, adherence levels, data completion and variance estimates, among others. For instance, in Skoretz *et al* study, the '... *primary objective was to determine the feasibility of using validated and objective interpretation measures for videofluoroscopy in conjunction with nasendoscopy to assess swallowing and upper airway physiology on prospectively enrolled CV [cardiovascular] surgery patients following prolonged intubation*' and the '... *secondary objective was to explore the tolerability and impact of this study on patients and nursing practice*' [17]. Accordingly, their outcome measurements included '*recruitment rate, patient participation, task completion durations, and the inter-rater reliability of VFS [videofluoroscopic swallowing study] measures using the intraclass correlation coefficient*'.

Some pilot studies may be performed to determine an appropriate endpoint for the main study; therefore, researchers may not be able to choose the most appropriate primary outcome for the main study until the pilot trial is completed. Of note, however, researchers should explicitly list that identifying the primary outcome for the main study as one of the pilot study objectives. Likewise, exploring learning curve effects may also be an important objective in surgical pilot studies. Learning curves are a well-known way to increase surgical proficiency over time, which consequently could distort comparisons between treatment groups [18, 19]. How to incorporate learning curve effects in surgical trials is an important issue that requires further investigation.

Sample Size

One key requirement for pilot studies is that they should ensure a sufficient sample to provide informative messages for feasibility of conducting a large-scale RCT. For pilot trials, sample size calculations should always be based on the feasibility objectives and scientific rationale. In many cases, pilot studies give a justified rationale as to the number in the sample without performing a formal sample size calculation. In other studies that have a primary objective of achieving an estimated recruitment, retention, or adherence rate, a desired degree of precision (variation, or confidence interval) around the estimated rate is usually needed to help calculate the sample size. We would refer readers to Thabane et al. publication about how to use the confidence interval approach to estimate sample size for a pilot study where rates are to be estimated [6].

Pilot studies may also provide some information about estimating variation of an effect size to inform the sample size calculation for a future main RCT. Readers can refer to relevant methodological publications for more detail [20, 21]. Nevertheless, caution is needed because findings from pilot studies may easily mislead sample size calculations for a main trial if the estimates are based on a small sample [22]. Other approaches in the literature include (1) discussion with health professionals for further supplemental information, (2) creating a sample size table with different variation estimates of an effect size to emphasize the uncertainty around the outcome of interest, and (3) running simulation studies to assess different scenarios and present a variety of results with estimates of variability [6].

Methods of Analysis

Pilot studies should not primarily focus on treatment effects and tests of effectiveness; instead, they are conducted to address the feasibility of conducting a main RCT. Therefore, statistical tests of significance may not be needed or necessary. Where hypothesis tests are performed a sample size calculation should have been carried out or some justification given. It is also helpful to include a cautionary caveat about the study being underpowered and therefore the results should be treated as preliminary [10]. Findings from pilot studies are usually summarized descriptively by means with standard deviations, and counts with percentages for each treatment group separately. Moreover, it is not uncommon to show the results of pilot studies qualitatively, for example, by using narrative descriptions. An example can be found in Forero et al. study, in which '*the feasibility outcomes were reported descriptively and narratively. For the clinical endpoints, only descriptive statistics, mean (standard deviation) for continuous outcomes and raw count (%) for categorical outcomes, were reported. Due to the nature of pilot designs, we chose not to conduct any informative statistical tests on the collected data*' [23].

Criteria of Success

Of note, pilot studies are not conducted to estimate an effect size or compare different treatment effects due to their small sample size and lack of generalizibility. However, it is good practice to draw up progression criteria before the pilot study begins that relate to objectives such as recruitment rates or adherence rates. As a rule of thumb, the criteria of success should be related to the primary feasibility objective(s). Therefore, feasibility findings from pilot trials can inform progression to a subsequent main RCT including whether a large RCT should be planned as is (main trial feasible, no modification needed), planned but with changes (main trial feasible, protocol amendments needed), or not planned (main trial not feasible, aborted completely). As mentioned above, aspects of the feasibility may include procedural, resource- or management-related, scientific and methodological considerations. In Pai et al. study, for example, the primary feasibility objective was to determine whether implementing the SENTRY (Strategies to Enhance Venous Thromboembolism Prophylaxis in Hospitalized Medical Patients) could be feasible and whether the strategies could improve appropriate thromboprophylaxis rates [24]. Therefore, the pilot study was considered *definitely feasible* if '*the proportion of at risk patients receiving appropriate prophylaxis in the intervention hospitals versus the usual care hospitals was > 25%*' [24].

Reporting of a Pilot Trial

Regarding the reporting of pilot studies, we would refer readers to the published CONSORT (Consolidated Standards of Reporting Trials) extension for pilot and feasibility trials [4]. The guideline provides instructions on how to transparently and adequately report abstracts and main texts of pilot studies with detailed examples and explanations. It also compares the standard CONSORT checklist items with the extension checklist items for pilot studies, with some items not applicable to pilot studies and some new items added. We suggest researchers who plan to design, conduct and report a pilot study should carefully refer to the reporting guideline and adhere to the checklist items as appropriate. It is important to note that the CONSORT extension checklist items are a very useful reference guide to consult at the design stage of the pilot study and many examples are given in the paper. It is also easily adapted to non-randomized studies by omitting the items that relate to randomization.

Key Resources for Further References

To assist with the implementation of pilot studies in surgery, Table 12.1 summarizes some key resources for readers. The table covers the aspects of surgical pilot studies including their general conduct (the what/why/how and common misconceptions), deficiencies in current practice, the IDEAL framework and recommendations, CONSORT extension reporting guideline, ethical issues, surgical pilot trial examples and examples of published protocols. For instance, Thabane et al. publication gives a straightforward tutorial on the what/why/how regarding a pilot trial; it also covers some aspects including the differences between pilot trials and proof-of-concept studies, some common confusions and misconceptions and some frequently asked questions, among others [6]. Ethical issues of pilot studies have not been appropriately addressed in the literature. We did a quick literature search of ethics guidelines for research, but did not find any detailed information on (1) whether a pilot study is ethical if its feasibility cannot be guaranteed, or (2) how to approach participants for their consent given the feasibility nature of pilot trials. However, we would refer readers to Thabane et al. publication [6] and the CONSORT reporting guideline by Eldridge et al. [5] that proposed some solutions to such ethical issues. Examples of surgical pilot trials [25, 26], as well as examples of published protocols [27, 28], can also be found in Table 12.1.

Returning to the Scenario

After reviewing the literature, you identified a pilot trial comparing the accelerated care with standard care in patients with a hip fracture [29].

Table 12.1 Some key resources for readers' further references to surgical pilot studies

Aspects of pilot studies	Key reference[a]
Definition	Eldridge, 2016 [4]; Eldridge, 2016 [5]
The what/why/how and common misconceptions	Thabane, 2010 [6]
Deficiencies in current practice	Lancaster, 2004 [10]; Arain, 2010 [11]
The IDEAL framework and recommendations	McCulloch, 2009 [13]; McCulloch, 2018 [14]
CONSORT extension—Reporting guideline	Eldridge, 2016 [4]
Ethical issues	Thabane, 2010 [6]; Eldridge, 2016 [4]
More examples of surgical pilot trials	Mason, 2015 [25]; Lim, 2018 [26]
Examples of published protocols of surgical pilot trials	Snee, 2016 [27]; Kearney, 2017 [28]

[a]Expressed as: first author, publication year [study reference]

Based on the CONSORT extension guideline to pilot trials, you appraise the article carefully. In general, the article was adequately conducted and well reported (Appendix Table 12.2 shows the items reported in the article according to the CONSORT checklist). All the feasibility objectives were met in the pilot trial; i.e. 60 patients were recruited, 80% of eligible patients underwent randomization and 100% of patients completed the follow-up assessments. The pilot trial was carried out in a similar setting to your own and suggested that a large scale trial would be feasible. You discover from colleagues that the authors have in fact gone ahead with a large scale definitive trial to answer the clinical question, which is currently recruiting. You decide to contact the team to see if you can become involved in the study.

Concluding Remarks

Pilot studies provide a platform to evaluate the feasibility and explore uncertainties of a subsequent large-scale RCT. In most cases, it is very important and necessary to perform a pilot study before running a main trial. However, some key elements have to be carefully considered when designing a pilot study. Moreover, researchers who plan to design, implement and report a pilot study are strongly recommended to refer to the CONSORT extension reporting guideline and adhere to the statement and checklist items as appropriate.

Appendix

See Table 12.2.

Table 12.2 CONSORT checklist of information reported in the HIP ATTACK pilot trial[a]

Section/Topic	Item No	Checklist item	Reported (Yes/No/NA)
Title and abstract			
	1a	Identification as a pilot or feasibility randomized trial in the title	Yes
	1b	Structured summary of pilot trial design, methods, results and conclusions (for specific guidance see CONSORT abstract extension for pilot trials)	Yes
Introduction			
Background and objectives	2a	Scientific background and explanation of rationale for future definitive trial, and reasons for randomized pilot trial	Yes
	2b	Specific objectives or research questions for pilot trial	Yes

(continued)

Table 12.2 (continued)

Section/Topic	Item No	Checklist item	Reported (Yes/No/NA)
Methods			
Trial design	3a	Description of pilot trial design (such as parallel, factorial) including allocation ratio	Yes
	3b	Important changes to methods after pilot trial commencement (such as eligibility criteria), with reasons	Yes
Participants	4a	Eligibility criteria for participants	Yes
	4b	Settings and locations where the data were collected	Yes
	4c	How participants were identified and consented	Yes
Interventions	5	The interventions for each group with sufficient details to allow replication, including how and when they were actually administered	Yes
Outcomes	6a	Completely defined pre-specified assessments or measurements to address each pilot trial objective specified in 2b, including how and when they were assessed	Yes
	6b	Any changes to pilot trial assessments or measurements after the pilot trial commenced, with reasons	NA
	6c	If applicable, pre-specified criteria used to judge whether, or how, to proceed with future definitive trial	NA
Sample size	7a	Rationale for numbers in the pilot trial	Yes
	7b	When applicable, explanation of any interim analyses and stopping guidelines	NA
Randomization			
Sequence generation	8a	Method used to generate the random allocation sequence	Yes
	8b	Type of randomization(s); details of any restriction (such as blocking and block size)	Yes
Allocation concealment mechanism	9	Mechanism used to implement the random allocation sequence (such as sequentially numbered containers), describing any steps taken to conceal the sequence until interventions were assigned	Yes
Implementation	10	Who generated the random allocation sequence, who enrolled participants and who assigned participants to interventions	Yes
Blinding	11a	If done, who was blinded after assignment to interventions (for example, participants, care providers, those assessing outcomes) and how	Yes
	11b	If relevant, description of the similarity of interventions	Yes
Statistical methods	12	Methods used to address each pilot trial objective whether qualitative or quantitative	Yes
Results			
Participant flow (a diagram is strongly recommended)	13a	For each group, the numbers of participants who were approached or assessed for eligibility, randomly assigned, received intended treatment, and were assessed for each objective	Yes
	13b	For each group, losses and exclusions after randomization, together with reasons	Yes
Recruitment	14a	Dates defining the periods of recruitment and follow-up	Yes
	14b	Why the pilot trial ended or was stopped	Yes

(continued)

Table 12.2 (continued)

Section/Topic	Item No	Checklist item	Reported (Yes/No/NA)
Baseline data	15	A table showing baseline demographic and clinical characteristics for each group	Yes
Numbers analysed	16	For each objective, number of participants (denominator) included in each analysis. If relevant, these numbers should be by randomized group	Yes
Outcomes and estimation	17	For each objective, results including expressions of uncertainty (such as 95% confidence interval) for any estimates. If relevant, these results should be by randomized group	Yes
Ancillary analyses	18	Results of any other analyses performed that could be used to inform the future definitive trial	Yes
Harms	19	All important harms or unintended effects in each group (for specific guidance see CONSORT for harms)	Yes
	19a	If relevant, other important unintended consequences	NA
Discussion			
Limitations	20	Pilot trial limitations, addressing sources of potential bias and remaining uncertainty about feasibility	Yes
Generalisability	21	Generalisability (applicability) of pilot trial methods and findings to future definitive trial and other studies	Yes
Interpretation	22	Interpretation consistent with pilot trial objectives and findings, balancing potential benefits and harms, and considering other relevant evidence	Yes
	22a	Implications for progression from pilot to future definitive trial, including any proposed amendments	Yes
Other information			
Registration	23	Registration number for pilot trial and name of trial registry	Yes
Protocol	24	Where the pilot trial protocol can be accessed, if available	NA
Funding	25	Sources of funding and other support (such as supply of drugs), role of funders	Yes
	26	Ethical approval or approval by research review committee, confirmed with reference number	Yes

Citation: Eldridge et al. [4]

[a]We strongly recommend reading this statement in conjunction with the CONSORT 2010, extension to randomized pilot and feasibility trials, Explanation and Elaboration for important clarifications on all the items. If relevant, we also recommend reading CONSORT extensions for cluster randomised trials, non-inferiority and equivalence trials, non-pharmacological treatments, herbal interventions and pragmatic trials. Additional extensions are forthcoming: for those and for up-to-date references relevant to this checklist, see www.consort-statement.org

References

1. Whitehead AL, Sully BG, Campbell MJ. Pilot and feasibility studies: is there a difference from each other and from a randomised controlled trial? Contemp Clin Trials. 2014;38(1):130–3.
2. Arnold DM, Burns KE, Adhikari NK, Kho ME, Meade MO, Cook DJ. The design and interpretation of pilot trials in clinical research in critical care. Crit Care Med. 2009;37(1 Suppl):S69–74.
3. Thabane L, Hopewell S, Lancaster GA, Bond CM, Coleman CL, Campbell MJ, et al. Methods and processes for development of a CONSORT extension for reporting pilot randomized controlled trials. Pilot feasibility Stud. 2016;2:25.
4. Eldridge SM, Chan CL, Campbell MJ, Bond CM, Hopewell S, Thabane L, et al. CONSORT 2010 statement: extension to randomised pilot and feasibility trials. BMJ (Clinical Research ed). 2016;355: i5239.
5. Eldridge SM, Lancaster GA, Campbell MJ, Thabane L, Hopewell S, Coleman CL, et al. Defining feasibility and pilot studies in preparation for randomised controlled trials: development of a conceptual framework. PLoS ONE. 2016;11(3): e0150205.
6. Thabane L, Ma J, Chu R, Cheng J, Ismaila A, Rios LP, et al. A tutorial on pilot studies: the what, why and how. BMC Med Res Methodol. 2010;10:1.
7. ClinicalTrials.gov [Internet]. Hamilton, Ontario (Canada): McMaster University. 2000 Feb. Identifer NCT01782755, Probiotics: Prevention of Severe Pneumonia and Endotracheal Colonization Trial (PROSPECT): A Feasibility Clinical Trial; 2013 Feb 4–2018 Mar 27 [cited 2018 Feb]; [about 8 screens]. Available from https://clinicaltrials.gov/show/NCT01782755.
8. Johnstone J, Meade M, Marshall J, Heyland DK, Surette MG, Bowdish DM, et al. Probiotics: prevention of severe pneumonia and endotracheal colonization trial-PROSPECT: protocol for a feasibility randomized pilot trial. Pilot Feasibility Stud. 2015;1:19.
9. Cook DJ, Johnstone J, Marshall JC, Lauzier F, Thabane L, Mehta S, et al. Probiotics: prevention of severe pneumonia and endotracheal colonization trial-PROSPECT: a pilot trial. Trials. 2016;17:377.
10. Lancaster GA, Dodd S, Williamson PR. Design and analysis of pilot studies: recommendations for good practice. J Eval Clin Pract. 2004;10(2):307–12.
11. Arain M, Campbell MJ, Cooper CL, Lancaster GA. What is a pilot or feasibility study? A review of current practice and editorial policy. BMC Med Res Methodol. 2010;10(1):67.
12. Loscalzo J. Pilot trials in clinical research: of what value are they? Circulation. 2009;119(13):1694–6.
13. McCulloch P, Altman DG, Campbell WB, Flum DR, Glasziou P, Marshall JC, et al. No surgical innovation without evaluation: the IDEAL recommendations. Lancet (London, England). 2009;374 (9695):1105–12.
14. McCulloch P, Feinberg J, Philippou Y, Kolias A, Kehoe S, Lancaster G, et al. Progress in clinical research in surgery and IDEAL. Lancet (London, England). 2018 January. [Epub ahead of print].
15. World Medical Association declaration of Helsinki. Recommendations guiding physicians in biomedical research involving human subjects. JAMA. 1997;277 (11):925–6.
16. Dingemans SA, Birnie MF, Backes M, de Jong VM, Luitse JS, Goslings JC, et al. Prophylactic negative pressure wound therapy after lower extremity fracture surgery: a pilot study. Int Orthop. 2018;42(4): 1–7.
17. Skoretz SA, Yau TM, Granton JT, Martino R. The feasibility of assessing swallowing physiology following prolonged intubation after cardiovascular surgery. Pilot Feasibility Stud. 2017;3:62.
18. Cook JA, Ramsay CR, Fayers P. Statistical evaluation of learning curve effects in surgical trials. Clin Trials (London, England). 2004;1(5):421–7.
19. Simpson AH, Howie CR, Norrie J. Surgical trial design—learning curve and surgeon volume: Determining whether inferior results are due to the procedure itself, or delivery of the procedure by the surgeon. Bone Joint Res. 2017;6(4):194–5.
20. Julious SA. Sample size of 12 per group rule of thumb for a pilot study. Pharm Stat. 2005;4(4):287–91.
21. Teare MD, Dimairo M, Shephard N, Hayman A, Whitehead A, Walters SJ. Sample size requirements to estimate key design parameters from external pilot randomised controlled trials: a simulation study. Trials. 2014;15:264.
22. Kraemer HC, Mintz J, Noda A, Tinklenberg J, Yesavage JA. Caution regarding the use of pilot studies to guide power calculations for study proposals. Arch Gen Psychiatry. 2006;63(5):484–9.
23. Forero M, Heikkila A, Paul JE, Cheng J, Thabane L. Lumbar transversus abdominis plane block: the role of local anesthetic volume and concentration-a pilot, prospective, randomized, controlled trial. Pilot Feasibility Stud. 2015;1:10.
24. Pai M, Lloyd NS, Cheng J, Thabane L, Spencer FA, Cook DJ, et al. Strategies to enhance venous thromboprophylaxis in hospitalized medical patients (SENTRY): a pilot cluster randomized trial. Implement Sci. 2013;8:1.
25. Mason JD, Blencowe NS, McNair AG, Stevens DJ, Avery KN, Pullyblank AM, et al. Investigating the collection and assessment of patient-reported outcome data amongst unplanned surgical hospital admissions: a feasibility study. Pilot Feasibility Stud. 2015;1:16.

26. Lim CP, Roberts M, Chalhoub T, Waugh J, Delegate L. Cadaveric surgery in core gynaecology training: a feasibility study. Gynecol Surg. 2018;15(1):4.
27. Snee M, McParland L, Collinson F, Lowe C, Striha A, Baldwin D, et al. The SABRTooth feasibility trial protocol: a study to determine the feasibility and acceptability of conducting a phase III randomised controlled trial comparing stereotactic ablative radiotherapy (SABR) with surgery in patients with peripheral stage I non-small cell lung cancer (NSCLC) considered to be at higher risk of complications from surgical resection. Pilot Feasibility Stud. 2016;2(1):5.
28. Kearney RS, Parsons N, Mistry D, Young J, Brown J, O'Beirne-Elliman J, et al. A protocol for a feasibility randomised controlled trial to assess the difference between functional bracing and plaster cast for the treatment of ankle fractures. Pilot Feasibility Stud. 2017;3(1):11.
29. Hip Fracture Accelerated Surgical Treatment and Care Track (HIP ATTACK) Investigators. Accelerated care versus standard care among patients with hip fracture: the HIP ATTACK pilot trial. CMAJ Can Med Assoc Journal (journal de l'Association medicale canadienne). 2014;186(1): E52–60.

Non-inferiority Randomized Controlled Trials

13

Yaad Shergill, Atefeh Noori, Ngai Chow and Jason W. Busse

Clinical Scenario

You are an oncologist attending the Canadian Conference on Ovarian Cancer Research, during which a keynote speaker and another attendee debate the use of primary chemotherapy versus primary surgery for newly diagnosed advanced ovarian cancer. You know the standard of care involves surgery followed by chemotherapy (primary surgery); however, the speaker refers to research suggesting chemotherapy before surgery (primary chemotherapy) is non-inferior to primary surgery for overall survival, and is associated with higher optimal debulking rates and lower risks of complications.

The next day, a 63-year-old engineer with newly diagnosed advanced ovarian cancer is awaiting a consult from you. Your patient is physically active, enjoys her career, and has a close support group. You discuss treatment options with your patient, and schedule a meeting to follow-up in 1 week. You recall the recent debate at the ovarian cancer conference, and decide to explore the evidence regarding primary surgery versus primary chemotherapy so that you can be prepared to discuss this issue when your patient returns to finalize a treatment plan.

Literature Search

To obtain the best evidence regarding primary chemotherapy or primary surgery for newly diagnosed advanced ovarian cancer, you begin a literature search according to the "Users' guide to the surgical literature: How to perform a literature search" [1]. You use the PICO format when identifying key words to use in your search process.

- Population: women with newly diagnosed advanced ovarian cancer
- Intervention: primary chemotherapy
- Comparator: primary surgery
- Outcomes: overall survival and quality of life

You access PubMed (www.ncbi.nlm.nih.gov/PubMed) on your computer. You combine the

Y. Shergill · A. Noori · N. Chow · J. W. Busse (✉)
Department of Health Research Methods, Evidence, and Impact, McMaster University, Hamilton, ON, Canada
e-mail: bussejw@mcmaster.ca

Y. Shergill
e-mail: yaad.shergill@gmail.com

J. W. Busse
Department of Anesthesia, McMaster University, Hamilton, ON, Canada

J. W. Busse
Michael G. DeGroote Institute for Pain Research and Care, McMaster University, Hamilton, ON, Canada

J. W. Busse
Michael G. DeGroote Centre for Medicinal Cannabis Research, McMaster University, Hamilton, ON, Canada

A. Thoma et al. (eds.), *Evidence-Based Surgery*,
https://doi.org/10.1007/978-3-030-05120-4_13

search terms "advanced ovarian cancer" and "primary chemotherapy" and "primary surgery" and limit the search to the "English-language studies carried out on human participants." Your search yields ten articles (Appendix), of which two are randomized controlled trials (RCTs) [2, 3]. The more recent 2015 CHORUS [2] trial, published in the Lancet, directly relates to your research question, and would seem to be the study referred to at the conference you attended. When you download the article and begin to read through it, you notice that the trial is labeled as a non-inferiority trial, and wonder how this differs from other trial designs.

Randomized Controlled Trials

RCTs remain the gold standard for evaluating the effectiveness of surgical interventions, as successful randomization ensures that patients in both treatment arms are prognostically similar at baseline and any differences in outcome can be attributed to the intervention. The experimental therapy is considered superior to the control intervention when the null hypothesis is rejected and shows a statistically significant difference in favor of the new treatment [4, 5]. For more information on RCTs, please see Chap. 11.

Non-inferiority RCT Design

Non-inferiority trials investigate whether a new surgical procedure is not worse than another procedure by more than an acceptable amount. The null hypothesis, which, if met will reject non-inferiority, if that the new surgical procedure is worse than the standard intervention by greater than an acceptable amount (delta, Δ), where Δ is the non-inferiority margin. The alternate hypothesis, which if met will demonstrate non-inferiority, is that the new surgical intervention is not worse than standard intervention for the condition by greater than Δ. A new surgical procedure that is non-inferior or "not unacceptably worse" than a standard procedure may be desirable when the new procedure is associated with fewer harms, favorable cost, or greater accessibility [6–8]. The rationale behind trialists' choice of their prespecified non-inferior margin is thus critical to providing readers with confidence in the validity of a study that has concluded non-inferiority.

The US Food and Drug Administration has suggested a strategy for setting non-inferiority margins based on the smallest plausible benefit of the existing standard therapy for the outcome under consideration [9]. This value is informed by identifying the most defensible estimate of effect from existing trials (or ideally, a systematic review) and the associated measure of precision; typically, the 95% confidence interval (95% CI). The smallest plausible benefit is the lower boundary of the 95% CI—the value closest to no effect. A new treatment should be similarly beneficial to conclude non-inferiority, and this is defined by many drug regulatory agencies as including at least 50% of the minimal plausible treatment effect [10].

For instance, an existing surgical procedure may show an absolute reduction of 4% in overall mortality, compared with nonsurgical care, with a 95% CI of 2–6%. The smallest plausible benefit is then a 2% reduction in overall mortality; half of this is 1%. If a non-inferiority trial testing an alternative surgical procedure shows a treatment effect with an associated measure of precision that includes no more than a 1% increase in overall mortality (e.g., a point estimate of no difference, with a 95% CI of −1 to 1%), then 50% of the 2% absolute reduction in absolute mortality is preserved and would satisfy the criteria for concluding non-inferiority. Estimates of precision associated with treatment effects that only include benefit versus the comparator demonstrated superiority and estimates of precision that exceeds the margin have shown inferiority to the comparator. Furthermore, 95% CIs that include the non-inferiority margin are inconclusive (e.g., a more precise estimate may or may not be non-inferior) (Fig. 13.1).

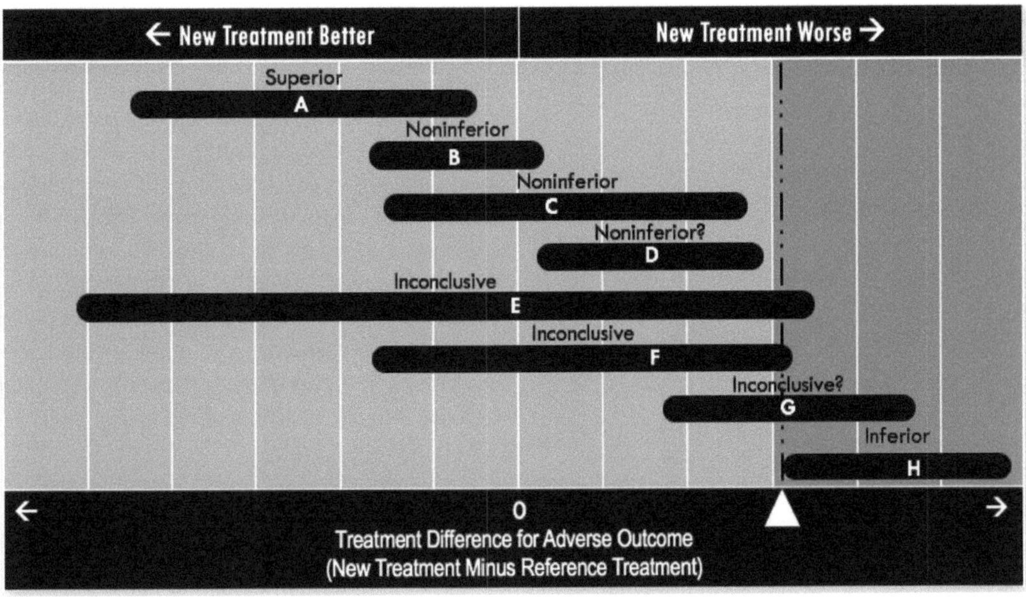

Fig. 13.1 Possible scenarios of observed treatment differences for adverse outcomes (harms) in non-inferiority trials. Bars indicate 2-sided 95% CIs. The dashed line at x = Δ refers to the non-inferiority margin, the light gray tinted region to the left of Δ refers to the zone of inferiority. A, if the CI lies to the left of zero, the new treatment is superior. B and C, if the 95%CI lies to the left of Δ and includes zero, the new treatment is non-inferior but not shown to be superior. D, if the 95% CI lies to the left of Δ and to the right of zero, the new treatment is non-inferior in the sense already defined but also inferior in the sense that a null treatment difference is excluded. E and F, if the 95% CI includes Δ and zero, the difference is nonsignificant but the result regarding non-inferiority is inconclusive. G, if the 95% CI includes Δ and is to the right of the zero, the difference is statistically significant but the result is inconclusive regarding possible inferiority of magnitude Δ or worse. H, if the 95% CI is above Δ, the new treatment is inferior. Adapted from Piaggio [11]

If non-inferiority trials choose overly generous margins (e.g., willing to cede considerable benefit), they may conclude non-inferiority when many informed patients would be unwilling to pursue the new procedure given the largest possible decreased effectiveness associated with its use. Unfortunately, many trialists do not adequately report and justify their choice of non-inferiority margin [12]. As a result, consumers of non-inferiority trials should use their judgement as to whether non-inferiority has been established, rather than relying solely on the conclusions of the study authors. You determine that the CHORUS trial [2] may be helpful to inform discussions with your patient, and you begin to critically appraise the article by using a framework set forth by previous users' guide articles (Box 1) [1, 13, 14].

Box 1. Critical Appraisal Framework for Non-inferiority Randomized Controlled Trial

Step 1: Are the results valid?

- Were the novel and standard surgical intervention groups prognostically similar at baseline?
- Was prognostic balance maintained as the trial progressed?
- Did investigators guard against an unwarranted conclusion of non-inferiority?
- Did investigators analyze patients according to the surgical treatment they received, as well as to the groups to which they were assigned?

- Did investigators justify their non-inferiority margin?

Step 2: What are the results?

Step 3: How can I apply the results to my patient or clinical practice?

- Were the study patients similar to my patients?
- Were all patient-important outcomes considered?
- Are the likely advantage of the novel surgical treatment worth the potential harm?

Step 1: Are the Results Valid?

The article you identified is an open-label, randomized, controlled, and non-inferiority trial that enrolled 552 patients from 87 hospitals in the United Kingdom and New Zealand. Eligible women with newly diagnosed advanced stage III or IV ovarian cancer were randomly assigned to either primary surgery followed by six cycles of chemotherapy (primary surgery group), or three cycles of chemotherapy, then surgery, and three more cycles of completion chemotherapy (primary chemotherapy group). The flow of study participants from the CHORUS trial [2] is summarized in Fig. 13.2.

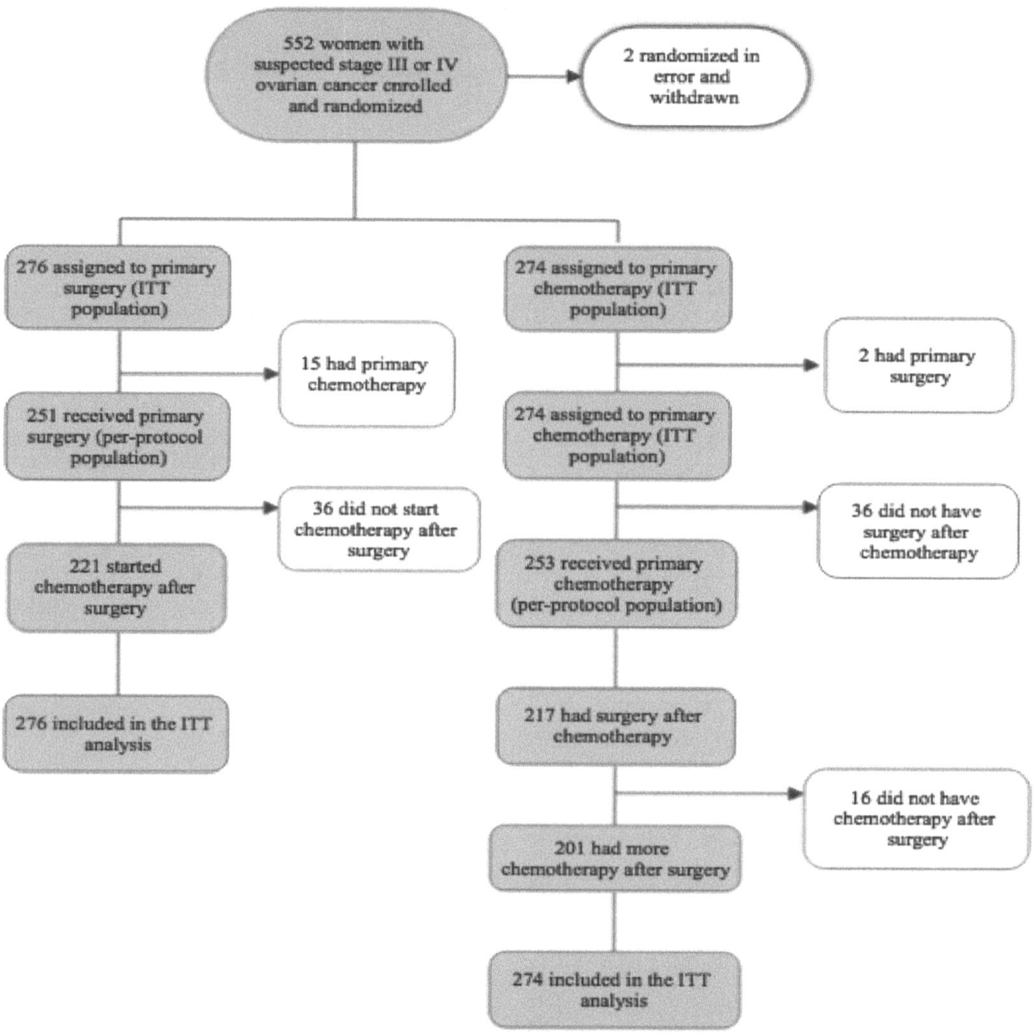

Fig. 13.2 Study flow of the CHORUS trial [2]

Were the novel and standard surgical intervention groups prognostically similar at baseline? Was prognostic balance maintained as the trial progressed?

Similar to superiority RCTs, non-inferiority trials can reduce the risk of bias by adequately randomizing patients to the different treatment arms; concealment of allocation; blinding of participants, healthcare providers, investigators, and outcome assessors; and minimizing loss to follow-up. Not all methodological safeguards against bias may be possible in surgical trials; for example, surgeons cannot be blinded in regard to which procedure they perform. Please see Chap. 11.

In the CHORUS [2] study, participants were centrally randomized by telephone using a minimisation method with a random element, and stratified according to randomizing center, tumor size, clinical FIGO stage, and prespecified chemotherapy regimen. Central randomization ensures concealment of allocation, and stratifying randomization by factors that may be associated with prognosis provides additional reassurances that treatment groups are prognostically similar at baseline. Review of the CHORUS trial's [2] table of baseline characteristics provides reassurance that randomization was successful (Table 13.1). Because of the nature of the interventions (primary surgery vs. primary chemotherapy), it was not possible to blind patients or clinicians; however, the primary outcome measure was overall survival which would not be influenced by lack of blinding [15]. The authors reported no loss to follow-up for their primary outcome, and no more than 7% missing data for secondary outcomes. No loss to follow-up over the course of the trial for the primary outcome ensures that prognostic balance between treatment arms was maintained throughout the study. You conclude that the trial is at low risk of bias.

Did investigators guard against an unwarranted conclusion of non-inferiority?

The CHORUS trial [2] provided both surgery and chemotherapy to both treatment arms; it was the order of approaches that were tested. The CHORUS trial [2] concluded that primary chemotherapy was non-inferior to primary surgery, a conclusion that rests—in part—on the assumption that the standard treatment (primary surgery) was delivered in an optimal manner. The investigators reported that all surgery was performed by accredited specialist gynecological oncologists, who operated on at least 15 patients with ovarian cancer each year, and whose work was regularly peer-reviewed. The CHORUS trial [2] predicted a 50% 3-year survival rate with primary surgery, consistent with previous trials [16], but found a much lower rate of 32%. This difference may be explained by an older median age of CHORUS patients [2] (65 years), and the high rate of poorly differentiated tumors (77%), but the lower than expected survival rate with primary surgery does pose some risk for a misleading finding of non-inferiority.

Did investigators analyze patients according to the surgical treatment they received, as well as to the groups to which they were assigned?

Randomization aims to balance prognostic factors between interventions; however, patients may not receive their allocated treatment. Trialists can address this issue by only analyzing those patients who adhered to the study protocol (a per-protocol analysis); however, this assumes that patients who deviated from protocol were prognostically similar to those who did not—an assumption that is often not met, as non-adherent patients are often sicker and destined to do worse. As such, per-protocol analyses are likely to lead to an overestimation of treatment effects in superiority trials. Using an intention-to-treat (ITT) analysis for superiority trials, where patients are analyzed according to the group to which they were randomized, provides a more conservative estimate of treatment effects [17].

In non-inferiority trials, however, ITT analysis may lead to a misleading conclusion of non-inferiority. Consider a non-inferiority trial in which the novel treatment is actually inferior, and patients are less adherent to the standard treatment. An ITT analysis that included all non-adherent patients would then reduce the apparent effectiveness of the standard therapy and facilitate the misleading conclusion of

Table 1 Baseline characteristics of participants from the CHORUS trial [2]

	Primary surgery (n = 276)	Primary chemotherapy (n = 274)	Total (n = 550)
Age			
Median age	66 (26–87, 57–72)	65 (34–88, 59–71)	62 (26–88, 58–72)
Tumor size			
Median tumor size (cm)	8 (0.7, 5–12)	8 (0.9–28, 5–12)	8 (0.7–30, 5–12)
≤ 2	13 (5%)	13 (5%)	26 (5%)
≤ 5	59 (21%)	60 (22%)	119 (22%)
≤ 10	111 (40%)	110 (40%)	221 (40%)
≤ 20	79 (29%)	79 (29%)	158 (29%)
>20	7 (3%)	7 (3%)	14 (3%)
Unmeasurable disease	7 (3%)	5 (2%)	12 (2%)
Clinical FIGO stage			
III	206 (75%)	206 (75%)	412 (75%)
IV	70 (25%)	68 (25%)	138 (25%)
CA125/CEA ratio			
>25	272 (99%)	268 (98%)	540 (98%)
≤ 25	4 (1%)	6 (2%)	10 (2%)
Prespecified chemotherapy regimen			
Single agent carboplatin	66 (24%)	63 (23%)	129 (23%)
Carboplatin + paclitaxel	207 (75%)	210 (77%)	417 (76%)
Carboplatin + other chemotherapy agent	3 (1%)	1 (<1%)	4 (1%)

Data are median (min–max, Q1–Q3) or n (%; percentages calculated for patients with non-missing data)
FIGO International Federation of Gynaecology and Obstetrics, *CA125* cancer antigen 125, *CEA* carcinoembryonic antigen

non-inferiority in comparison with the new approach. As such, a per-protocol analysis is the more conservative approach for non-inferiority trials. Investigators that present both ITT and pre-protocol analyses provide further confidence in a conclusion of non-inferiority when the results between both approaches are concordant. Of note, the choice of analysis may have limited impact on results in most cases. A review of 117 non-inferiority comparisons in which both an ITT and per-protocol analysis were reported found differing conclusions in 7 (4%) of cases [12]. The CHORUS study [2] reported both ITT and per-protocol analyses and found similar results.

Did investigators justify their non-inferiority margin?

Non-inferiority trials are undertaken on the basis that a new approach is either safer, less costly, or more readily available, and the issue is not whether the new approach is more effective than standard care, but only that it is similarly effective (not much worse). The CHORUS [2] investigators reported that historical trials of primary surgery for advanced ovarian cancer have found a 3-year survival rate of 50%, and they believed that most patients would be willing to accept up to 6% less survival with primary chemotherapy. This meant that non-inferiority could be concluded if the upper limit of the 90% CI for the hazard ratio for the effect of primary surgery versus primary chemotherapy on overall mortality was less than 1.18. The authors' of CHORUS selected their non-inferiority margin based on "consideration of the size of differences noted in similar trials and clinical consensus" [2]. Their rationale is therefore vague, and it is not possible to derive the non-inferiority margin from the details provided. Moreover, it is not clear whether or not patients with advanced ovarian cancer would accept a 6% loss of survival at 3 years follow-up. The information provided in the trial registry does not include any further details (http://www.isrctn.com/ISRCTN74802813).

This is lack of detail is, unfortunately, not unusual. In their systematic review of 163 non-inferiority trials, Aberegg and colleagues found that only 25% provided clear justification for their selected margin, 58% provided no rationale, and 17% reported vague reasoning [12]. The choice of non-inferiority margin also informs the required sample size, and the 550-patient CHORUS trial had 65% power for comparison between the treatment groups [2]. The authors addressed this concern by combining their results with another trial which would increase power to 90% [18].

Step 2: What Are the Results?

Treatment of advanced ovarian cancer focusses on survival, but other important outcomes are quality of life and adverse events associated with therapy. Pursuing chemotherapy before surgery may reduce tumor size, facilitate more successful debulking surgery, and—with less extensive surgery required—reduce postoperative complication rates; however, delaying surgery may also decrease survival rates.

The CHORUS trial [2] found a nonsignificant pattern for greater overall 3-year survival that favored primary chemotherapy versus primary surgery (34% vs. 32%), but they did not report an associated measure of precision for the absolute difference of 2%. In an ITT analysis, the hazard ratio (HR) for overall 3-year survival was 0.87 with an associated estimate of precision (95% CI: 0.72–1.05) for which the upper boundary fell below the non-inferiority margin of 1.18 (this would correspond to scenario C in Fig. 13.1). A per-protocol analysis was consistent with these results (HR 0.89; 95% CI: 0.78–1.01).

The planned meta-analysis for overall survival moved the point estimate closer to no effect, and improved precision (HR 0.93; 95% CI: 0.82–1.05) (Fig. 13.3). Improvement in quality of life, measured by the EORTC quality of life questionnaire and the ovarian cancer-specific quality of life questionnaire, at 6 and 12 months was not significantly different between treatment groups, but did favor primary chemotherapy (63% vs.

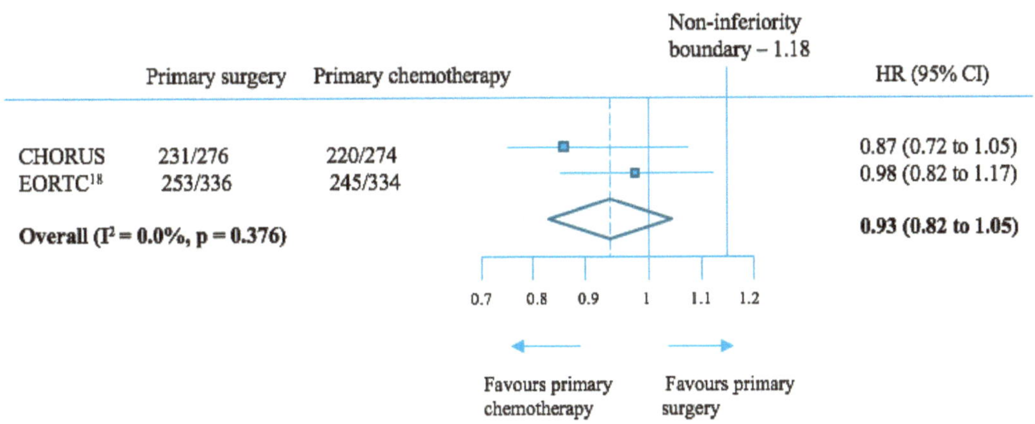

Fig. 13.3 Forest plot of overall survival in CHORUS [2] and EORTC studies [18]

55% and 61% vs. 44%, respectively) [18]. The primary surgery group had more grade 3 or 4 adverse events – most commonly serious bleeding—than primary chemotherapy (24% vs. 14%), and fewer women were discharged from the hospital within 14 days after surgery if they were allocated to the primary surgery arm (80% vs. 93%).

Step 3: How Can I Apply the Results to My Patient or Clinical Practice?

Were the study participants similar to my patient?

Your patient is similar to the baseline demographics provided in Table 13.1 of the CHORUS study [2]. If this patient had been approached by the CHORUS study [2], you are confident that she would have met inclusion criteria. You conclude that your patient is similar to the study participants in the CHORUS study and that results would apply to her.

Were all patient-important outcomes considered?

The investigators selected overall survival as the primary outcome. This clinical trial endpoint has been supported by the Society of Gynecologic Oncology in a consensus statement [19]. The CHORUS trial [2] also explored quality of life and adverse events as secondary outcomes, which are important endpoints in advanced ovarian cancer [20]. You are satisfied that all major patient-important outcomes were considered.

Are the likely advantages of the novel surgical treatment worth the potential harm and costs?

The CHORUS trial [2], including pooled effects with the EORTC trial [18], demonstrated less adverse events and faster discharge from hospital with primary chemotherapy versus primary surgery, with similar results on overall mortality, disease-free progression, and quality of life. Thus, pursuit of the novel approach (primary chemotherapy) appears supported by the evidence.

Conclusion

Non-inferiority trials are an appropriate study design to explore whether a novel approach that has advantages in cost, harms, or availability is similarly effective to the existing standard. Criteria for assessing validity include those used for conventional RCTs, but also include consideration of whether the conventional approach was delivered optimally and if findings are robust to both an ITT and per-protocol analysis. Moreover, clinicians, in consultation with their patients, should determine whether the loss in effectiveness suggested by the upper boundary of the 95% CI associated with the treatment effect of the novel approach is acceptable, regardless of a specific trial's non-inferiority threshold.

Appendix

1. Kehoe S, Hook J, Nankivell M, Jayson GC, Kitchener H, Lopes T, et al. Primary chemotherapy versus primary surgery for newly diagnosed advanced ovarian cancer (CHORUS): an open-label, randomised, controlled, non-inferiority trial. Lancet. 2015;386(9990):249–57.
2. Ledermann JA. Primary chemotherapy: the future for the management of advanced ovarian cancer? Int J Gynecol Cancer. 2010;11(Suppl 2):S17–9.
3. Kayikcioglu F, Kose MF, Boran N, Caliskan E, Tulunay G. Neoadjuvant chemotherapy or primary surgery in advanced epithelial ovarian carcinoma. Int J Gynecol Cancer. 2001;11(6):466–70
4. Milam MR, Tao X, Coleman RL, Harrell R, Bassett R, Dos Reis R, et al. Neoadjuvant chemotherapy is associated with prolonged primary treatment intervals in patients with advanced epithelial ovarian cancer. Int J Gynecol Cancer. 2011;21(1):66–71.
5. Munstedt K, Franke FE. Role of primary surgery in advanced ovarian cancer. World J Surg Oncol. 2004;2:32.

6. Hegazy MA, Hegazi RA, Elshafei MA, Setit AE, Elshamy MR, Eltatoongy M, et al. Neoadjuvant chemotherapy versus primary surgery in advanced ovarian carcinoma. World J Surg Oncol. 2005;3:57.
7. Alberts DS, Hannigan EV, Liu PY, Jiang C, Wilczynski S, Copeland L, et al. Randomized trial of adjuvant intraperitoneal alpha interferon in stage III ovarian cancer patients who have no evidence of disease after primary surgery and chemotherapy: an intergroup study. Gynecol Oncol. 2006;100(1):133–8.
8. Eisenhauer EL, Tew WP, Levine DA, Lichtman SM, Brown CL, Aghajanian C, et al. Response and outcomes in elderly patients with stages IIIC-IV ovarian cancer receiving platinum–taxane chemotherapy. Gynecol Oncol. 2007;106(2):381–7.
9. Drews F, Bertelli G, Lutchman-Singh K. Management of advanced ovarian cancer in South West Wales—a comparison between primary debulking surgery and primary chemotherapy treatment strategies in an unselected, consecutive patient cohort. Cancer Epidemiol. 2017;49:85–91.
10. Jarnagin WR, Dematteo RP, D'Angelica MI, Barakat RR, Chi DS. The addition of extensive upper abdominal surgery to achieve optimal cytoreduction improves survival in patients with stages IIIC-IV epithelial ovarian cancer. Gynecol Oncol. 2006;103(3):1083–90.

References

1. Cadeddu M, Farrokhyar F, Levis C, Cornacchi S, Haines T, Thoma A. users' guide to the surgical literature. Understanding confidence intervals. Can J Surg. 2012;55(3):207–11.
2. Kehoe S, Hook J, Nankivell M, Jayson GC, Kitchener H, Lopes T, et al. Primary chemotherapy versus primary surgery for newly diagnosed advanced ovarian cancer (CHORUS): an open-label, randomised, controlled, non-inferiority trial. Lancet. 2015;386(9990):249–57.
3. Alberts DS, Hannigan EV, Liu PY, Jiang C, Wilczynski S, Copeland L, et al. Randomized trial of adjuvant intraperitoneal alpha-interferon in stage III ovarian cancer patients who have no evidence of disease after primary surgery and chemotherapy: an intergroup study. Gynecol Oncol. 2006;100(1):133–8.
4. Bothwell LE, Greene JA, Podolsky SH, Jones DS. In: Malina D, editor. Assessing the gold standard—lessons from the history of RCTs. N Engl J Med. 2016;374(22):2175–81.
5. Altman DG, Schulz KF, Moher D, Egger M, Davidoff F, Elbourne D, et al. The revised CONSORT statement for reporting randomized trials: explanation and elaboration. Ann Intern Med. 2001;134 (8):663–94.
6. Hahn S. Understanding noninferiority trials. Korean J Pediatr. 2012;55(11):403–7.
7. Temple R, Ellenberg SS. Placebo-controlled trials and active-control trials in the evaluation of new treatments. Part 1: Ethical and scientific issues. Ann Intern Med. 2000;133(6):455–63.
8. Ellenberg SS, Temple R. Placebo-controlled trials and active-control trials in the evaluation of new treatments. Part 2: Practical issues and specific cases. Ann Intern Med. 2000;133(6):464–70.
9. U.S. Department of Health and Human Services Food and Drug Administration Center for Drug Evaluation and Research, Center for Biologics Evaluation and Research. Non-inferiority clinical trials to establish effectiveness: guidance for industry. [internet]. 2016. [cited 2018 July 5]. Available from https://www.fda.gov/downloads/Drugs/Guidances/UCM202140.pdf.
10. Althunian TA, de Boer A, Groenwold RHH, Klungel OH. Defining the noninferiority margin and analysing noninferiority: an overview. Br J Clin Pharmacol. 2017;83(8):1636–42.
11. Piaggio G, Elbourne DR, Pocock SJ, Evans SJW, Altman DG, For the CONSORT Group. Reporting of noninferiority and equivalence randomized trials. JAMA. 2012;308(24):2594–604.
12. Aberegg SK, Hersh AM, Samore MH. Empirical consequences of current recommendations for the design and interpretation of noninferiority trials. J Gen Intern Med. 2018;33(1):88–96.
13. Thoma A, Farrokhyar F, Bhandari M, Tandan V, Evidence-Based Surgery Working Group. Users' guide to the surgical literature. How to assess a randomized controlled trial in surgery. Can J Surg. 2004;47(3):200–8.
14. Thoma A, Farrokhyar F, Waltho D, Braga LH, Sprague S, Goldsmith CH. Users' guide to the surgical literature: how to assess a noninferiority trial. Can J Surg. 2017;60(6):426–32.
15. Anthon CT, Granholm A, Perner A, Laake JH, Møller MH. No firm evidence that lack of blinding affects estimates of mortality in randomized clinical trials of intensive care interventions: a systematic review and meta-analysis. J Clin Epidemiol. 2018;100:71–81.
16. Seidman JD, Yemelyanova A, Cosin JA, Smith A, Kurman RJ. Survival rates for international federation of gynecology and obstetrics stage III ovarian

carcinoma by cell type. Int J Gynecol Cancer. 2012;22(3):367–71.
17. Gupta SK. Intention-to-treat concept: a review. Perspect Clin Res. 2011;2(3):109–12.
18. Vergote I, Tropé CG, Amant F, Kristensen GB, Ehlen T, Johnson N, et al. Neoadjuvant chemotherapy or primary surgery in stage IIIC or IV ovarian cancer. N Engl J Med. 2010;363(10):943–53.
19. Herzog TJ, Armstrong DK, Brady MF, Coleman RL, Einstein MH, Monk BJ, et al. Ovarian cancer clinical.
20. Shimokawa M, Kogawa T, Shimada T, Saito T, Kumagai H, Ohki M, et al. Overall survival and post-progression survival are potent endpoint in phase III trials of second/third-line chemotherapy for advanced or recurrent epithelial ovarian cancer. J Cancer. 2018;9(5):872–9.

14 Expertise-Based Randomized Controlled Trials

Daniel Waltho, Kristen Davidge and Cagla Eskicioglu
and for the Evidence-Based Surgery Working Group

Clinical Scenario

You are an orthopedic surgeon in the community seeing a 25-year-old, male, right-hand dominant, hockey player in your clinic. He has been diagnosed with recurrent, traumatic, anterior glenohumeral instability of his right shoulder, which followed a hockey-related injury 5 years ago. The patient reports multiple episodes of his right shoulder 'popping out' since the injury (approximately two episodes per year). Being quite proficient with the open repair technique for shoulder stabilization, you offer this procedure to the patient. However, the patient remarks that a friend of his with the same condition was treated at a tertiary care hospital with an arthroscopic repair of his shoulder. Your patient asks you which of the two procedures will result in a better overall result in terms of his quality of life. Having only performed the open repair in your practice, you are unsure of the answer and so you consult the literature.

Introduction

The randomized controlled trial (RCT) is an experimental study design, which randomly assigns participants typically into two arms: experimental group (typically a novel intervention) and a control group (typically the current standard intervention). Ideally, the intervention (s) and comparator(s) are carried out by the same party to ensure consistency and standardization between groups (See Chap. 11: Randomized Controlled Trial Comparing Surgical Interventions). However, in certain cases, these treatments differ significantly in terms of the skills required to implement them. This issue represents a large factor dissuading non-pharmacological RCTs. RCTs involving surgical intervention(s) are one such example, wherein surgeons with a specific expertise and skill set may need to be selectively involved in the treatment of one group. These circumstances represent a challenge when conducting an RCT of this nature.

Novel surgical interventions can have a learning curve that may be difficult for all participating surgeons to overcome. To address this

D. Waltho
Department of Surgery, Division of Plastic Surgery, McMaster University, 1280 Main Street West, Hamilton, ON L8S 4L8, Canada
e-mail: Daniel.waltho@medportal.ca

K. Davidge
Department of Surgery, Division of Plastic Surgery, University of Toronto, 555 University Ave, 5th floor Black Wing, Toronto, ON M5G1X8, Canada
e-mail: Kristen.davidge@sickkids.ca

C. Eskicioglu (✉)
Department of Surgery, Division of General Surgery, McMaster University, 50 Charlton Avenue East, Hamilton, ON L8N 4A6, Canada
e-mail: eskicio@mcmaster.ca

A. Thoma et al. (eds.), *Evidence-Based Surgery*,
https://doi.org/10.1007/978-3-030-05120-4_14

dilemma, an expertise-based RCT (EBRCT) design has been proposed, wherein two unique sets of health professionals possessing a relatively similar expertise with one of the study treatments are assigned to that respective intervention group. This method was first proposed in 1980 by Van der Linden and has been applied sparingly since then [1].

This design allows for comparable skill in executing the therapies in question and may also lend itself to improved participation and compliance amongst surgeons. As such, EBRCTs have emerged as an effective study design in the surgical literature and remain the standard for RCTs comparing surgery versus medical management or comparing two or more distinct surgical techniques [2]. Indeed, their use in surgical settings has been increasing over the past decade [2]. It is prudent for surgeons to be familiar with this design when attempting to answer their clinical or research questions. The surgeon, however, must exercise caution when interpreting the results of an EBRCT. Careful consideration of the methodology used in these RCTs is critical to making appropriate clinical decisions.

This chapter provides the readers with the tools to appraise EBRCTs in surgery. The framework for this appraisal is found in Box 1. Because the EBRCT is a modified RCT, some of the appraisal items in Box 1 are similar to those found in Chap. 11. More attention, however, will be spent on the differences between the two study designs.

Box 1. Guidelines how to assess an expertise-based RCT

A. **Are the results valid?**

(i) Was the learning curve taken into consideration?

(a) Sufficient level of expertise in each treatment group objectively determined and clearly stated
(b) Matching of equally skilled surgeons between each treatment group
(c) Sufficient number of surgeons in each treatment group
(d) Sufficient level of expertise in each treatment group objectively determined and clearly stated

(ii) Were the subjects randomized?
(iii) Was the randomization con cealed?
(iv) Were the experimental and control group similar in terms of prognostic factors?
(v) Were the subjects stratified?
(vi) Were subjects analysed in the group they were initially randomized into at enrolment?
(vii) Was follow-up complete?

B. **What are the results?**

(i) How were the results of the trial being measured?
(ii) How large is the treatment effect?

C. **Are the results applicable to my patients?**

(i) Does the study represent my patient population?
(ii) Does the trial consider all relevant patient-important outcomes?
(iii) Do the benefits of the procedure outweigh any potential risks and costs?

Literature Search

To identify the best evidence and inform our patient a literature search was performed according to the Users' Guide for Surgical Literature: How to perform a high-quality literature search [3]. In this case, the best level of evidence would be a high-quality RCT or preferably a meta-analysis thereof. Designing our research question, using the PICOT format (Box 2), allows us to choose important key words for our search. Your clinical question relevant to this scenario would be as follows.

Box 2: Stating the Research Question Using the PICOT Format

Population: males with recurrent, traumatic, anterior glenohumeral instability
Intervention: open shoulder repair
Comparison: arthroscopic shoulder repair
Outcome: disease or condition-specific quality of life
Time Horizon: long-term post-operative period

Using the PICOT Format above, the research question would look like: 'What is the quality of life of males with recurrent, traumatic, anterior glenohumeral instability after an open shoulder repair, as compared to those who receive an arthroscopic shoulder repair?' To answer your research question you search PubMed Clinical Queries with the search terms 'glenohumeral instability' AND 'open' AND 'arthroscopic' AND 'quality of life'. You identify a RCT, entitled 'A randomized clinical trial comparing open and arthroscopic stabilization for recurrent traumatic anterior shoulder instability: two-year follow-up with disease-specific quality-of-life outcomes', by Mohtadi et al. [4]. In this RCT, an expertise-based methodology was used. Patients were randomized to either open or arthroscopic shoulder repairs, and further randomized to a surgeon with sufficient experience in that chosen technique. Important to this design, surgeons in the trial were assigned to their preferred technique a priori.

Table 14.1 Key methodological features of the Mohtadi et al. [4] article

Study period	2001–2008
Source of sample	University of Calgary Sports Medicine Centre
Source of funding	Calgary Orthopaedic Research and Education Fund Calgary Regional Health Authority Research and Development Fund Hip Hip Hooray! (Canadian Orthopaedic Foundation)
Sample size	Open repair: $n = 98$ Arthroscopic repair: $n = 98$ • Statistically significant increase in % of cases with dominant shoulder involvement • Statistically significant increase in mean time from injury to repair • Age, sex, contact sport involvement, dislocations and # anchors used statistically not significant
Analysis	Independent sample *t* tests were used to compare mean quality of life scores groups at 2 years post-operatively
	Adjusted Bonferroni comparisons and repeated-measures analyses of mean quality of life scores were conducted with use of a mixed-model analysis of variance (ANOVA) for treatment group and time of assessment
	Intention to treat was utilized for all patients
	Chi-square analysis was used to compare recurrence rates between groups
	Logistic regression analysis was performed to assess the independent predictors of recurrence
	Sensitivity analysis was performed on loss to follow-up/withdrawal

Key methodological features of this study are outlined in Table 14.1.

Are the Results Valid?

In this section, we will determine whether the methodology used for this EBRCT was robust, such that we can be confident that any differences, or lack thereof, between treatment groups are more likely to be true. Thus, we will be asking the following questions:

(i) Was the learning curve taken into consideration?
(ii) Were the subjects randomized?
(iii) Was the randomization concealed?
(iv) Were the experimental and control group similar in terms of prognostic factors?
(v) Were the subjects stratified?
(vi) Were subjects analysed in the group they were initially randomized into at enrolment?
(vii) Was follow-up complete?

Was the Learning Curve Taken Into Consideration?

This aspect of validity is a common pitfall in surgical RCTs and is a primary focus of optimization in the EBRCT. When an RCT comparing two surgical interventions is performed without an expertise-based design, the experimental group is often a relatively novel procedure, with which many surgeons may not have sufficient experience. The presence of a learning curve will likely create a discrepancy between the surgeon's proficiency and their ultimate degree of success with the newer surgical treatment. This discrepancy may translate into a systematic difference in outcomes between groups favouring the older procedure. The EBRCT design assigns patients to an intervention group where only surgeons who are well experienced in that specific surgical procedure perform the intervention. Further this design can match patients based on surgeon's level of experience. In other words, if one patient randomized to the experimental treatment arm receives their respective procedure by a surgeon with a certain degree of experience in that technique, he/she will be matched to a patient randomized to the comparison arm who receives their respective procedure from another surgeon with a similar degree of experience in the comparison technique. Therefore, this design allows the surgeons to perform their preferred surgical technique, which in turn increases validity and feasibility of the trial.

To ensure validity in this category, one must ensure that the expertise-based protocol was carried out appropriately. Therefore, this chapter proposes the following sub-criteria that must be fulfilled to determine validity:

(a) Sufficient level of expertise in each treatment group objectively determined and clearly stated
(b) Matching of equally skilled surgeons between each treatment group
(c) Sufficient number of surgeons in each treatment group

(a) *Sufficient level of expertise in each treatment group objectively determined and clearly stated*
Level of surgeon expertise is at the crux of this RCT design. To conclude that the trial results are valid, it must first be determined that the surgeons performing the treatment(s) are adequately trained, such that resultant outcomes (i.e. Success, complications, etc.) are not attributable to poor surgical technique. Therefore, the study should provide an objective metric for each surgeon based on expertise in their assigned operative treatment. There is evidence to suggest that for many procedures, at least 5 years of experience is required to reach the plateau of the learning curve [2]. In the Mohtadi et al. [4] trial, one surgeon in each group had 10 years of experience, while the remaining surgeons in each group had 2–5 years of experience. No sensitivity analysis was done on the study outcomes based on expertise level. Moreover, the authors are assuming that each surgeon has performed a similar number of cases in their respective technique. Whereas, a surgeon could, in theory, have performed only one open procedure a year for the past 10 years and another surgeon could have performed 100 arthroscopic procedures a year for 10 years. A more

appropriate metric for measuring expertise may be the total number of a particular procedure performed.

(b) *Matching of equally skilled surgeons between each treatment group*
Another critical component of the EBRCT protocol is matching of surgeons based upon their level of expertise in their respective treatment group. In the above sub-criterion, we identify a diversity of skill level with the surgeons involved in the trial. While it is important to enlist surgeons in all treatment groups who have sufficient training to be considered 'experts' in a given surgical procedure, these surgeons still exist on a spectrum in terms of how seasoned they are in that technique. Therefore, further matching of surgeons based on their level of expertise is indicated to control for any variation in outcomes that may be attributed to how many of these procedures a surgeon has performed. In the Mohtadi et al. [4] trial, surgeons were matched by experience based on the approximate number of years they were performing their preferred technique. This ensures that for every patient randomized to a surgeon who has performed the arthroscopic technique for a certain number of years, a patient would also be randomized to a surgeon who has performed the open technique for the same number of years. However, as mentioned above, the number of years may not necessarily correspond to the number of procedures performed and matching would be more suitably performed based on the later metric.

(c) *Sufficient number of surgeons in each treatment group*
To further optimize the execution of the EBRCT design, the trial must ensure an adequate number of surgeons in each treatment group, thereby limiting the number of incidences where patients may cross over to the other group. The number of surgeons required is contingent upon both the volume and priority of cases. There is likely to be increased difficulty with respect to the availability of any surgeon in the desired group when the cases are frequent and need to be done on an emergent basis. In the case of the Mohtadi et al. [4] trial, cases were done on an elective basis and a total of 226 eligible patients were included in expertise-based randomization between 2001 and 2008. Throughout the trial period, two surgeons performed open repairs and three surgeons performed arthroscopic repairs. Only one patient, who was randomized to open repair, crossed over. Therefore, we can conclude that there were an adequate number of surgeons in both groups to support this trial.

Based on these criteria, we can conclude that a fairly robust expertise-based design was carried out throughout the trial, however caution must be taken when interpreting the results as true expertise of the surgeons involved is not clearly reported.

Were the Subjects Randomized?

In this trial, the allocation was determined using computer-generated, variable-block-size randomization. Block randomization is simply randomization of participants within blocks such that equal numbers of patients are assigned to each treatment. Variable-block-sizes decreases predictability in the allocation process by varying the number of patients assigned to a given block throughout the allocation process. In the Mohtadi et al. [4] trial, appropriate randomization is utilized. Because this trial is an expertise-based design, allocation determined both the technique and surgeon as discussed above. Patients would then meet with their assigned surgeon, who discussed the technique, confirmed eligibility, and addressed any concerns. Randomization was, therefore, sufficiently executed in this trial.

Was the Randomization Concealed?

Above all, concealment of allocation should apply to those enrolling a patient into the trial, as it ensures that systematic selection bias associated with decisions to enrol certain patients into each treatment arm is limited. In the Mohtadi et al. [4] RCT, the allocation was concealed with consecutively numbered opaque envelopes. Assuming no tampering occurred, we can be satisfied that allocation concealment was sufficient for those enrolling patients initially. However, because the trial is based upon two significantly different surgical approaches, open versus arthroscopic, which incorporate different incisional patterns, blinding of patients is difficult to achieve. Mohtadi et al. [4] were unable to sufficiently blind the patients to the treatment selection. Furthermore, the authors state that the research assistant performing the clinical examinations for evaluation of treatments was aware of the treating surgeon. This is due to both the difference in incisional patterns indicated above, as well as the expertise-based nature of surgeon allocation. Finally, while concealment of allocation is impossible to achieve for the surgeons providing treatment, it is highly unlikely to introduce bias in this case. In traditional surgical RCTs, where the same surgeon performs both interventions, there is a concern that if a surgeon strongly believes in the superiority of one of the two interventions, then either consciously, or subconsciously, patients may be treated differently (for example obtaining more meticulous hemostasis) or introducing co-interventions. However, the use of the EBRCT study design avoids these concerns especially if this is a pragmatic expertise-based RCT.

Were the Experimental and Control Groups Similar in Terms of Prognostic Factors?

To ensure validity, we need to determine if differences in outcomes between treatment groups may be attributable to differences between patient populations in each group. Randomization attempts to minimize this by limiting systematic biases that may cause certain patients to fall into one of the arms and not the other. Care should be taken to observe the initial demographic data of each group. Ideally, no statistically significant differences should exist between key demographic information that may change outcomes, such as age, gender or comorbidities ($p > 0.05$). According to the authors, there was no statistically significant difference between groups in terms of age, gender, collision/contact sport involvement, number of previous dislocations or the number of suture anchors used intraoperatively. However, baseline characteristics differed significantly between treatment groups in two categories. First was the proportion of dominant shoulders being treated, wherein a significantly larger proportion of open repairs were done on the patient's dominant shoulder. Second was the length of time from initial injury, wherein a significantly longer period from injury occurred with the open group. A relative increase in the time from injury with the open repairs could skew the results in favour of the arthroscopic procedure, as a greater time until repair typically yields poorer results. Shoulder dominance is less clear, as a dominant shoulder repair group may lead those patients to be more motivated or capable of post-operative therapy and recovery or may also cause post-operative injury due to over-exertion. Moreover, because this primary outcome was based on a quality of life measurement, perceived improvement in disease-specific quality of life may be greater if surgery is performed on a dominant shoulder injury. In the Mohtadi et al. [4] trial, it is not clear whether this baseline characteristic discrepancy affects validity. Needless to say, key patient demographics remain, for the most part, uniform between groups.

Were the Subjects Stratified?

The further subdivision of subjects beyond the treatment administered is called stratification. Stratification attempts to ensure equal allocation of subgroups of participants based on a desire for uniform populations between groups as described in the previous section. This exercise, therefore, limits systematic differences that may skew results in favour of one treatment.

Stratification can be based on gender, age or other demographic factors. In keeping with an expertise-based design, in the Mohtadi et al. [4] trial, stratification occurred at the level of the surgeon, wherein surgeons of a similar level of expertise in their respective technique were matched. The authors comment on the randomization of patients being stratified accordingly, however do not specify the patient characteristics for which stratification was based upon. Based on the demographic information discussed in the previous section, we can be satisfied with homogeneous strata between both treatment arms.

Were Subjects Analysed in the Group They Were Initially Randomized into at Enrolment?

Intention-To-Treat (ITT) analysis is a method wherein all patients enrolled and randomly allocated to a treatment are analysed in that group to which they were randomized, regardless of deviations that occur after randomization (e.g. protocol violations, loss to follow-up/ withdrawal, patient non-compliance). This practice optimizes validity by ensuring that the study population remains uniform between study groups, thus avoiding crossover of participants to a group, to which they were not randomized. In the Mohtadi et al. [4] RCT, all patients were analysed on an ITT basis so we can conclude that validity has been optimized in this regard.

Was Follow-Up Complete?

To capture treatment effects, patients must be followed up both frequently and for a sufficient duration. Ideally, multiple patient follow-ups for a patient's lifetime would provide the most accurate data, however feasibility must be considered. Therefore, the surgeon should identify the duration and frequency of follow-up that would be practical based on the disease and treatment being studied. These follow-up periods usually correspond to the surgeon's typical follow-up routine in their clinical practice. In addition to a sufficient follow-up period, a sufficient proportion of patients in the study should complete follow-up to ensure validity. In the Mohtadi et al. [4] RCT, follow-up occurred at 3 months, 6 months, 1 year and 2 years post-operatively. The authors report that 19 patients in the open repair group and 14 patients in the arthroscopic repair group were lost to follow-up at 2 years. To optimize validity, a study should aim to have less than 20% of subjects lost to follow-up [5]. In this case, 85% of patients initially randomized remained in the trial throughout the 2-year follow-up. Therefore, we can conclude that there are no major concerns regarding follow-up in this RCT.

What are the Results of the Trial?

Once the validity of the trial has been established, we must determine the magnitude of the treatment effect. In this section, we will further understand the results of the trial by answering the following questions:

(i) How were the results of the trial being measured?
(ii) How large is the treatment effect?

How Were the Results of the Trial Being Measured?

Study outcomes should be measured using an objective tool that ideally has been appropriately validated and shown to be reliable. The primary outcome was disease-specific quality of life. The authors utilize a Patient-Reported Outcome (PRO) measure to address this outcome. The Western Ontario Shoulder Instability Index (WOSI) was chosen. It uses a 100 mm visual analog scale response format. Patients completed the WOSI at baseline, at 3 and 6 months post-operatively, and at 1 and 2 years post-operatively. Evaluating the original psychometric study on this PRO, we determine that it is both validated and reliable in this category [6].

The secondary outcome was shoulder function, including both patient-reported and clinician-reported measures. The American Shoulder and Elbow Surgeons (ASES) scale, a shoulder-specific functional assessment tool is a PRO assessing shoulder function. The score was determined based on patient evaluation of pain, instability and activities of daily living and utilized a 0–100 scale. Once again, exploring the psychometric literature, we are assured that this outcome is both valid and reliable in the study population [7]. Furthermore, clinical assessment of shoulder range of motion was performed by trained, independent research assistants using a standardized tool (i.e., gonio meter). Clinical assessment was presumably also used to measure adverse events/complications and recurrence rates. Based on this article, we can conclude that this method of clinical assessment is both valid and reliable. Recurrent instability was another secondary outcome, however details surrounding how this was assessed were not disclosed by the authors.

How Large Is the Treatment Effect ?

In our clinical scenario, we ask which of the two treatments is superior. In order to answer our initial clinical question, we must first determine whether there are statistically significant differences between the two techniques. Assessing the Mohtadi et al. [4] article with respect to the primary outcome, no statistically significant difference was found between the two treatments in terms of disease-specific quality of life (mean WOSI scores). Further, no statistically significant difference was found between the two treatments in terms of shoulder function (ASES scores and active ROM). However, recurrence rates at two years were significantly different, with 11% in the open group and 23% in the arthroscopic group ($p = 0.05$). No statistical analysis was performed based on adverse events/complications, presumably because there were no clinically significant results in these categories. Based on this data, we can only conclude that a difference between the two procedures exists based on the recurrence of instability.

Are the Results Applicable to Clinical Practice?

According to Guyatt et al., in order to accept that the evidence in a particular study is applicable to your patient(s), three critical questions must be addressed [8]:

(i) Does the study represent my patient population?
(ii) Does the trial consider all relevant patient-important outcomes?
(iii) Do the benefits of the procedure outweigh any potential risks and costs?

Does the Study Represent My Patient Population?

Prior to applying the results of a study to your patient(s), you should review the study population to ensure that the patient demographics are in line with that of your patient(s). The authors presumably included all-comers with recurrent traumatic anterior shoulder instability. However, those patients with glenoid fracture or bone loss seen on pre-operative X-ray were excluded. Assessing the demographic breakdown of patients, mean age was 27.8 and 27.2 between the open and arthroscopic group, respectively, with an 82% male predominance in both groups. Based on these fundamental demographics, we can conclude that the study population is representative of our patient from the clinical scenario. Furthermore, approximately half of these patients injured their shoulder in a contact sport, while a third to a half of the shoulder instability in the study involved the dominant shoulder. Finally, shoulder injuries were around the 6-year mark at the time of both treatments. Therefore, we are confident that our patient's clinical scenario is relatively well reflected in the study.

Does the Trial Consider All Relevant Patient-Important Outcomes?

Looking at our clinical scenario, the main outcome in question was quality of life. Indeed, this is likely to be the most important outcome for the patient, as it provides a practical culmination of symptoms and functional aspects germane to the condition and procedure. The Mohtadi et al. [4] RCT addresses disease-specific quality of life as a primary outcome. In addition, the authors include shoulder function, including recurrent instability, and safety outcomes secondarily. Shoulder function provides appropriate data to confirm the mechanism of any quality of life improvements that may have been found in the study. Safety outcomes, including complications and adverse outcomes, are critical in deciding whether to adopt or endorse a particular surgical intervention. The authors presumably study all complications and adverse outcomes throughout the follow-up period. Overall, the included outcomes are both clinically important and comprehensive in assessing the two treatment arms.

Do the Benefits of the Procedure Outweigh Any Potential Risks and Costs?

Another practical argument for deciding upon a treatment is the risks and costs to the patient, healthcare system and society. A significant benefit in a particular treatment decision should outweigh potentially undue risks to the patient or excessive costs that may be associated with a novel surgery. There were no significant complications reported within this study. Both treatment arms had a small number of cases of transient nerve dysfunction which resolved spontaneously. The authors did not include a cost analysis within their study. Costs can be dichotomized into direct and indirect and can be further divided into costs to the healthcare system, the patient and to society. In this case, if we review the literature, we come across a recent cost-effectiveness study by Min et al. [9] According to this study, the average direct cost of surgery for the arthroscopic shoulder repair was $20,385 and the average cost of surgery of the open repair was $21,389.10 The authors conclude that both the arthroscopic and the open are highly cost-effective but the arthroscopic procedure is more cost-effective due to a lower health utility state after a failed open procedure [9]. However, this study does not incorporate indirect costs to patient or society and further costs are based on a single institution. Further research would be indicated to determine true risk and benefit ratio, however there appears to be similarity between the groups so as not to dissuade the surgeon or patient from either procedure.

Conclusion

The expertise-based RCT is a promising answer to the challenges that are faced when applying the RCT design to surgical interventions. By obviating the issue of learning curve, the surgeon can be more confident that differences between treatment groups are not attributable to surgeon inexperience. Furthermore, concerns of surgeons personally believing in the superiority of a specific surgical procedure and potentially introducing bias, either consciously or subconsciously, is not an issue in this type of study design. However, care must still be taken when interpreting the results, ensuring that the RCT methodology is rigorous. The EBRCT design represents an ideal approach to the surgical trial. Presently, this design is not prominent in the literature, however appears to be growing more frequent in the past decade. Knowledge in how to identify an appropriately designed EBRCT, and analyse and interpret the methodology and results, will no doubt be critical to evidence-based surgery moving forward.

Resolution of Scenario

In follow-up with your patient, you present the results of the Mohtadi et al. [4] paper. You explain that according to the best level of evidence, there is no significant difference between the two treatments in terms of quality of life based on a follow-up of 2 years. Furthermore, you explain that the function of the shoulder is similar between the open and arthroscopic treatments. However, you caution the patient that recurrence of shoulder instability can occur approximately twice as frequently in patients undergoing arthroscopic repair. Following this discussion, the patient wishes to proceed with an open repair of his right shoulder.

References

1. Van der Linden W. Pitfalls in randomized surgical trials. Surgery. 1980;87:258–62.
2. Devereaux PJ, Bhandari M, Clarke M, Montori VM, Cook DJ, Yusuf S, et al. Need for expertise based randomised controlled trials. BMJ. 2005;330(7482):88 Review.
3. Waltho D, Kaur MN, Haynes RB, Farrokhyar F, Thoma A. Users' guide to the surgical literature: how to perform a high-quality literature search. Can J Surg. 2015;58(5):349–58.
4. Mohtadi NG, Chan DS, Hollinshead RM, Boorman RS, Hiemstra LA, Lo IK, et al. A randomized clinical trial comparing open and arthroscopic stabilization for recurrent traumatic anterior shoulder instability: two-year follow-up with disease-specific quality-of-life outcomes. J Bone Joint Surg Am. 2014;96(5):353–60.
5. Oleckno W. Epidemiology: concepts and Methods. Am J Epidemiol. 2008;168(11):1339–40.
6. Kirkley A, Griffin S, McLintock H, Ng L. The development and evaluation of a disease-specific quality of life measurement tool for shoulder instability. The Western Ontario Shoulder Instability Index (WOSI). Am J Sports Med. 1998;26(6):764–72.
7. Kocher MS, Horan MP, Briggs KK, Richardson TR, O'Holleran J, Hawkins RJ. Reliability, validity, and responsiveness of the American shoulder and elbow surgeons subjective shoulder scale in patients with shoulder instability, rotator cuff disease, and glenohumeral arthritis. J Bone Joint Surg Am. 2005;87(9):2006–11.
8. Guyatt G, Rennie D, Meade M, Cook D. Users' guides to the medical literature: a manual for evidence-based clinical practice 3rd ed. New York: McGraw-Hill; 2015.
9. Min K, Fedorka C, Solberg MJ, Shaha SH, Higgins LD. The cost-effectiveness of the arthroscopic Bankart versus open Latarjet in the treatment of primary shoulder instability. J Shoulder Elbow Surg. 2018;27(6S):S2–9.

The Surgeon's Guide to Systematic Review and Meta-Analysis

15

Andrea Copeland, Lucas Gallo and Noor Alolabi

Introduction

As the body of surgical literature expands, the need to summarize research in the form of high-quality reviews and meta-analyses is increasing. Review articles represent an efficient way to digest and summarize the body of available literature to facilitate up-to-date, evidence-based clinical practice [1–3].

Many types of review articles exist, notably traditional narrative reviews, systematic reviews and meta-analysis. However, these vary with regard to their methodological rigour, their susceptibility to bias, and the accuracy of their results (Table 15.1) [1].

While traditional narrative reviews provide a general overview of a particular topic or question [1], systematic reviews attempt to address a focused clinical question and utilize an explicit and reproducible strategy to identify, appraise and summarize the primary literature [3]. In meta-analyses, quantitative results are then synthesized to produce a single best estimate of effect. Systematic reviews and meta-analyses are typically restricted to a specific population, intervention, comparator and outcome—for example, the use of nailing versus plating in the management of humeral neck fractures in trauma patients and its effect on post-operative complications rates at specific times [1].

Systematic reviews and meta-analyses are generally at the top of the level of evidence (LOE) hierarchy but do still have limitations [6–8]. Their quality is dependent on the quality of the primary studies being reviewed, and therefore their value, as a summary of the primary literature, is limited by the input: colloquially, 'garbage in, garbage out' [9].

This chapter seeks to familiarize surgeons with the basic techniques for critically appraising systematic reviews and meta-analyses as presented in the surgical literature.

Clinical Scenario

You are a plastic surgeon and are asked to see a 55-year-old commercial pilot who presents following a fall onto his dominant right hand with pain localized to the anatomical snuffbox. After completing your history and physical examination, you suspect the patient may have an acute

A. Copeland (✉) · L. Gallo
Department of Surgery, Division of Plastic and Reconstructive Surgery, McMaster University, Hamilton, ON, Canada
e-mail: andrea.copeland@medportal.ca

L. Gallo
e-mail: lucas.gallo@medportal.ca

N. Alolabi
Department of Orthopedics, Division of Hand and Microvascular Surgery, Mayo Clinic, Rochester, MN, USA
e-mail: noor.alolabi@medportal.ca

A. Thoma et al. (eds.), *Evidence-Based Surgery*,
https://doi.org/10.1007/978-3-030-05120-4_15

Table 15.1 Differences between traditional narrative reviews, systematic reviews and meta-analyses* [1, 4–7]

	Narrative review	Systematic review	Meta-analysis
Research question	Broad	Focused	Focused
Literature search	Not reported, or not comprehensive	Explicit, reproducible	Explicit, reproducible
Article selection criteria	Not reported	Criterion-based, complete	Criterion-based, complete
Quality assessment	Not reported	Methodology assessed	Methodology assessed
Result summary	Qualitative	Qualitative	Quantitative

scaphoid fracture. Radiographs demonstrate a non-displaced scaphoid waist fracture. You communicate the results to the patient and discuss potential management options. The patient expresses that he is eager to quickly return to work and asks whether surgery will shorten his recovery time. You are uncertain whether cast immobilization or surgical fixation better quickens return to work (RTW) outcomes. You place the patient in a thumb spica splint and arrange follow-up to discuss the available evidence.

Finding the Evidence

This scenario can be structured in PICOT format as in Table 15.2.

This can then be summarized into the following research question: 'Among adult patients with acute, non-displaced scaphoid waist fractures, does operative management decrease the time to RTW compared to non-surgical management?' A large systematic review and meta-analysis or a large randomized controlled trial are preferable, as they lie at the top of the hierarchy of scientific evidence [10].

To find the evidence to your question, you perform a literature search. You limit your search to the following inclusion criteria: (1) English language articles, (2) systematic reviews or RCTs published within the last 10 years, (3) adult (age $\geq$ 18 years) population and (4) articles that assess RTW outcomes following surgical versus non-surgical management of acute non-displaced scaphoid fractures. You exclude the following: (1) nonrandomized observational studies, and (2) studies which evaluate outcomes following displaced scaphoid fractures.

Searching the MEDLINE database from the National Library of Medicine, you derive your keywords from the clinical question. You enter the terms 'Surgical' AND 'Cast Immobilization' AND 'Scaphoid Fracture' AND 'Return to Work'; which yields 15 results—Appendix 1. You limit the search to 'Systematic Reviews', narrowing it to two articles. One article [11] assesses the intervention of interest; however, it restricts its patient group to high demand manual workers between 16 and 40 years of age. Therefore, the patient group being studied is significantly younger and not consistent with the patient described in the clinical scenario. The remaining article by Alnaeem et al. [12] is titled 'A Systematic Review and Meta-Analysis Examining the Differences Between

Table 15.2 Clinical question demonstrated in PICOT format

Population	Patients with non-displaced scaphoid fractures
Intervention	Surgery
Comparison	Cast immobilization
Outcome	Return to work
Time horizon	All time horizons

Table 15.3 Users' guide for how to review systematic reviews

Are the results valid? - Did the review address a sensible clinical question? - Was the search for relevant studies detailed and exhaustive? - Was publication bias assessed? - Were the primary studies of high methodological quality? - Were assessments of studies reproducible?
What are the results? - Were the results similar from study to study? - What are the overall results of the review? - How precise were the results?
Can I apply the results to patient care? - How can I best interpret the results and apply them to my patients? - Were all patient-important outcomes considered? - Is the benefit worth the potential costs and risks?

Adapted from Bhandari et al. [1]

Nonsurgical Management and Percutaneous Fixation of Minimally and Nondisplaced Scaphoid Fractures' [12]. It adequately addresses the question posed in the clinical scenario and you decide to conduct a critical appraisal. You use the following guide, adapted from Bhandari et al. [1], to help guide your analysis (Table 15.3).

Are the Results Valid?

Did the Review Address a Sensible Clinical Question?

A good research question is both focused and clinically relevant [13]. A focused question yields a consistent treatment effect across the range of Population, Intervention, Comparison, Outcomes, and Time Horizons (the 'PICOT elements'). Consider the hypothetical example of a systematic review that pools the results from all therapies, both operative and non-operative, for all types of upper extremity fractures, to generate a single estimate of the effect on union rates. Clinicians would universally agree that this question is too broad and the results would not be useful [6]. Conversely, asking a question with very narrow inclusion and exclusion criteria may produce too few primary studies to review, and decreases the generalizability of the results [2].

A clinically relevant question, as described by Thoma et al. [14] in their article 'Forming the Research Question', meets at least one of the following four criteria:

1. The intervention is novel;
2. The intervention consumes large health care resources;
3. There is a controversy on the effectiveness of the novel procedure as compared with the existing procedure or;
4. There is a large cost difference between two prevailing interventions.

For a complete description on forming a surgical research question, please refer to Chap. 3.

Alnaeem et al. [12] study addresses an appropriately focused clinical question with a well-defined population (patients greater than 15 years of age with isolated, acute, non-displaced or minimally displaced scaphoid fractures), intervention (percutaneous or mini-open screw fixation), control (non-operative treatment with cast immobilization), and primary (time to return to work) and secondary (time to union and complication rate) outcomes. In addition, the answer to this clinical question appears to be uncertain in the current body of literature and is therefore clinically relevant. Therefore, you feel that Alnaeem et al. [12] addresses a sensible clinical question, as per the criteria listed above [14].

Was the Search for Relevant Studies Detailed and Exhaustive?

The ultimate goal of a search strategy for a systematic review is to include the entire body of evidence that is relevant for a given research question [15]. The published and unpublished literature should be searched, including English and non-English journals [2]. The inclusion of journals in multiple languages reduces the risk of language bias, whereby studies with positive results are preferentially accepted to English language journals, and therefore may result in an overestimation of treatment effect in the systematic review. It also strengthens the generalizability of the results [3, 7].

Most investigators will search common bibliographic databases such as MEDLINE, EMBASE and Cochrane Controlled Trials Register (see the article by Haines et al. [2] for descriptions and uses of these databases). However, there is controversy regarding the inclusion of unpublished literature in systematic reviews. Since unpublished studies are more likely to be methodologically weak, their inclusion may compromise the validity of the meta-analysis. Conversely, omitting them may lead to publication bias (see the following section). Therefore, it is preferable to include unpublished studies in the search strategy and subsequently perform subgroup analysis to determine whether publication impacts the results. Unpublished studies can be identified by hand searching conference proceedings and contacting experts in the field [2, 6, 16]. Consulting a medical librarian helps reassure the reader that the search was exhaustive [2, 3]. Publishing the search strategy also ensures transparency and reproducibility.

Moreover, investigators may also choose to evaluate the completeness of a literature search through the use of Capture-Mark-Recapture (CMR) techniques as a means to estimate the population of articles available for a given topic, known as a horizon estimation [17]. While the specifics of CMR methodology may extend beyond the scope of this chapter, it requires that study authors establish a priori search stopping criteria (% of total article estimate), perform a search of likely databases and complete screening to final inclusion, calculate the horizon estimate using CMR techniques and subsequently compare article retrieval with the established horizon estimate to determine whether the initial search stopping criteria is satisfied [17]. This technique encourages authors to continue to search additional sources and therefore guide efficient search strategies [17].

Finally, two or more independent investigators should be involved in article selection and data abstraction to minimize errors and limit selection bias. In a recent meta-analysis of systematic reviews, 48.4% of systematic reviews used two or more independent data extractors [7].

Alnaeem et al. [12] used a defined time frame (1974–2015), identified their primary databases (PubMed MEDLINE, Ovid MEDLINE, EMBASE, SCOPUS, Cochrane central register of controlled trials and Cochrane bone, joint and muscle trauma registry), listed their search terms ('scaphoid', 'navicular' or 'hand fracture'; 'percutaneous or screw fixation'; 'conservative', 'immobilization' or 'cast'; 'miniopen' or 'minimally invasive'), and provided the complete search strategy in an Appendix 1, making it adequately reproducible. Additionally, Alnaeem et al. [12] screened all articles using two independent reviewers ('H.A. and J.K.'), ultimately limiting the potential for errors and minimizing selection bias. However, you notice that the authors did not mention if their literature search was performed with the help of a medical librarian. Furthermore, non-English articles and the unpublished literature were excluded and there is no estimate of search completeness using CMR techniques.

Was Publication Bias Assessed?

Publication bias is 'the selective publication of research findings based on the magnitude, direction or statistical significance of the study result' [18]. Small studies with negative results are less frequently submitted or accepted for publication. In a systematic review that excludes the unpublished literature, publication bias may, therefore, lead to an overestimation of treatment effect and potentially a false-positive result [2, 16, 19, 20].

Publication bias is frequently explored with a funnel plot. As demonstrated by Tseng et al. [21], this diagram plots the effect size (x axis) against the sample size (y axis) of individual studies. In studies with larger sample sizes, shown at the top of the plot, the scattered dots are closer together representing higher precision. Smaller studies, at the bottom of the plot, are located more peripherally, representing over- or under-estimation of a treatment effect. If there is no publication bias, the dots create a symmetrical, inverted funnel shape. If, however, there is a paucity of small studies with negative findings, the plot will appear asymmetrical at the bottom, implying publication bias [21]. To complement this qualitative representation, a statistical test (e.g. rank correlation test) should be utilized, though it has limited power where the meta-analysis is small (<25 studies) [4, 16, 20].

In the study by Alnaeem et al. [12], publication bias was not addressed.

Were the Primary Studies of High Methodological Quality?

To avoid duplication and promote greater transparency, the PROSPERO database was developed in 2011 for authors of systematic reviews and meta-analyses to prospectively register research protocols where there are at least one health-related outcome [22]. It is recommended that authors publish their protocols as it allows readers to compare it to its completed review and assess for any discrepancies, ultimately minimizing the opportunity for reporting bias [22].

Additionally, the Preferred Reporting Items for Systematic reviews and Meta-Analysis (PRISMA) statement [23] is a 27-item checklist and flow diagram that was originally published in 2009 to help authors improve the reporting quality of their systematic reviews and meta-analyses. While not considered to be a quality assessment instrument, the PRISMA statement can be referenced to critically appraise academic review articles published within the literature [23].

The quality of a systematic review is only as sound as that of its primary articles, thus the methodological quality of primary articles should be assessed. In one study, 35.3% of systematic reviews published in the plastic surgery literature evaluated the methodological quality of the primary studies, and 30% factored this into their conclusions [7].

At present, there is no single, universally endorsed assessment instrument to evaluate the methodological quality of primary studies referenced within systematic reviews and meta-analyses [6]. While several composite scoring tools exist (i.e. checklists and scales), the three-item Jadad score [24], which can be used for the assessment of RCTs (i.e. randomization, double-blinding and participant withdrawal), and the 12-item MINORs score [25], which can be used for the evaluation of nonrandomized trials, are common examples.

While composite scoring tools are commended for their ease of use, they are often criticized for simply recording whether or not methodological safeguards (i.e. allocation concealment) were reported rather than assess whether they were performed appropriately within a trial (see Voineskos et al. [26]). Domain-based evaluations such as the Cochrane Collaboration's Risk of Bias tool [27], assesses and reports each quality component individually. This 'component approach' gives a more transparent analysis of methodological quality and should be utilized [20, 27–30].

Instead of excluding primary studies that are found to have poor methodological quality, investigators should perform a subgroup analysis to determine the impact of the quality score on the results [1].

In the chosen article by Alnaeem et al. [12] methodological quality of the primary studies was appropriately assessed. For RCTs, both the Cochrane Collaboration's tool and the Jadad score [24] were used; however, only the Jadad score was reported in the results section. For observational studies, the MINORS score [25] was used. Overall, the authors concluded that the quality of included studies was 'satisfactory'. However, you notice that they did not use the quality scores to include or exclude any of the studies, nor did they perform subgroup analysis to compare the effect of methodological quality on treatment effect. Furthermore, assessing and reporting the components of methodological quality individually is more transparent and useful than using scales that simply produce a summative score [6, 26].

Were Assessments of Studies Reproducible?

Systematic reviews must have a reproducible selection process. Eligibility criteria and data to be extracted should be listed. The selection process can be visually represented in the form of a

PRISMA flow diagram [31]. Each stage should be conducted by two or more independent reviewers to minimize error and bias. Interobserver agreement, such as the kappa statistic, should then be measured. If there is good chance-correlated agreement between investigators, the reader will have more confidence in the results of the review [6, 13]. In addition to the kappa statistic, it is useful to report the variables on which the reviewers most often disagreed. This adds another level of transparency to the selection and data extraction process [21].

The process of study selection by Alnaeem et al. [12] was systematic and the process was appropriately documented in a PRISMA flow diagram (Appendix 2). Two independent reviewers were involved in title and abstract screening, full-text review, and quality assessment of primary studies and disagreements were resolved by consensus. However, the degree of interobserver agreement (i.e. the kappa statistic) was not reported.

What Are the Results?

Were the Results Similar From Study To Study?

A meta-analysis creates a single summary estimate of treatment effect by combining individual studies as though their sample size were all part of one larger study. However, the effect size of each study should be similar enough to justify combining them. Some variation is expected between studies due to chance. The question becomes, then to what extent are the observed differences in effect size greater than one would expect by chance.

This question can be answered both visually, by inspecting the point estimates and confidence intervals on a Forest plot, and statistically, by using tests of heterogeneity. In the context of systematic reviews and meta-analyses, heterogeneity refers to the differences in the effect sizes appreciated (intervention outcomes) across included studies. Specifically, similar point estimates and greatly overlapping confidence intervals indicate less heterogeneity and make the pooled summary estimate more meaningful [6, 16].

While visual inspection of the Forest plot gives the reader a rough estimate of heterogeneity, statistical tests like the *I* squared statistic (I^2) are important to quantify heterogeneity. *I* squared (I^2) describes the percentage of total variation attributable to underlying differences in effect (i.e. heterogeneity) rather than chance [32]. A value above 50% represents substantial heterogeneity. Another test assessing heterogeneity is Cochrane's *Q* test (measured with a chi-square test). A low *p*-value (<0.1) indicates that the observed differences are unlikely to be due to chance. Unfortunately, these tests may lack power to detect statistically significant heterogeneity when the review includes too few studies with few patients in each study [2, 20, 21].

In summary, widely different point estimates, non-overlapping confidence intervals, a high *I* squared (I^2) value, and a low *p*-value associated with the chi square test should raise concern about pooling results across studies into a single summary estimate.

If substantial heterogeneity exists between studies, authors should look for explanations by performing a subgroup analysis [16], since combining two differing subgroups could lead to misleading conclusions [2, 3]. Other potential sources of heterogeneity may include differences in study groups, interventions, controls, outcome reporting, time horizons and research methodology. These hypotheses of potential sources of heterogeneity should be made a priori, to reduce the likelihood of false-positive findings.

Finally, the degree of heterogeneity between studies should direct the choice of statistical effect estimate model. While random-effects models account for variation both within studies and between studies, fixed-effects models assume there is one true effect size underlying all studies and hence do not consider between-study variation. They are, therefore, only appropriate for meta-analyses with a large number of homogenous studies (typically *I* squared (I^2) $<25\%$). If any degree of heterogeneity is suspected, a random-effects model, while it will produce larger confidence intervals, is the more conservative choice. The reader should be suspicious of a fixed-effect model in the surgical literature, given the inevitable heterogeneity demonstrated by surgery [2, 16].

Alnaeem et al. [12] chose the time to RTW as the primary end point. A random-effects model was appropriately chosen. The individual studies had similar point estimates and overlapping CIs. Heterogeneity was tested using the chi-square test, which was statistically significant ($p = 0.0008$), and the I squared statistic (I^2), calculated at 79%. This suggests that 79% of the observed variability cannot be explained by chance alone, indicating high heterogeneity. This heterogeneity may be attributable to differences in the study groups (e.g. athletes may be more motivated to return to work), intervention (e.g. variations in surgical technique and post-operative regimen), control (e.g. different durations of cast immobilization) or outcomes (e.g. different methods of measuring return to work—insurance forms vs. patient reported). No attempt to identify reasons for heterogeneity with subgroup analysis was reported in the Alnaeem et al. [12] article.

What Are the Overall Results of the Review?

After completing the systematic review, if the primary studies are of poor quality or are too heterogeneous, the data should be presented qualitatively. However, a meta-analysis is performed if the data are appropriate for pooling. The rationale for pooling should be also stated.

Not all studies need to be pooled. For example, nonrandomized data could be included in the systematic review but excluded from the meta-analysis. Alternatively, all studies could be included in the meta-analysis, but the RCTs could be analyzed separately from the non-RCTs [3].

Results from a meta-analysis are typically displayed graphically as Forest plots (Fig. 15.1). Outcomes for dichotomous variables are expressed as ratios, while continuous outcome measures are expressed as weighted or standard mean differences. Individual study results are presented in rows. A box represents the study's effect estimate and its associated whiskers represent the confidence interval (CI). The longer the whiskers, the less precise the estimate. If the CI crosses the 'line of no effect', it is considered not statistically significant. This is also expressed as a probability value (p value) in the 'test for overall effect'. The weighting of an individual study is represented by the size of its box and is typically determined by its sample size and the precision of its results [33]. Occasionally, studies are also weighted by their methodological quality [1]. At the bottom of the Forest plot, the data are pooled from the weighted averages of the study results and is depicted as a diamond, where the centre of the diamond indicates the overall effect estimate and the width of the diamond depicts the overall CI [33].

Finally, the pooled effect size should ideally be represented in units that are easy to interpret and meaningful to clinicians and patients. Dichotomous outcomes should be reported as absolute risk reduction and number needed to treat (see Chap. 6). Continuous outcomes should reference a patient-important effect size, such as minimal important difference [34].

In the selected study [12], ten articles were included in qualitative analysis and six were selected for meta-analysis, excluding four case series. Five of these six articles measured the primary outcome (time to return to work). The calculated pooled mean difference was 38.64 days (95% CI, 27.9–49.48), indicating that patients who underwent percutaneous surgical fixation returned to work 38.64 days earlier than those who were treated non-operatively. There was no reference made to minimal important difference, which makes the pooled mean difference of 38.64 days somewhat less meaningful; however, one must consider the 'importance' of all outcomes in the context of the individual patient, ultimately considering their stated goals and beliefs.

How Precise Were the Results?

Precision of results is determined by the size of the CI around its point estimate. A small sample size and a wide standard deviation both widen the CI. A narrow CI indicates a more precise summary estimate [6].

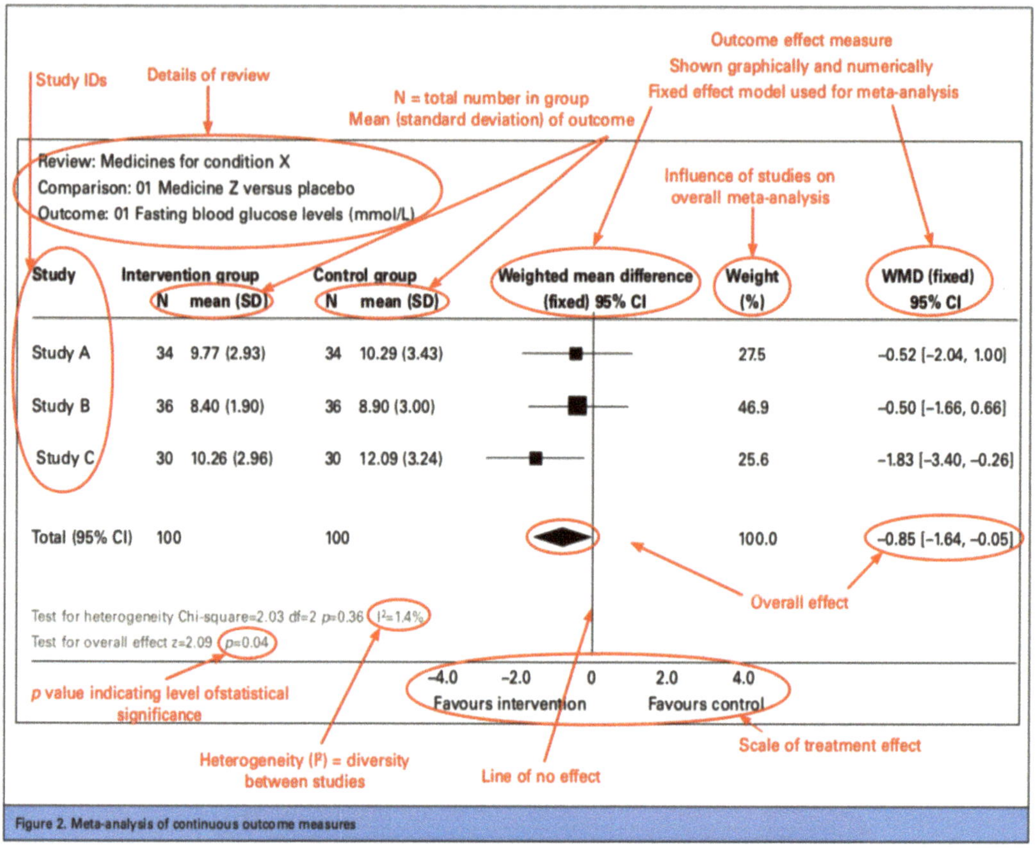

Fig. 15.1 Meta-analysis of continuous outcome measures

In the Alnaeem et al. article [12], the CI informs us that we can be certain with 95% probability that the true benefit of surgical fixation is a faster return to work that lies between 27.9 and 49.48 days. This relatively narrow CI indicates a precise result. It does not cross the line of no effect and the p value is <0.00001, indicating statistical significance.

Can I Apply the Results to My Patients?

How Can I Best Interpret the Results and Apply Them to My Patients?

While a systematic review or meta-analysis may support the use of a particular intervention, it is the responsibility of the surgeon to ensure that the findings are applicable to his or her patient. After assessing the internal validity of the study, surgeons should review treatment settings, inclusion/exclusion criteria, and patient characteristics to ensure adequate external validity that will demonstrate similar outcomes to their patient population [21].

The study by Alnaeem et al. [12] included English articles published prior to 2015 with $n > 10$, that assessed percutaneous fixation (or miniopen technique) of isolated, acute, non-displaced scaphoid fractures in patients older than 15 years of age. Your patient—a 55-year-old male commercial pilot presenting with an acute non-displaced scaphoid waist fracture—fits the inclusion criteria and study characteristics. The study has appropriate external validity for the results to be applied to your patient.

Were All Patient-Important Outcomes Considered?

Along with a defined primary outcome, other relevant outcomes must be considered when informing clinical decisions. Specifically, the effectiveness of an intervention should be derived by measuring 'patient-important outcomes'—the clinical events deemed relevant to a specific patient population [5, 35]. These outcomes may include the occurrence of stroke, death or quality of life outcomes. For example, potential patient-important outcomes of percutaneous fixation for scaphoid fracture include the risk of infection, reoperation, and neurovascular injury. A focused review of the evidence may provide an accurate result of the effect of fixation on each of these outcomes, but an informed clinical decision requires that all outcomes be considered. As a result, the ideal systematic review will present a series of reviews for each patient-important outcome [6, 20].

A limitation of most systematic reviews and meta-analyses remains that they frequently do not report all relevant patient-important outcomes [1]. While reasons for this may vary, one explanation is that individual studies often measure outcomes differently, or not at all, making it difficult to pool and summarize results [1, 6]. To address this, the implementation of core outcome sets (COS) has been proposed. COS have been defined within the literature as an agreed upon set of outcomes that should be reported at a minimum in all studies assessing a particular condition [36, 37]. This initiative, referred to as Core Outcome Measures in Effectiveness Trials (COMET), seeks to improve homogeneity in outcome reporting to improve outcome-pooling in the form of systematic reviews and meta-analyses [32]. Authors and readers of systematic reviews are encouraged to review COMET resources to identify whether a set of 'core outcomes' exist for their condition of interest.

In addition to time to return to work, Alnaeem et al. [12] also evaluated the adverse effects of therapy, which is considered a patient-important outcome. They found a higher complication rate in the operative group (14% vs. 7%) but this was not statistically significant ($p = 0.2$). Again, this outcome must be considered in the context of the patient's own stated goals and beliefs; while not statistically significant, this may represent a clinical and patient-important difference. Quality of life outcome measures were not assessed as they were inconsistently reported in the primary studies.

Is the Benefit Worth the Potential Costs and Risks?

Either explicitly or implicitly, it is the responsibility of surgeons to make recommendations by weighing the potential costs and benefits of an intervention in the context of the patient's values and preferences [6]. For example, a manual labourer may deem continued observation to be an unacceptable management strategy and may instead opt for prompt surgical intervention. As a result, systematic reviews should avoid specific care recommendations as they are unable to account for specific patient circumstances and values that can only be determined through direct consultation with the patient [21].

In the chosen example, the patient's primary concern was returning to work. Complication rates and time to union should also be discussed. Overall, given that the results for RTW and radiographic union statistically favour the surgical group with no significant difference in complication rate, one can infer based on the available evidence that surgical intervention provides a benefit. However, it is important to note the significant heterogeneity for time to RTW and time to union, with I squared (I^2) values of 79 and 88%, respectively. When this is considered in the context of the patient's expressed preference to RTW, one can conclude that the potential benefits of surgical intervention may outweigh the costs and risks for this particular patient; however, the results should be interpreted with caution and must be considered in the context of the patient's own beliefs given the increased complication risk associated with undergoing surgical intervention.

Resolution of the Clinical Scenario

At the follow-up appointment, you report your findings to the patient. You conclude that the statistically significant results presented in the study by Alnaeem et al. [12] have adequate internal and external validity and ultimately support the use of percutaneous pinning to improve RTW outcomes and union rates. You inform the patient that surgical fixation demonstrated an increased prevalence of complications, although not statistically significant. The patient reaffirms his desire to return to work as soon as possible despite this risk and the decision is made to pursue surgical management.

Conclusion

While systematic reviews and meta-analyses represent the top of the level of evidence hierarchy, they are not without limitations. Consequently, surgeons must possess the skills to interpret the results of review articles to recognize the potential for bias and appropriately assess their application to clinical practice.

Appendix 1: Search Results

1. Arora R, Gschwentner M, Krappinger D, Lutz M, Blauth M, Gabl M. Fixation of nondisplaced scaphoid fractures: making treatment cost effective. Arch Orthop Trauma Surg. 2006;127(1):39–46.
2. Schernberg F. Recent scaphoid fractures (within the first three weeks). Chir Main. 2005;24(3, 4):117–31.
3. Geurts G, Van Riet R, Meermans G, Verstreken F. Volar percutaneous transtrapezial fixation of scaphoid waist fractures: surgical technique. Acta Orthop Belg. 2012;78 (1):121–5.
4. Majeed H. Non-operative treatment versus percutaneous fixation for minimally displaced scaphoid waist fractures in high demand young manual workers. J Orthop Traumatol. 2014;15(4):239–44.
5. Alnaeem H, Aldekhayel S, Kanevsky J, Neel O. A systematic review and meta-analysis examining the differences between nonsurgical management and percutaneous fixation of minimally and nondisplaced scaphoid fractures. J Hand Surg. 2016;41(12):1135–44.
6. Drexier M, Haim A, Pritsch T, Rosenblatt Y. Isolated fractures of the scaphoid: classification, treatment and outcome. Harefuah. 2011;150(1):50–5.
7. Bond C, Shin A, McBride M, Dao K. Percutaneous screw fixation or cast immobilization for nondisplaced scaphoid fractures. J Bone Joint Surg Am. 2001;83(4):483–8.
8. Schädel-Höpfner M, Marent-Huber M, Sauerbier M, Pillukat T, Eisenschenk A, Siebert H. Operative versus conservative treatment of non-displaced fractures of the scaphoid bone. Results of a controlled multicenter cohort study. Unfallchirurg. 2010;113(10):804–13.
9. Fowler J, Ilyas A. Headless compression screw fixation of scaphoid fractures. Hand Clin. 2010;26(3):351–61.
10. Yinusa W, Adetan O, Odatuwa-Omagbemi D, Eyo M. Bilateral simultaneous fracture of the carpal scaphoid successfully treated with conservative cast immobilisation: a case report. West Afr J Med. 2010;29(6):425–8.
11. Haddad F, Goddard N. Acute percutaneous scaphoid fixation: a pilot study. J Bone Joint Surg. 1998;80(1):95–9.
12. Soubeyrand M, Even J, Mansour C, Gagey O, Molina V, Biau D. Cadaveric assessment of a new guidewire insertion device for volar percutaneous fixation of nondisplaced scaphoid fracture. Injury. 2009;40(6):645–51.
13. Noaman H, Shiha A, Ibrahim A. Functional outcomes of nonunion scaphoid fracture treated by pronator quadratus pedicled bone graft. Ann Plast Surg. 2011;66(1):47–52.
14. McQueen M, Gelbke M, Wakefield A, Will E, Gaebler C. Percutaneous screw fixation versus conservative treatment for fractures of the waist of the scaphoid. J Bone Joint Surg Br. 2008;90(1):66–71.
15. Yin Z, Zhang J, Kan S, Wang P. Treatment of acute scaphoid fractures. Clin Orthop Relat Res. 2007;460(1):142–51.

Appendix 2: Prisma Flow Diagram [23, 38]

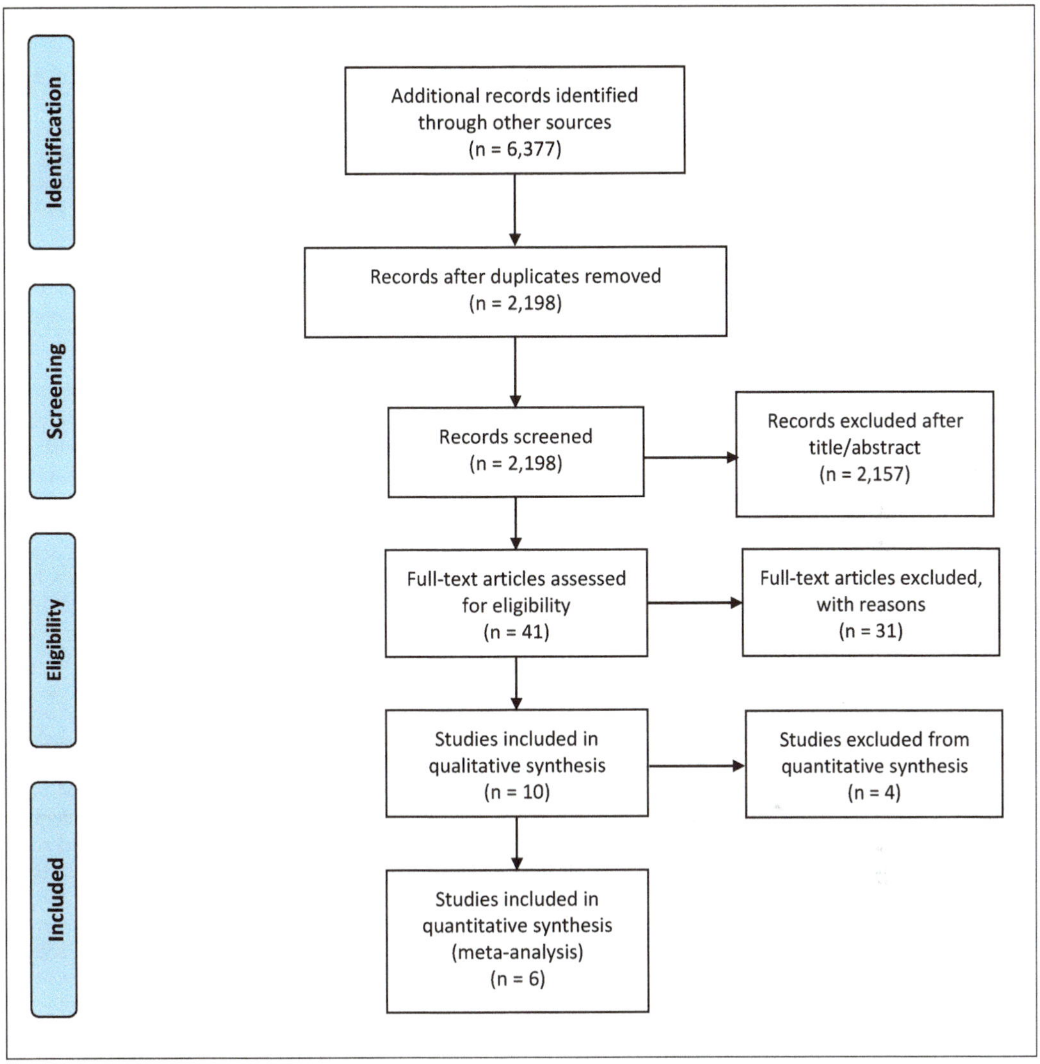

References

1. Bhandari M, Devereaux PJ, Montori V, Cinà C, Tandan V, Guyatt GH, et al. Users' guide to the surgical literature: how to use a systematic literature review and meta-analysis. Can J Surg. 2004;47(1):60–7.
2. Haines T, McKnight L, Duku E, Perry L, Thoma A. The role of systematic reviews in clinical research and practice. Clin Plast Surg. 2008;35(2):207–14.
3. Kelley BP, Chung KC. Developing, conducting, and publishing appropriate systematic review and meta-analysis articles. Plast Reconstr Surg. 2018;141(2):516–25.
4. Begg CB, Mazumdar M. Operating characteristics of a rank correlation test for publication bias. Biometrics. 1994;50(4):1088–101.
5. Fleming TR, DeMets DL. Surrogate end points in clinical trials: are we being misled? Ann Intern Med. 1996;125(7):605–13.
6. Guyatt G, Rennie D, Meade M, Cook D, editors. Users' guides to the medical literature: a manual for evidence-based clinical practice, vol. 706. Chicago, Illinois: McGraw-Hill Education.

7. Samargandi OA, Hasan H, Thoma A. Methodologic quality of systematic reviews published in the plastic and reconstructive surgery literature: a systematic review. Plast Reconstr Surg. 2016;137(1):225e–36e.
8. Sprague S, McKay P, Thoma A. Study design and hierarchy of evidence for surgical decision making. Clin Plast Surg. 2008;35(2):195–205.
9. Egger M, Smith GD, Sterne JA. Uses and abuses of meta-analysis. Clin Med. 2001;1(6):478–84.
10. Petrisor BA, Bhandari M. The hierarchy of evidence: levels and grades of recommendation. Indian J Orthop. 2007;41(1):11–5.
11. Majeed H. Non-operative treatment versus percutaneous fixation for minimally displaced scaphoid waist fractures in high demand young manual workers. J Orthop Traumatol. 2014;15(4):239–44.
12. Alnaeem H, Aldekhayel S, Kanevsky J, Neel OF. A systematic review and meta-analysis examining the differences between nonsurgical management and percutaneous fixation of minimally and nondisplaced scaphoid fractures. J Hand Surg. 2016;41(12):1135–44.
13. Thoma A, Eaves FF III. What is wrong with systematic reviews and meta-analyses: if you want the right answer, ask the right question! Aesthetic Surg J. 2016;36(10):1198–201.
14. Thoma A, McKnight L, McKay P, Haines T. Forming the research question. Clin Plast Surg. 2008;35(2):189–93.
15. Waltho D, Kaur MN, Haynes RB, Farrokhyar F, Thoma A. Users' guide to the surgical literature: how to perform a high-quality literature search. Can J Surg. 2015;58(5):349–58.
16. Zlowodzki M, Poolman RW, Kerkhoffs GM, Tornetta P III, Bhandari M, International Evidence-Based Orthopedic Surgery Working Group. How to interpret a meta-analysis and judge its value as a guide for clinical practice. Acta Orthop. 2007;78(5):598–609.
17. Lane D, Dykeman J, Ferri M, Goldsmith C, Stelfox H. Capture-mark-recapture as a tool for estimating the number of articles available for systematic reviews in critical care medicine. J Crit Care. 2013;28(4):469–75.
18. Montori V, Smieja M, Guyatt G. Publication bias: a brief review for clinicians. Mayo Clin Proc. 2007;75(12):1284–8.
19. Cook DJ, Guyatt GH, Ryan G, Clifton J, Buckingham L, Willan A, et al. Should unpublished data be included in meta-analyses? Current convictions and controversies. JAMA. 1993;269(21):2749–53.
20. Montori VM, Swiontkowski MF, Cook DJ. Methodologic issues in systematic reviews and meta-analyses. Clin Orthop Relat Res. 2003;413:43–54.
21. Tseng TY, Dahm P, Poolman RW, Preminger GM, Canales BJ, Montori VM. How to use a systematic literature review and meta-analysis. J Urol. 2008;180(4):1249–56.
22. Booth A, Clarke M, Dooley G, Ghersi D, Moher D, Petticrew M, et al. PROSPERO at one year: an evaluation of its utility. Syst Rev. 2013;2(1):1–7.
23. Moher D, Liberati A, Tetzlaff J, Altman D. Preferred reporting items for systematic reviews and meta-analyses: the PRISMA statement. PLoS Med. 2009;6(7):e1000097.
24. Jadad A, Moore R, Carroll D, Jenkinson C, Reynolds D, Gavaghan D, et al. Assessing the quality of reports of randomized clinical trials: is blinding necessary? Control Clin Trials. 1996;17(1):1–12.
25. Slim K, Nini E, Forestier D, Kwiatkowski F, Panis Y, Chipponi J. Methodological index for non-randomized studies (MINORS): development and validation of a new instrument. ANZ J Surg. 2003;73(9):712–6.
26. Voineskos SH, Coroneos CJ, Ziolkowski NI, Kaur MN, Banfield L, Meade MO, et al. A systematic review of surgical randomized controlled trials: part I. Risk of bias and outcomes common pitfalls plastic surgeons can overcome. Plast Reconstr Surg. 2016;137(2):696–706.
27. Higgins JP, Green S, editors. Cochrane handbook for systematic reviews of interventions (version 5.1. 0). London, UK: The Cochrane Collaboration; 2016.
28. Jüni P, Altman DG, Egger M. Assessing the quality of controlled clinical trials. BMJ. 2001;323(7303):42–6.
29. Jüni P, Witschi A, Bloch R, Egger M. The hazards of scoring the quality of clinical trials for meta-analysis. JAMA. 1999;282(11):1054–60.
30. Moher D, Jadad AR, Nichol G, Penman M, Tugwell P, Walsh S. Assessing the quality of randomized controlled trials: an annotated bibliography of scales and checklists. Control Clin Trials. 1995;16(1):62–73.
31. Liberati A, Altman DG, Tetzlaff J, Mulrow C, Gøtzsche PC, Ioannidis JP, et al. The PRISMA statement for reporting systematic reviews and meta-analyses of studies that evaluate health care interventions: explanation and elaboration. PLoS Med. 2009;6(7):e1000100.
32. Higgins JP, Thompson SG, Deeks JJ, Altman DG. Measuring inconsistency in meta-analyses. BMJ. 2003;327(7414):557.
33. Ried K. Interpreting and understanding meta-analysis graphs: a practical guide. Aust Fam Physician. 2006;35(8):635–8.
34. Evaniew N, van der Watt L, Bhandari M, Ghert M, Aleem I, Drew B, et al. Strategies to improve the credibility of meta-analyses in spine surgery: a systematic survey. Spine J. 2015;15(9):2066–76.
35. Gallo L, Eskicioglu C, Braga LH, Farrokhyar F, Thoma A. Users' guide to the surgical literature: how

to assess an article using surrogate end points. Can J Surg. 2017;60(4):280.

36. Prinsen CA, Vohra S, Rose MR, King-Jones S, Ishaque S, Bhaloo Z, et al. Core Outcome Measures in Effectiveness Trials (COMET) initiative: protocol for an international Delphi study to achieve consensus on how to select outcome measurement instruments for outcomes included in a 'core outcome set'. Trials. 2014;15(1):247.
37. Potter S, Holcombe C, Ward JA, Blazeby JM, BRAVO Steering Group. Development of a core outcome set for research and audit studies in reconstructive breast surgery. Br J Surg. 2015;102 (11):1360–71.
38. Preferred reporting items for systematic reviews and meta-analyses: the PRISMA statement [Internet]. Equator-network.org. 2018 [cited 2018 Sep 10]. Available from: http://www.equator-network.org/reporting-guidelines/prisma/.

16 Prospective and Retrospective Cohort Studies

Ramy Behman, Lev Bubis and Paul Karanicolas

Introduction

Cohort studies are a type of observational study that follows samples of at-risk individuals forward in time to examine associations between measured exposures and future outcomes. Exposures may include surgical techniques, medical interventions, patient characteristics or health-system factors [1].

Cohort studies are classified as prospective or retrospective. In prospective cohort studies, enrolment of the cohort and determination of exposure status occur before any subjects experience the outcome—with subjects subsequently followed forward in real time. Retrospective cohort studies, by contrast, are designed after outcomes have occurred. Investigators conducting retrospective cohort studies look backward in time to identify a cohort of at-risk individuals and ascertain their exposure status, then look ahead towards the present to determine if they experienced the outcome. In general, retrospective cohort studies are less costly and time-consuming compared with prospective studies. However, retrospective studies often rely on data sources designed for other purposes.

Compared to cohort studies, randomized controlled trials (RCTs) generally provide a higher level of evidence about the effectiveness of interventions owing to their lower risk of bias [2]. Nevertheless, cohort studies have an essential role in evidence-based surgery. Cohort studies are the optimal study design to evaluate prognostic factors; allowing for efficient longitudinal follow-up of large, representative study samples—including subgroups often excluded or under-sampled in RCTs [3–5]. Cohort studies are also invaluable for the study of multiple exposures, rare exposures, exposures with known risks to which it would be unethical to allocate study subjects, or in situations where there is a long duration of time between exposure and outcome.

Clinical Scenario

You are the resident on call at a busy academic hospital, where you are assessing a 78-year-old woman presenting with abdominal pain, nausea, vomiting and obstipation. Her medical history is notable for an open hysterectomy for uterine fibroids. Findings on CT scan are consistent with

R. Behman · L. Bubis
Department of Surgery, University of Toronto, Toronto, ON, Canada
e-mail: ramy.behman@main.utoronto.ca

L. Bubis
e-mail: lev.bubis@mail.utoronto.ca

P. Karanicolas (✉)
Department of Surgery, University of Toronto, Sunnybrook Health Sciences Centre, Sunnybrook Research Institute, Toronto, ON, Canada
e-mail: paul.karanicolas@sunnybrook.ca

A. Thoma et al. (eds.), *Evidence-Based Surgery*,
https://doi.org/10.1007/978-3-030-05120-4_16

your clinical diagnosis of adhesive small bowel obstruction (aSBO). There is no indication for urgent surgical exploration, so you admit the patient for a trial of non-operative management. The following morning at handover, the attending surgeon asks if you administered a water-soluble contrast study. You explain that you have never used this technique. The attending surgeon suggests you review this intervention, stating there is evidence of both diagnostic and therapeutic benefit [6].

Literature Search

That evening (5 June 2018), you search Medline. Entering 'adhesive small bowel obstruction AND contrast', your search strategy yields 96 results. Reviewing these, you find a recently published titled 'Multi-institutional, prospective, observational study comparing the Gastrografin challenge versus standard treatment in adhesive small bowel obstruction' to begin your literature review [7]. You elect to begin your literature review with this article, as you believe its large sample size, recruitment from large academic medical centres, and recency of completion make it likely to be relevant to your practice setting.

Article Summary

The article by Zielinski and colleagues describes a multicenter prospective cohort study evaluating whether a standardized aSBO treatment protocol incorporating a routine water-soluble contrast study decreases operative interventions, length of stay and complications compared to an aSBO protocol without contrast studies [7]. In a cohort of 316 aSBO patients, the adjusted odds of operative exploration for those receiving contrast studies was statistically significantly lower than for those who did not. Length of stay was also lower in the contrast study group, but complications were similar. The authors concluded that oral contrast challenges provide therapeutic benefit for the management of a patient with aSBO. An outline of the study reported by Zielinski and colleagues [7] is provided in Table 16.1.

Using the study by Zielinski and colleagues [7] as a case study, in the following chapter, we present a practical guide for the appraisal of cohort studies in surgery (Box 1). Our aim is to provide practicing surgeons and trainees with a framework for the evaluation of the methodological quality and applicability of cohort studies.

Box 1. Guide to interpretation of cohort studies in surgery [8]

1. **What are the study's research question and clinical relevance?**
2. **Are the results valid?**

   I. What is the study population?
   IIA. Are the data sources reliable?
   IIB. Are the data collection methods sound?
   III. Do the authors provide clear and justifiable definitions of the primary and secondary outcomes?
   IV. Have the authors accounted for potential sources of bias?
   V. Is the statistical analysis (a) valid and (b) described clearly?

3. **What are the results?**

   I. Are baseline characteristics of the exposure groups clearly reported and accounted for?
   II. Are the results and relevant statistics clearly stated?
   III. How precise were estimates of effect size?
   IV. Are results robust to planned sensitivity analyses?
   V. Were subgroup analyses used? If so, were these specified a priori and is the issue of multiple testing addressed?

Table 16.1 Outline of the prospective cohort study conducted by Zielinski et al. [7]

Study element	Summary
Population and setting	316 patients with aSBO without signs of bowel strangulation, hernia, history of abdominal or pelvic malignancy, or abdominal surgery within 6 weeks presenting to 1 of 14 academic medical centres in the United States
Exposure/comparators and allocation	*Exposure*—aSBO treatment protocol with or without oral contrast challenge *Allocation*—selection of aSBO treatment protocol at discretion of treating surgeon (except at institutions without availability of oral contrast agent)
Results	*Rate of surgical exploration*—20.8% in oral contrast group versus 44.1% in non-contrast group ($p < 0.0001$). On adjusted analysis receipt of oral contrast study was associated with significantly lower odds of operative exploration (aOR 0.23, 95% CI 0.12–0.43) *Overall complication rate*—12.5% in oral contrast group versus 17.9% in non-contrast group ($p = 0.22$) *Length of stay*—median 4 days (Q1–Q3: 2–7 days) in oral contrast group versus median 5 days (Q1–Q3: 2–13 days) in non-contrast group ($p = 0.036$)
Authors' conclusions	Patients managed with an aSBO protocol incorporating routine oral contrast studies had lower rates of surgical exploration and shorter hospital length of stay, without an increase in risk of complications compared to no contrast. Incorporation of an oral contrast study is of benefit in the care of aSBO patients presenting without indications for immediate surgical exploration

Abbreviations aSBO—adhesive small bowel obstruction; aOR—adjusted odds ratio; Q1—first quartile; Q3—third quartile; AUROC—area under the receiver operating characteristic curve

4. **How can I interpret these results in the context of my clinical practice?**
   I. Are the results of the study placed in the broader context of the clinical question?
   II. Is there a description of the existing literature?
   III. Were all clinically important outcomes considered?
   IV. Are limitations of the study clearly described?

This list was modified from Thoma et al. [8].

What are the Study's Research Question and Clinical Relevance?

Study objectives and hypotheses should be described clearly and supported by a coherent rationale, which outlines the clinical importance of the topic. It is important to note that cohort studies are vulnerable to the problematic practices of data dredging and selective reporting [9, 10]. In reading a cohort study, it is often impossible to know whether research questions or methods were altered during the research conduct or if additional unreported analyses were undertaken. As such, protocol registration prior to the commencement of research bolsters the validity of studies. In the article under review, Zielinski and colleagues [7] appropriately described the rationale for conducting their study, the limits of existing evidence and clearly state their a priori hypothesis: that incorporation of contrast challenges into an aSBO protocol will decrease rates of operative exploration, length of stay and complications compared to aSBO protocols without contrast challenges.

Are the Results Valid?

What is the Study Population?

The population of interest should be explicitly specified. A detailed description of the inclusion and exclusion criteria for cohort entry is essential for readers to evaluate to whom the study results apply. Sample size calculations based on anticipated effect sizes in comparative effectiveness studies are valuable to ensure studies are adequately powered to detect clinically meaningful difference between interventions, should they truly exist. In their article, Zielinski et al. [7] appropriately describe study inclusion and exclusion criteria, and provide a sample size calculation based on historic rates of their primary outcome of surgical exploration for aSBO.

Are the Data Sources Reliable?

There should be a clear description of data sources. In retrospective cohort studies, data may be obtained from primary sources (i.e. from chart abstraction and prospective institutional databases) or secondary sources designed for alternate purposes (i.e. from administrative, demographic and physician claims databases) [11]. Some studies have demonstrated poor accuracy of secondary data for surgical outcomes assessment [12, 13]. However, retrospective chart abstraction or creation of institutional databases require a large amount of resources and are unfeasible for large population-based studies. For research using administrative databases, validity may be bolstered through conduct of preliminary studies assessing their accuracy [14, 15]. In prospective studies, data may be obtained via active data collection processes specific to the study or through linkage to routinely collected data from external sources such as registries or population-based databases. For prospective studies using active data collection, reliability may be bolstered by creating clear data collection protocols inclusive of detailed variable definitions prior to study conduct.

Are the Data Collection Methods Sound?

Authors should report on the methods of data collection as well as the extent of missing data. Missing data may compromise the validity of study results. As such, considerable effort should be made to minimize missing data and the method of handling missing data in statistical analyses should be described. In addition, where multiple contributors participate in data collection, assessment of consistency (e.g. inter-rater reliability) is important to assure the quality of data collection [16]. Zielinski et al. [7] do not describe data collection methods used in their study, nor do they describe whether any data was missing. Consequently, readers cannot assess whether data collection methods or missing data impacts the validity of study results.

Do the Authors Provide Clear and Justifiable Definitions of the Primary and Secondary Outcomes?

The outcomes measured in surgical cohort studies should address the key aspects of the clinical question under study. When applicable, authors should justify their designation of primary and secondary outcomes. Methods of outcome ascertainment must be carefully planned and reported with sufficient clarity to be replicable. Zielinski et al. [7] did not explicitly specify primary and secondary outcomes. However, the authors provide a power calculation to determine the sample size required to detect a significant difference in the rate of operative exploration between the contrast and non-contrast groups. Other outcomes reported include length of hospital stay and complications. In addition, Zielinski et al. [7] report the diagnostic accuracy of the oral contrast challenge for prediction of need for operative exploration.

In studies of surgical interventions, the timeframe of outcomes assessment is a key consideration. A high proportion of postoperative complications are diagnosed only after hospital discharge. Data sources that are limited to the index hospitalization may, therefore, substantially undercount postoperative adverse events [12, 17]. In this regard, a limitation of the study conducted by Zielinski et al. [7] is that the timeframe for assessment of the secondary outcomes of complications is not specified. It is possible that study groups may have differing risks of short-term (i.e. in-hospital) and longer term (i.e. 30-day) complications. Therefore, a clear description of timeframes for outcome assessment is imperative to allow readers to fully understand the study results.

Have the Authors Accounted for Potential Sources of Bias?

Bias in observational studies refers to the occurrence of systematic errors in study design or conduct. Compared to random error, which is variable and unpredictable, bias results in systematic deviations from the estimation of true values. The internal validity of a study denotes the extent to which its causal conclusions are justified and rests upon the minimization of bias. There are myriad subtypes of bias [18, 19]. In general, sources of bias can be classified into the following categories: (a) selection bias, (b) information bias, and (c) confounding [20, 21].

Selection Bias

Selection bias refers to systematic errors that arise from the selection of subjects for inclusion in the study. Selection bias may occur when factors related to inclusion of study subjects are associated with exposures or outcomes leading to distortion of effect estimates or unrepresentativeness of the study sample relative to the target population [22].

Cohort studies in surgery may be especially prone to certain types of selection bias. Immortal person-time bias occurs in instances where exposure status is assigned after the onset of follow-up. Assignment to one exposure group, therefore, may be conditional on survival from the time of study onset [23]. Confounding by indication is another important source of bias in cohort studies comparing alternative treatments. Confounding by indication refers to situations where treatment group allocation is dependent upon prognostic factors, which may not all be measured in a cohort study [24].

In the study reported by Zielinski et al. [7], allocation to study groups was based on surgeon selection and institution. While measured baseline variables of the two study groups were similar, unmeasured patient- and disease-related factors may influence allocation by surgeon judgment, leading to selection bias. In addition to the introduction of bias, it does not state in the article if the surgeons had any training, or experience in selection. In contrast to RCTs, in which random allocation produces balance between measured and *unmeasured* covariates, the problem of selection bias is never wholly surmountable in cohort studies. Readers must judge whether the most important covariates for a clinical question are measured and addressed.

Information Bias

Information bias refers to systematic errors in the classification or measurement of variables. Information bias is differential if the error in variable classification is dependent on the value of the outcome or exposure of interest; otherwise, it is non-differential [21]. In theory, information bias should be non-differential in cohort studies if consistent data collection practices are applied across all study subjects. However, in practice, this may not be the case, leading to observer bias or interviewer bias.

Observer bias occurs when outcome ascertainment is influenced by assessors' knowledge of subjects' exposures. Observer bias can be minimized by blinding outcome assessors, having multiple outcome assessors review each subject, using objective outcome measures and by allowing differential levels of certainty for outcome ascertainment (i.e. outcome 'possible', 'probable', or 'definite') [22]. Interviewer bias occurs in prospective studies using personalized interviewers. If interviewers are un-blinded to exposure status, they risk consciously or subconsciously obtaining answers which accord with their preconceptions [22]. In addition to ensuring blinding of study interviewers, measures such as standardized data collection forms and interview scripts may reduce interviewer bias.

Zielinski et al. [7] used an objective primary outcome (operative exploration). However, outcome assessors and the mechanisms for outcome ascertainment are not comprehensively described. Lack of blinding of assessors or divergent methods of outcome assessment at alternate sites in this multicentre study may lead to bias through differential ascertainment of secondary outcomes that are potentially influenced by assessors' judgment (e.g. pneumonia, surgical site infection).

Confounding

Confounding occurs when an apparent association between two factors is distorted by extraneous factors [25]. This distortion occurs when there is an extraneous factor that is independently associated with both the exposure and the outcome of interest [25, 26]. The effect of the exposure on an outcome may be mixed with or mistaken for the effect of an extraneous variable that has not been accounted for (Fig. 16.1).

A classic example of confounding is the association between yellow fingernails and lung cancer. A confounder (smoking) is associated with both the exposure (yellow fingernails) and the outcome (lung cancer). Without appropriately identifying and accounting for potential confounding, a distorted relationship between the exposure and the outcome (that yellow fingernails cause lung cancer) may have been concluded. Similarly, studies of surgical outcomes must consider potential confounders of associations between surgical interventions and clinical outcomes.

Confounding may be divided into two groups: measured confounding and unmeasured confounding [27]. Measured confounding describes potential factors that were measured in the study that can be accounted for in the analysis. Unmeasured confounding refers to potential confounders that were not captured in data collection.

In cohort studies, accounting for potential confounding is often limited to the analysis phase through a variety of statistical approaches. Broadly, these approaches include matching (including propensity score techniques), stratification by potential confounders, and regression (e.g. multivariable models) [28–30]. In the article by Zielinski et al. [7], the authors use multivariable regression to estimate the association between contrast studies and outcomes of interest while adjusting for potential confounders. Chapter 31 describes approaches to confounding in more detail.

Is the Statistical Analysis (a) Valid and (b) Described Clearly?

A description of the statistical analysis should be provided in sufficient detail that, given the dataset, one could replicate the analysis and find identical results. A clear and detailed description of the statistical analysis not only allows for reproducibility but is also necessary to evaluate the validity of a study's methods.

Readers should consider whether the statistical approaches are (1) appropriate for the variables of interest, and (2) account for potential confounding in a suitable manner. Many considerations are necessary to evaluate the validity

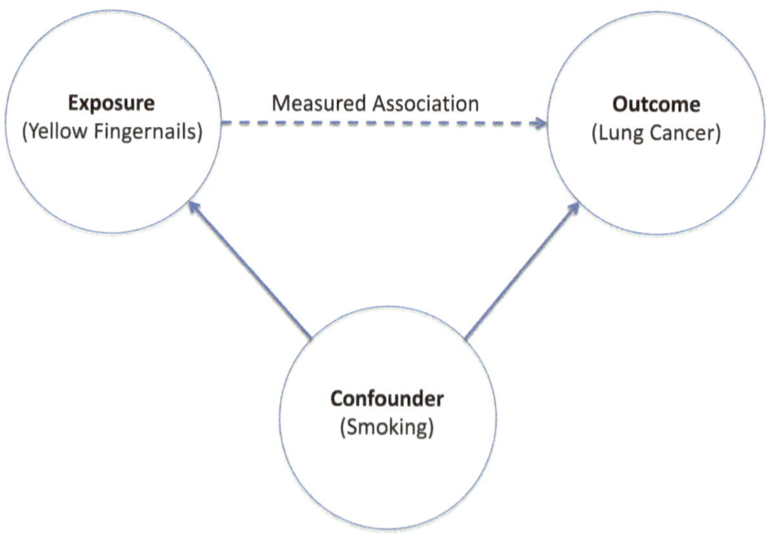

Fig. 16.1 Directed acyclic graph (DAG) illustrating confounding of observed relationship between yellow fingernails and lung cancer by an extraneous factor (smoking)

of an analytical approach; these are discussed in greater detail in Chaps. 27–31.

In the study by Zielinski et al. [7], the final paragraph of the Methods section describes the different variable types, how they were presented and which statistical methods were used to compare them. The authors clearly describe how potentially subjective clinical and radiological variables such as obstipation, mesenteric edema and SB faeces sign were defined for this study.

The covariates selected by the authors for multivariable analysis are valid to the question of interest, albeit not an exhaustive list of potential confounders. Interestingly, the authors elect to include CT findings in the multivariable model for operative exploration, but do not include physiologic or biochemical findings in this model and do not give an explanation as to why these were excluded. While CT findings provide information regarding the degree of bowel obstruction, physiologic and biochemical findings also contribute valuable information that guides clinical decision-making.

What Are the Results?

Are Baseline Characteristics of the Exposure Groups Clearly Reported and Accounted For?

Cohort studies are inherently subject to selection bias, which may distort findings. A clear description of differences in baseline characteristics between treatment groups provides important contextual information with which subsequent results may be interpreted. In the article under study, the baseline characteristics were similar in the two treatment groups, suggesting comparability. However, readers of observational studies should not allow similarity of baseline characteristics to make them confident in a study's results, since unmeasured or unreported baseline characteristics may be different between exposure groups.

When baseline characteristics differ significantly between exposure groups, there should be concern about selection bias. In these instances, analytic methods such as matching or multivariable regression may be used to account for these differences in baseline characteristics. The article by Zielinski et al. [7] reported the baseline characteristics of the two exposure groups in Table 16.1, demonstrating that the groups were similar. The authors included many of the important demographic, clinical and radiological characteristics for patients treated for adhesive SBO. Several potentially relevant baseline characteristics were not described, including duration of symptoms, number of previous admissions for SBO, admitting service (medical vs. surgical), and admission septic status.

It is unclear why the authors include CT findings in Table 1 by Zielinski et al. [7] as 'Baseline Characteristics' but report physiologic and biochemical findings separately. Physiologic and biochemical findings are compared between the two exposure groups separately in Table 2 by Zielinski et al. [7].

Are the Results and Relevant Statistics Clearly Stated?

Results should be clearly described according to the analytical approach outlined in the Methods section of the study. Readers of the study should be able to identify which statistical test yielded the results being described. In addition to the results, the study should report the appropriate statistics (e.g. *p*-value, standardized difference, confidence interval) in a manner that is appropriate to the statistical test and is consistent throughout the study.

In the study by Zielinski et al. [7], univariate analyses (proportions, comparison of means/medians) were reported using *p*-values and multivariable analyses were reported using odds ratios and 95% confidence intervals. The results are clearly stated and the reporting is consistent. Readers are easily able to identify a description of the corresponding analytical approach in the Methods section.

How Precise Were Estimates of Effect Size?

Effect estimates may be reported in a variety of ways, depending on the outcomes of interest. Reporting can vary from simple differences in proportions to absolute/relative risk ratios to odds ratios and hazard ratios. Confidence intervals should be reported to allow readers to determine the precision of effect estimates; similarly, if variability estimates were included the reader could have calculated confidence intervals to determine precision.

Confidence intervals provide important information with which effect sizes should be interpreted. Wide confidence intervals suggest a high degree of uncertainty and that effects should be interpreted with caution; narrow confidence intervals suggest a high degree of certainty of the reported effect size [31, 32]. *P*-values, while not specifically reflecting the precision of effect sizes, are a measure of the type I error—the probability that an observed effect is due to chance. Both confidence intervals and *p*-values are dependent on sample size and error [31–33].

In the article under study, the authors clearly describe the key results, dividing these into diagnostic outcomes and therapeutic outcomes. With respect to the diagnostic ability of water-soluble contrast studies, the authors report the positive-predictive value, negative-predictive value, and estimate the area under the receiver operating characteristic (AUROC) curve (a measure of a test's diagnostic ability) of water-soluble contrast studies. The authors did not report likelihood ratios, which should be reported in evaluations of diagnostic ability in addition to positive- and negative-predictive values. The authors report the primary therapeutic outcome (rates of surgical exploration) using univariate and multivariable analyses, reporting proportions with chi-square *p*-values and odds ratios with 95% confidence intervals, respectively. Rates of bowel resections and complications are also reported as proportions with chi-square *p*-values and median length of stay and median time to operative exploration are reported described with interquartile ranges and compared using Mann–Whitney *U* tests. It should be noted that the authors of this study incorrectly reported the interquartile range, which is a single number that represents the difference between the first and third quartiles.

Are Results Robust to Planned Sensitivity Analyses?

Sensitivity analyses are used to evaluate the validity of study results by testing whether an effect is consistent under alternate study conditions [34]. By introducing or eliminating some of the inherent uncertainty that existed in the original study design, investigators can test how much of the measured effect size was a result of the independent variables of interest, and how much was a product of uncertainty or potential confounders [34].

A careful reading of the results of sensitivity analyses is critical. Results that differ substantially from the primary analysis reduce confidence in the conclusions. In this article, the authors did not perform sensitivity analyses.

Were Subgroup Analyses Used? If So, Were these Specified a Priori and is the Issue of Multiple Testing Addressed?

Unlike sensitivity analyses, which are performed to test assumptions that have been made by investigators, subgroup analyses are used to determine if the relationship between an exposure and an outcome differs across levels of a third variable [30]. To perform a subgroup analysis, the study population is divided into levels of the third variable and patients are compared across groups. The subgroups should be specified prior to the analysis of data, and not be the result of conclusions that are found during data analysis [35]. In the article under study, the authors did not perform any subgroup analyses.

Readers of studies that include subgroup analyses should be aware of issues with multiplicity in which, when multiple subgroup analyses are performed, the probability of false positive results increase [30]. For more information about subgroup analysis, please see Chap. 30.

How Can I Interpret these Results in the Context of My Clinical Practice?

Are the Results of the Study Placed in the Broader Context of the Clinical Question?

The aim of cohort studies is to use a sample of patients for whom data are available to answer a clinical question that applies to the broader referent patient population. The extent to which results from a study sample may be generalized to the overall population is the external validity or applicability of the study. A careful evaluation of study design, setting and analytical approach is necessary to identify sources of bias and confounding that may limit a study's internal validity—a prerequisite for external validity [36].

Investigators should frame their study in the context of a larger clinical question and should clearly indicate how their results may be generalized to the overall population that their cohort aims to represent. The readers of a study then have a responsibility to question whether it is appropriate to do so. Differences in patient population or setting may limit the applicability a study's results to the reader's own practice. Unfortunately, Zielinski et al. [2] do not discuss how closely their patient population and study setting reflect the population and setting of patients with small bowel obstruction in general.

Is There a Description of the Existing Literature?

A description of the existing literature about a clinical topic and a discussion of how the results of a study fit into the body of literature provides important information to a reader. A study in which the findings are supported by previously published studies increases confidence in the conclusions, as the previously published studies may be performed in different settings and with different patients. Alternatively, a study that contradicts the existing literature or for which there is a paucity of comparable studies should be considered with caution and the generalizability of its findings carefully explored.

The authors of the present study thoroughly discuss how their findings correlate with the existing literature and how this study might fill gaps in current knowledge. It should be noted that selective reporting of literature that supports a study's findings is common and readers of cohort studies should be cautious. For example, Zielinski et al. [7] report in detail the findings of studies that support their own, including the odds ratios and confidence intervals for operative exploration associated with the use of water-soluble contrast studies. In contrast, the authors do not describe the results of the studies with conflicting results, including a Cochrane Systematic Review and Meta-Analysis that suggests there is no difference in the rate of operative exploration associated with water-soluble contrast studies [37].

Were All Clinically Important Outcomes Considered?

The effect of an intervention on any single outcome is typically only a small part of the relevant clinical picture. Particularly in studies of surgical interventions, important corollary outcomes invariably exist (e.g. complications rates, peri-operative mortality, length of stay, readmission rate, quality-of-life). Without this broader clinical picture, application of a study's results to a clinical setting is challenging and potentially dangerous. For example, in the article by Zielinski et al. [2], the authors reported rates of specific complications such as acute kidney injury and pneumonia as these were potentially relevant outcomes for routine water-soluble contrast use in aSBO. The authors do not report on several important clinical outcomes, including peri-admission mortality, readmission and recurrence of SBO.

Are Limitations of the Study Clearly Described?

Authors should clearly describe the limitations of their study and how these limitations may impact the study's interpretation and application. Potential limitations in any study include those associated with study setting and study design. Issues such as selection bias, information/measurement bias, and measured and unmeasured confounding are present to some extent in every cohort study. The potential impact of these factors on the interpretation study results should be clearly described in the Discussion section, as exemplified by Zielinski and colleagues [7] in the paper under review. Specifically, the authors highlight the risk of treatment-selection bias resulting from lack of randomization and blinding as well as deviations from study protocol. They describe how they attempted to mitigate these limitations as well as how these limitations may have affected the study findings. The authors do not discuss other important limitations including unmeasured confounding and the absence of relevant biochemical data from the multivariable model of the primary therapeutic outcome.

Resolution of the Clinical Scenario

The study by Zielinski et al. [7] provides evidence supporting the use of water-soluble contrast studies in patients with adhesive small bowel obstruction. The study design and the analytic approach used are appropriate for the clinical outcome of interest and the large, multi-institutional study population is likely generalizable to the SBO population of interest. The authors demonstrate that management with a protocol that includes water-soluble contrast studies is associated with significantly lower rates of operative exploration and shorter length of stay, with no significant difference in complication rates relative to no contrast. In addition to these therapeutic benefits, the findings of this study suggest a diagnostic role for water-soluble contrast studies in predicting a need for operative exploration.

The patient with SBO that you admitted the night before seems to be a suitable candidate for this intervention and after discussion with your team, you elect to incorporate water-soluble contrast studies into your management of patients with adhesive SBO.

Conclusion

The article by Zielinski et al. [7] exemplifies many of the strengths and weaknesses of cohort studies. The authors are mindful of many of the limitations of cohort studies and, where possible, take appropriate steps to mitigate them. The authors also take care to describe the current state of knowledge and how the present study fits into the broader clinical question.

While cohort studies cannot replace randomized controlled trials in terms of the quality of evidence, they play an important role in the surgical literature. Cohort studies are valuable in settings in which randomized trials may be unethical or unfeasible. Studies of rare diseases, studies of prognosis rather than therapy, and studies with extremely long-term outcomes are particularly well suited to a cohort-study design. As with all medical literature, readers should be discerning and critical. Certain biases and the risks of confounding will always exist in cohort studies. The interpretation of these studies and their application to patient populations should be mindful of these risks.

References

1. Exposure. In: Porta M, editor. A dictionary of epidemiology. Oxford: Oxford University Press; 2008.
2. Murad MH, Asi N, Alsawas M, Alahdab F. New evidence pyramid. Evid Based Med. 2016;21(4):125–7.
3. Laupacis A, Wells G, Richardson WS, Tugwell P. Users' guides to the medical literature. V. How to use an article about prognosis. Evidence-Based Medicine Working Group. JAMA. 1994;272(3):234–7.
4. Schiphorst AH, Pronk A, Borel Rinkes IH, Hamaker ME. Representation of the elderly in trials of laparoscopic surgery for colorectal cancer. Colorectal Dis. 2014;16(12):976–83.
5. Unger JM, Hershman DL, Albain KS, Moinpour CM, Petersen JA, Burg K, et al. Patient income level and cancer clinical trial participation. J Clin Oncol. 2013;31(5):536–42.

6. Ceresoli M, Coccolini F, Catena F, Montori G, Di Saverio S, Sartelli M, et al. Water-soluble contrast agent in adhesive small bowel obstruction: a systematic review and meta-analysis of diagnostic and therapeutic value. Am J Surg. 2016;211(6):1114–25.
7. Zielinski MD, Haddad NN, Cullinane DC, Inaba K, Yeh DD, Wydo S, et al. Multi-institutional, prospective, observational study comparing the Gastrografin challenge versus standard treatment in adhesive small bowel obstruction. J Trauma Acute Care Surg. 2017;83(1):47–54.
8. Thoma A, Farrokhyar F, Bhandari M, Tandan V, Evidence-Based Surgery Working G. Users' guide to the surgical literature. How to assess a randomized controlled trial in surgery. Can J Surg. 2004;47 (3):200–8.
9. Cole P. The hypothesis generating machine. Epidemiology. 1993;4(3):271–3.
10. Loder E, Groves T, Macauley D. Registration of observational studies. BMJ. 2010;340:c950.
11. Registries for evaluating patient outcomes: a user's guide. Rockville (MD): Agency for Healthcare Research and Quality (US); 2014. Available from: https://www.ncbi.nlm.nih.gov/books/NBK208611/. Accessed 20 Jul 2018.
12. Lawson EH, Louie R, Zingmond DS, Brook RH, Hall BL, Han L, et al. A comparison of clinical registry versus administrative claims data for reporting of 30-day surgical complications. Ann Surg. 2012;256(6):973–81.
13. Cima RR, Lackore KA, Nehring SA, Cassivi SD, Donohue JH, Deschamps C, et al. How best to measure surgical quality? Comparison of the Agency for Healthcare Research and Quality Patient Safety Indicators (AHRQ-PSI) and the American College of Surgeons National Surgical Quality Improvement Program (ACS-NSQIP) postoperative adverse events at a single institution. Surgery. 2011;150(5):943–9.
14. Mason SA, Nathens AB, Byrne JP, Fowler R, Gonzalez A, Karanicolas PJ, et al. The accuracy of burn diagnosis codes in health administrative data: a validation study. Burns. 2017;43(2):258–64.
15. Lee DS, Stitt A, Wang X, Yu JS, Gurevich Y, Kingsbury KJ, et al. Administrative hospitalization database validation of cardiac procedure codes. Med Care. 2013;51(4):e22–6.
16. Shiloach M, Frencher SK Jr, Steeger JE, Rowell KS, Bartzokis K, Tomeh MG, et al. Toward robust information: data quality and inter-rater reliability in the American College of Surgeons National Surgical Quality Improvement Program. J Am Coll Surg. 2010;210(1):6–16.
17. Bilimoria KY, Cohen ME, Ingraham AM, Bentrem DJ, Richards K, Hall BL, et al. Effect of postdischarge morbidity and mortality on comparisons of hospital surgical quality. Ann Surg. 2010;252(1):183–90.
18. Sackett DL. Bias in analytic research. J Chronic Dis. 1979;32(1–2):51–63.
19. Delgado-Rodriguez M, Llorca J. Bias. J Epidemiol Community Health. 2004;58(8):635–41.
20. Grimes DA, Schulz KF. Bias and causal associations in observational research. Lancet. 2002;359 (9302):248–52.
21. Rothman KJ, Greenland S, Lash TL. Modern epidemiology, 3rd ed. Philadelphia: Wolters Kluwer Health/Lippincott Williams & Wilkins; 2008. 758 p.
22. Tripepi G, Jager KJ, Dekker FW, Wanner C, Zoccali C. Bias in clinical research. Kidney Int. 2008;73 (2):148–53.
23. Gail MH. Does cardiac transplantation prolong life? A reassessment. Ann Intern Med. 1972;76(5):815–7.
24. Tripepi G, Jager KJ, Dekker FW, Zoccali C. Selection bias and information bias in clinical research. Nephron Clin Pract. 2010;115(2):c94–9.
25. Greenland S, Morgenstern H. Confounding in health research. Ann Rev Public Health. 2001;22(1):189–212.
26. Mamdani M, Sykora K, Li P, Normand S-LT, Streiner DL, Austin PC, et al. Reader's guide to critical appraisal of cohort studies: 2. Assessing potential for confounding. BMJ. 2005;330 (7497):960–2.
27. Fewell Z, Davey Smith G, Sterne JAC. The impact of residual and unmeasured confounding in epidemiologic studies: a simulation study. Am J Epidemiol. 2007;166(6):646–55.
28. Normand S-LT, Sykora K, Li P, Mamdani M, Rochon PA, Anderson GM. Readers guide to critical appraisal of cohort studies: 3. Analytical strategies to reduce confounding. BMJ. 2005;330(7498):1021–3.
29. Austin PC. The performance of different propensity-score methods for estimating differences in proportions (risk differences or absolute risk reductions) in observational studies. Stat Med. 2010;29(20):2137–48.
30. Wang R, Lagakos SW, Ware JH, Hunter DJ, Drazen JM. Statistics in medicine—reporting of subgroup analyses in clinical trials. N Eng J Med. 2007;357:2189–94.
31. Nakagawa S, Cuthill IC. Effect size, confidence interval and statistical significance: a practical guide for biologists. Biol Rev Camb Philos Soc, 5 ed. 2007:82(4):591–605.

32. Gardner MJ, Altman DG. Confidence intervals rather than P values: estimation rather than hypothesis testing. Br Med J (Clin Res Ed). 1986;292 (6522):746–50.
33. Button KS, Ioannidis JPA, Mokrysz C, Nosek BA, Flint J, Robinson ESJ, et al. Power failure: why small sample size undermines the reliability of neuroscience. Nat Rev Neurosci. 2013;14(5):365–76.
34. Schneeweiss S. Sensitivity analysis and external adjustment for unmeasured confounders in epidemiologic database studies of therapeutics. Pharmacoepidemiol Drug Saf. 2006;15(5):291–303.
35. Yusuf S, Wittes J, Probstfield J, Tyroler HA. Analysis and interpretation of treatment effects in subgroups of patients in randomized clinical trials. JAMA. 1991;266(1):93–8.
36. Calder BJ, Phillips LW, Tybout AM. The concept of external validity. J Consum Res. 1982;9(3):240–4.
37. Abbas S, Bissett IP, Parry BR. Oral water soluble contrast for the management of adhesive small bowel obstruction. Cochrane Database Syst Rev. 2007:(3): CD004651.

Case-Control Studies

17

Achilles Thoma, Jenny Santos, Jessica Murphy,
Eric K. Duku and Charles H. Goldsmith

Introduction

As explained in Chap. 5, the preferred method to determine the effects of a surgical intervention is a randomized controlled trial (RCT). However, while RCTs can minimize common research biases, there are situations where performing an RCT is not feasible. Two such occasions include (1) Ethical consideration of randomization and (2) The ability to detect the outcome of interest. Clinical trials in surgery aim to compare the effectiveness of novel procedures or interventions to the standard of care. A precondition to undertaking an RCT is the assumption that the novel intervention is not harmful, and we are in a state of "equipoise", which means genuine uncertainty of the benefits of the novel intervention. Ethical issues arise when a patient is placed in potential danger; for example, we cannot ethically randomize a patient into a research arm that we suspect may cause harm, or is potentially less effective than another option.

In terms of outcome detection, issues can occur if the outcome of interest is rare or takes a long period of time to develop. In these situations, an RCT would not be suitable as it would be both time-consuming and expensive, while the outcome may not occur within the timeframe of the study [1]. These issues leave clinicians with the choice of using a cohort or case-control study design.

While cohort and case-control studies are both forms of observational research, they have individual differences, advantages and disadvantages; these differences are summarized in Table 17.1. They are also explained in more detail in Chap. 16. Well-known examples of case-control studies include (1) the 1926 study revealing that breast cancer risk increased with low fertility rates [2];

A. Thoma (✉) · J. Santos · J. Murphy
Department of Surgery, Division of Plastic Surgery, McMaster University, Hamilton, ON, Canada
e-mail: athoma@mcmaster.ca

J. Santos
e-mail: santoj8@mcmaster.ca

J. Murphy
e-mail: murphj11@mcmaster.ca

E. K. Duku
Department of Psychiatry and Behavioural Neurosciences, Offord Centre for Child Studies, McMaster University, Hamilton, ON, Canada
e-mail: duku@mcmaster.ca

A. Thoma · C. H. Goldsmith
Department of Health Research Methods, Evidence and Impact, McMaster University, Hamilton, ON, Canada
e-mail: cgoldsmi@sfu.ca

C. H. Goldsmith
Faculty of Health Sciences, Simon Fraser University, Burnaby, BC, Canada

C. H. Goldsmith
Department of Occupational Science and Occupational Therapy, Faculty of Medicine, The University of British Columbia, Vancouver, BC, Canada

A. Thoma et al. (eds.), *Evidence-Based Surgery*,
https://doi.org/10.1007/978-3-030-05120-4_17

Table 17.1 Comparison of cohort and case-control studies

	Cohort study	Case control study
Advantages	– Gather data regarding the sequence of events, therefore can assess causality – Examine multiple outcomes for an exposure – Good for investigating rare exposures – Can calculate rate of disease in exposed and unexposed	– Good for rare outcomes or outcomes with long latency periods – Relatively quick and inexpensive – Require comparatively fewer patients – Can utilize existing records – Can examine multiple exposures/risk factors
Disadvantages	– Large numbers of patients required – Susceptible to selection bias – Susceptible to recall bias or information bias* – Less control over variables* – May be expensive and require longer duration for follow-up** – Susceptive to loss to follow-up**	– Susceptible to recall or information biases – Validation of information is difficult – Possible incomplete ability to control for extraneous variables – Possible difficulty selecting appropriate comparison group – Rates of diseased in exposed and unexposed individuals cannot be determined
Procedure	1. Take disease-free (at risk) population 2. Identify exposed and unexposed cohort groups 3a. Identify diseased subjects by interview or written records* 3b. During follow-up identify the diseased subjects (incident cases)** 4. Analyze differences (i.e.: incidence or relative risk) among the exposed and unexposed	1. Identify the cases (those who have the outcome of interest) 2. Select controls, which, may be matched to cases 3. Measure exposure or risk factors of interest 4. Compare the presence or absence of exposure in the cases and controls
Direction of investigation	– *From present to past – **From present to future	From present to past

*Retrospective Cohort Studies; **Prospective Cohort Studies
Created with information from Song and Chung [2]

(2) the association between smoking and lung cancer [2] and (3) the association between the limb malformation, phocomelia, and thalidomide ingestion during pregnancy [1].

Clinical Scenario

At the paediatric surgical rounds, an uncommon case of chylothorax was presented in a 3-month-old child who had heart surgery via a sternotomy incision. A previous heart surgery through a thoracotomy incision was unsuccessful. A discussion ensued as to the risk of chylothorax in this case. One paediatric cardiac surgeon claimed that this was due to the complexity of the congenital heart surgery performed whereas another claimed that this was due to the repeat surgery. The head of the service asks the paediatric cardiac fellow to review the literature on the association between chylothorax and repeat paediatric cardiac surgery.

Literature Search

As stated in previous chapters, the first step to finding the best available evidence is to formulate a research question based on the PICOT format (see Chap. 3):

- **P**opulation: Paediatric Population
- **I**ntervention: Cardiac surgery OR Redo Cardiac Surgery
- **C**omparative intervention: None
- **O**utcomes: Chylothorax
- **T**ime: Any Time After Surgery

Using the PICOT format terms, your clinical research question could be one of two:

"In paediatric patients undergoing cardiac surgery, what is the risk of chylothorax following surgery?" OR "In paediatric patients undergoing a redo cardiac surgery, what is the risk of chylothorax following surgery".

Next, you use the above terms to perform a thorough literature search (see Chap. 4). Using the terms: "Paediatric" AND "Cardiac Surgery" AND "Chylothorax" you perform a literature search in the Cochrane Library to determine if there are any acceptable randomized control trials. The search yields two articles, however, neither are relevant to your research question (see Appendix 1). You try performing another literature search on Cochrane using "Redo Cardiac Surgery" in place of "Cardiac Surgery" and this search yields no results. Since your search on Cochrane Library was not successful, you perform a literature search using PubMed using "Paediatric" AND "Cardiac Surgery" AND "Chylothorax". Your search yields 84 publications, so you decide to narrow your search to those published in 2018 and utilize the "best match" sorting feature; this new filter yields nine publications (see Appendix 2). Eight of these articles focused on the management of chylothorax or elements of this condition. One of these articles, by Day et al. [3] titled "Chylothorax following paediatric cardiac surgery: A case-control study" seemed promising. It is a matched case-control study investigating the association between numerous factors on the risk of chylothorax.

Appraisal of the Selected Article

When reviewing the article, you realize you are somewhat unfamiliar with the methodology and analysis used in case-control studies. As you want to be confident in the results that you will present to your colleagues, you search for a resource to help you better understand this study design. You find an article by Thoma et al. [1] that you feel can help you appraise this article before presenting it to your colleagues. The Thoma et al. [1] article provides appraisal questions specific to case-control studies where harm to a patient is involved; these questions are summarized in Box 17.1.

Box 17.1. Guidelines for the Appraisal of an Article in the Surgical Literature Using a Case-Control Study Design [1]

A. **Are the results valid?**

(i) Were cases and controls similar with respect to the indication or circumstances that would lead to exposure?
(ii) Were the circumstances and methods for determining exposure similar for cases and controls?
(iii) Was the correct temporal relationship demonstrated?
(iv) Was there a dose-response relationship?

B. **What were the results?**

(i) How strong is the association between exposure and outcome?
(ii) How precise was the estimate of risk?

C. **Will the results help me in caring for my patients in my practice?**

(i) Was the follow-up sufficiently long?
(ii) Is the exposure similar to what might occur in my patient?
(iii) What is the magnitude of risk?
(iv) Are there any benefits known to be associated with the exposure?
(v) Were the patients in the appraised study similar to the patient in my practice?

Are the Results Valid?

i. *Were cases and controls similar with respect to the indication or circumstances that would lead to exposure?*

The study by Day et al. [3] reviewed health records of all paediatric patients who received cardiac surgery at the Royal Children's Hospital (Australia). The authors used a 48-month window from January 2008 to January 2012, as the inclusion criteria for review. They authors identified 121 cases (diagnosed with chylothorax). The comparison (control) group was formed by identifying 121 patients who had also received heart surgery, within the same time period, but did not develop chylothorax. The control group was matched to the cases by (1) Age (within three months if younger than one year of age or within one year for older patients); (2) Date of surgery (within one year); and (3) Sex. The matching of cases and controls is often performed in case-control studies to better control for confounding (the confusion of the effect of a risk factor on the outcome of interest, which is actually due to some other factor not accounted for in the study) as well as to provide a control group that better represents the target population. While the authors controlled for these three factors, they did not explicitly check, with statistical testing, to ensure that the matching process worked for these variables.

The objective of the Day et al. [3] study, was to explore the risk of developing chylothorax following surgery associated with a number of identified influencing factors. To explore this association the cases and controls cannot be matched for these factors; the following factors have been identified as influencing the development of chylothorax following surgery and were explored by Day et al. [3]: (1) genetic risk factors; (2) the annual hospital volume [4]; (3) weight; (4) RACHS-1 score; (5) arch surgery; (6) open or closed heart; (7) incision site; and (8) surgery type (redo or virgin).

ii. *Were the circumstances and methods for determining exposure similar for the cases and controls?*

When selecting cases, Day et al. [3] used the diagnostic criteria of (1) a pleural fluid lymphocyte count of >80% or (2) a triglyceride level > 1.1 mmol/L. Having predetermined diagnostic criteria helps to reduce misclassification bias, or the error associated with misidentifying a patient's disease status [1]. The authors then found a matched control group that had undergone cardiac surgery within the same time period but did not develop chylothorax. For both the case and control groups, the Cardiobase database from the Royal Children's Hospital in Melbourne was used.

iii. *Was the correct temporal relationship established?*

Establishing a temporal relationship, meaning that the exposure occurred before the outcome, is important in determining whether there is an association. In the Day et al. [3] study, the authors do not give any information on the date of surgery as compared to the date of diagnosis. The absence of these data may likely be due to the fact that the objective of this study was to determine the diagnosis of chylothorax post-surgery, therefore, one would assume that the diagnosis date (outcome) would have come after the re-do surgery date (exposure). While you understand why this information may not be provided, you feel it would have been helpful to be given the dates of surgery and the date of diagnosis. This information could have been beneficial to compare both the impact of the length of time between surgeries on risk, and the length of time past from surgery to diagnosis between the cases and controls.

iv. *Was there a dose-response relationship?*

Determining a dose-response relationship can be difficult in surgery; it is much easier, for example, to find a dose-response relationship between smoking (number of packs per year) and lung cancer [1]. Previous work in the area of cardiac surgery and chylothorax have suggested a possible dose-response relationship between number of surgeries and the development of chylothorax. Both Ismail et al. [5] and Mery et al. [4] found that there was an increased incidence rate in redo cardiac surgery cases. In the Day et al. [3] article, results indicate that there is an increased risk with redo surgery; therefore this may be suggesting that there is a dose-response relationship in regard to number of interventions and chylothorax risk.

However, concluding a dose-response relationship the study by Day et al. [3] may not be realistic as the authors did not use a measure detailing the specific number of redo surgeries in the analysis. The redo surgery variable was classified as "none" or "at least 1 redo".

What Are the Results?

i. *How strong is the association between exposure and outcome?*

In a case-control study, those individuals who have the outcome of interest are known prior to the study beginning, therefore, a relative risk estimate cannot be used [1]. Instead, the odds ratio (OR) is more appropriate to measure the association of the exposure on the outcome [1]. An OR represents a ratio of the odds having the outcome in an "exposed" or case group relative to the odds of having the outcome in an "unexposed" or control group [6].

Day and colleagues matched the cases to the controls, and therefore a matched analysis method was used to calculate the OR as opposed to the standard method [1]. The standard approach for the OR is calculated using the number of individuals within both case and control groups who were or were not exposed to any risk factor(s) of interest for an unmatched study [1]. These numbers are best visualized by using 2 × 2 tables. This type of table is appropriate for unmatched studies because cases are independent from controls. Table 17.2 illustrates the basic format of a 2 × 2 table, to facilitate the calculation of an OR for every risk factor (exposure) included in an *unmatched* study. It is also important to note that calculating an OR by hand in this manner does not account for potential confounding by other factors (genetic risk factors, the annual hospital volume [4], weight at time of surgery, RACHS-1 score, arch surgery, open or closed heart, and incision site [3].

Using the format of this basic 2 × 2 table, an OR can be calculated using the following formula:

$$\text{Odds Ratio} = \frac{a/b}{c/d} = \frac{ad}{cb}$$

In the Day et al. [3] article, the exposure of interest was re-do congenital cardiac surgery, while the outcome of interest was postoperative chylothorax. The authors included various risk factors for chylothorax following cardiac surgery including the risk adjustment for congenital heart surgery (RACHS-1) score, arch surgery, open or closed heart, incision site and incision type (redo or virgin). A univariable OR is then calculated for each risk factor. For example, Table 17.3 illustrates what the 2 × 2 table for "Virgin surgery" versus "Redo surgery" would look like, using data from Day et al. [3], had the study been *unmatched* [3].

$$\begin{aligned}\text{Odds Ratio} &= \frac{ad}{cb}\\ &= \frac{(36)(112)}{(85)(9)}\\ &= 5.27\end{aligned}$$

An OR of less than 1 represents a "protective" effect of the risk factor increasing the odds of the target group developing the target outcome [1]. In comparison, an OR of greater than 1 represents a "hazardous" effect [1]. For the above-mentioned scenario, you are interested in the OR associated with the repeat surgery. Using a multivariable conditional logistic regression model, Day et al. [3] reported an OR of 20.7 (95% CI: 4.24–100) for redo surgeries. This means that the odds of chylothorax developing in those exposed to a redo surgery is 20.7 times greater than those who are having a surgery for the first time after controlling for other confounding variables.

However, as cases and controls were matched by date of surgery, age at surgery and sex and Day et al. [3] used a matched analysis, the basic format of the 2 × 2 table above would be slightly changed and the study results would have resulted from a different method of calculation. In a matched case-control, numbers of exposed and unexposed patients are illustrated by how many PAIRS had different exposure statuses (Table 17.4). Contrary to the traditional method, cases and controls are no longer independent groups and the unit of analysis is the matched case-control pair.

In turn, the formula shown above for an *unmatched* case-control study is also slightly changed to calculate the OR in a *matched* study:

$$\text{Odds Ratio} = \frac{b}{c}$$

In Table 17.4, the cells describe how many patients, within each *matched* pair (121 in total) were exposed or unexposed (redo or virgin surgery). For a matched case-control design, cells b and c are the only cells that would apply to calculate an OR, as you can be confident that the odds of having the outcome due to the exposure or not having the outcome due to not being exposed would be comparable between cases and controls in a matched sample.

In this particular situation, it is not possible to calculate the OR that would represent the dependent nature of cases and controls as the study does not provide information for matched pairs and just lists information by group for cases and controls. Again, calculating an OR in this manner does not account for potential confounding by other factors such as the risk factors listed previously.

Tables 17.2, 17.3 and 17.4 are purely for illustrative purposes, to show how you might go about getting a raw/unadjusted OR to measure the risk between the exposure and outcome in your study. This type of analysis is referred to as a univariable analysis. The univariable model in the Day et al. [3] article yielded an OR of 10.0, between redo surgeries and the risk of chylothorax. As this was significant at the 10% level

Table 17.2 Basic format of a 2 × 2 table used in case-control studies

	Outcome	
Exposure	Yes (Cases)	No (Controls)
Yes	a	b
No	c	d

Table 17.3 Format of a 2 × 2 table that could have been used in the Day et al. [3] study had the design been *unmatched*

	Chylothorax	
Surgery type	Cases	Controls
Redo	36	9
Virgin	85	112

Table 17.4 Format of a 2 × 2 table that should be used in the Day et al. [3] study due to its *matched* design

	Control pair member	
Case pair member	Exposed	Not exposed
Exposed	a	b
Not exposed	c	d

in this analysis [3] (this is often used in univariable models to determine which risk factors may be cofounding the results), it was one of the risk factors to be included in the subsequent multivariable model.

In this multivariable model, used to account for confounding by other factors, Day et al. [3] found an OR of 20.7, between redo surgeries and the risk of chylothorax. As the risk became greater in this model, this means that confounding factors had an effect on the relationship between chylothorax and "redo" surgeries, so it was appropriate to include those factors in the multivariable model.

ii. *How precise was the estimate of risk?*

The precision of an OR estimation can be judged by the confidence interval, which, is strongly impacted by the sample size of a study.

Day et al. [3] used two methods of calculating the OR, a univariable conditional logistic regression model and a multivariable conditional logistic regression model. When looking at the univariable model, the "redo" group had an OR of 10.0 with a 95% confidence interval of 3.05–32.8 [3]. In the multivariable model, the "redo" surgery group had an OR of 20.7 with a 95% confidence interval of 4.24–100 [3]. As a multivariable model accounts for other factors that can affect the relationship between an outcome and exposure, any conclusions should be based on the results from a multivariable model (OR = 20.7; 95% CI: 4.24–100).

The confidence intervals are quite wide, and most likely due to the low number of patients ($n = 45$) who had "redo" surgeries. While there are no set criteria to determine if a confidence interval is "too wide", we can look at previous studies in the same area. Day et al. [3] state that their study is the second largest study in the area identifying 121 cases of chylothorax, second only to a multi-site study [3]. Additionally, one should consider the fact that chylothorax is a relatively rare condition, therefore the absolute risk is quite low, and there is a smaller chance of this event occurring within a specific time interval. Therefore, while the estimate of the risk of chylothorax may not be overly precise, due to the small sample size, Day et al. [3] did have an adequate number of patients, as compared to other work in the area. Additionally, this shows that "redo" surgeries are quite rare in this particular study.

How Can I Apply the Results to My Patients in a Clinical Practice?

i. *Was the follow-up sufficiently long?*

Determining if the length of follow-up was sufficient in a case-control study is different than in a prospective RCT or a cohort study [1]. As previously stated, the outcome of interest has already occurred in case-control studies before the onset of the investigation. Day et al. [3] included records in this study up to 48-months from January 2008, which is equivalent to approximately 4 years, or January 2012. A study period of 3 years seems sufficient for the outcome of interest; although some outcomes take time to develop, chylothorax has been found to develop on average, eight days following surgery [8].

When comparing the current article to the literature, chylothorax studies seem to have a follow-up period varying from 2 to 7 years [7–10]. Further, Day et al. [3] identify 121 cases, making it the second largest study of its kind. Given the fact that the outcome has occurred prior to the commencement of the study, the similar follow-up interval to other studies, and the large number of cases identified, you are confident in concluding that the follow-up in the Day et al. [3] study was sufficient.

ii. *Is the exposure similar to what might occur in my patient?*

Where the exposure in the Day et al. [3] study is cardiac surgery, the exposure of interest in our scenario is redo heart surgery. Given that both exposures (cardiac surgery or redo heart surgery) are standardized procedures used for specific diseases or in specific situations, there is no reason to believe that there would be a difference between the exposure of your own patient, and the patients in the Day et al. [3] article.

iii. *What is the magnitude of the risk?*

As previously explained, the Odds Ratio (OR) measures association between an exposure and an outcome. Additionally, the OR can also be used to compare the magnitude of the exposure for an outcome [10]. Box 17.2 summarizes how OR can demonstrate the effect of an exposure on an outcome.

Box 17.2. The Meaning of Different OR

OR = 1	The exposure does not affect the odds of the outcome occurring
OR > 1	The exposure is associated with higher odds of the outcome occurring
OR < 1	The exposure is associated with lower odds of the outcome occurring

Created using information from [10]

In the Day et al. [3] article, an OR of 20.7 was seen in the multivariable model, and an OR of 10.0 was seen in a univariate model. Both of these ORs demonstrate an increased risk of chylothorax with repeat cardiac surgery. In addition to the OR, confidence intervals can be used to measure the magnitude of association. While the confidence interval is used to determine precision, it can also identify the presence of statistical significance [10]. The 95% confidence interval can be used as a proxy for significance if the confidence interval does not include 1, or the "null value" [10]. Figure 17.1 illustrates the OR and confidence interval for each model; in both cases, neither confidence interval includes the null value, implying significance.

iv. *Are there any benefits that are known to be associated with the exposure?*

In this specific case, the "exposure" is a second surgery. Literature within cardiac surgery has discussed the common need for re-operation to address left-over or recurring defects from prior surgeries or to manage the breakdown or outgrowth of grafts [11]. In fact, an analysis of the Congenital Heart Surgery Database reporting that one-third of operations in the database were for re-operative cardiac surgery, for patients with congenital heart disease [11]. While it has been questioned over the years if re-operation is the cause for morbidity and operative mortality, studies over the past 20 years have concluded that there is minimal risk [11]. These minimal-risks are due to enhancements in the quality of surgical techniques and peri-operative care.

For chylothorax specifically, Day and colleagues [3] reviewed nine studies and reported that the incidence of chylothorax following a cardiac surgery varied from 0.85 to 15.8%. In the Day and colleagues [3] report an incidence rate of 5.23%. However, this is more of a prevalence rate; one cannot truly determine incidence from a case-control study as the outcome has already occurred before commencement and therefore includes both new and existing cases of infection. However, we can still ascertain that the overall risk for chylothorax seems quite low.

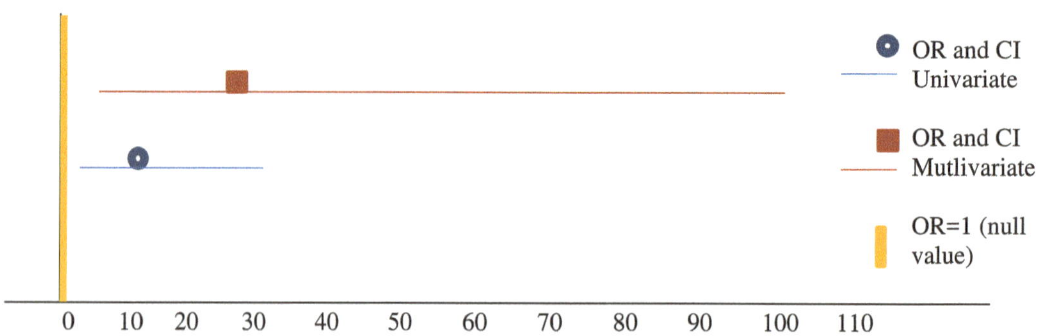

Fig. 17.1 Odds ratio and confidence interval for univariate and multivariable model

Due to this low risk, the apparent commonality and mandatory nature of second surgeries you believe that there are benefits of this exposure to the patient.

v. *Were the patients in the appraised study similar to the patient in my practice?*

In the Day et al. [3] study, the median age for the case and control groups was 0.23 and 0.25 years, respectively. The patient in our scenario is 3 months old (or 0.25 years), the authors mention that those under 12 months of age are at higher risk and therefore, the results can likely be applied to our patient [3]. Additionally, this study was performed in Australia, which does not have any drastic differences in terms of healthcare, access to services and lifestyle compared to the Canadian population [7]. Due to these similarities, you are confident that the information from the Day et al. [3] article could be generalized to your patient.

Resolution of the Scenario

Based on the evidence presented in the Day et al. [3] article, the Paediatric cardiac fellow presents her conclusions to her staff. Chylothorax has odds 10× as likely to occur with repeat cardiac surgery than a single previous surgery. She also acknowledges that the Day et al. [3] article also incriminates the complexity of the cardiac surgery especially around the arch of the aorta as carrying a higher risk for chylothorax. In this regard, both staff were correct.

Additional Information for the Reader

Appraising epidemiological studies usually involves piecing together numerous components. The Graphical Appraisal Tool for Epidemiological studies (GATE) framework can help to organize these different elements of a study [12]. Figure 17.2 is our interpretation of this

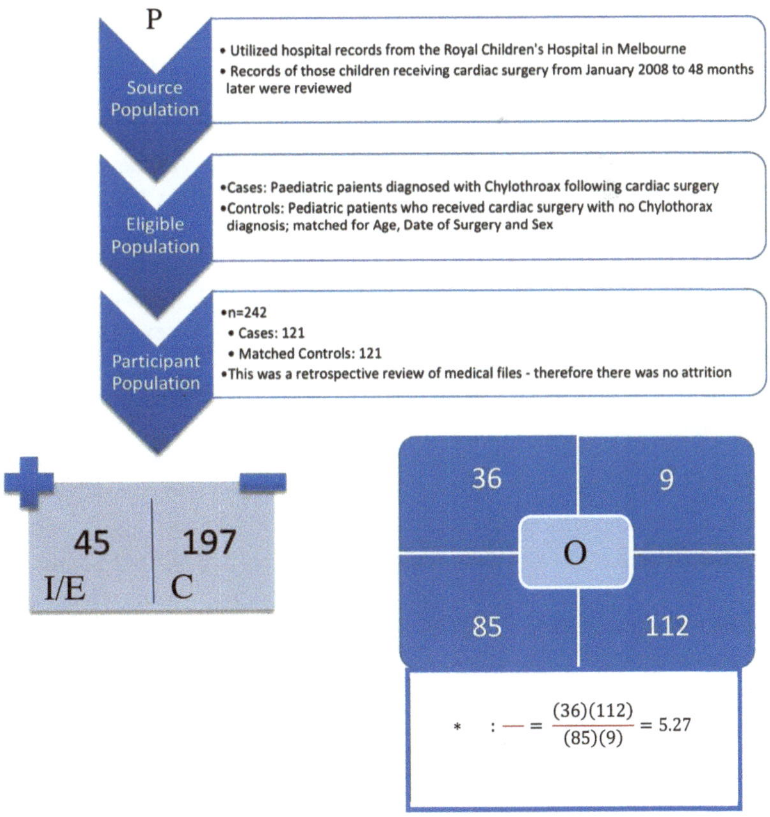

Fig. 17.2 GATE framework [12] interpretation for the Day et al. [3] article appraisal. P Population; I Intervention; E Exposure; C Comparison; OR Odds Ratio. * This calculation represents an OR using data from the Day et al. [3] study, had it been unmatched

framework, as it relates to the Day et al. [3] article. The original framework was developed by The Evidence-Based Medicine (EBM) Working group to help students conceptualize a study as a whole, as well as by its individual parts [4].

We have taken this framework and adjusted it to represent the variables that were looked at for this particular scenario. In our version of this framework, we used "Redo surgery" as the exposure/intervention and "Virgin surgery" as the comparison. We then explain the odds ratio calculation to show the risk associated with developing chylothorax (cases) following a "Redo surgery" (exposure). For this recreation of the framework, the time horizon was left out as there was no specific time horizon, other than just "following surgery" for this scenario. We encourage the reader to review the GATE framework as it offers a clear and concise format to summarize and appraise epidemiological studies [12].

Appendix 1

Search Results Using Cochrane Library: "Paediatric", "Cardiac Surgery", "Chylothorax"

1. Das A, Shah PS. Octreotide for the treatment of chylothorax in neonates. Cochrane Database of Systematic Reviews. 2010;9: CD006388.
2. Mosalli R, AlFaleh K. Prophylactic surgical ligation of patent ductus arteriosus for prevention of mortality and mobidity in extremely low birth weight infants (Review). Cochrane Database of Systematic Reviews. 2008;1:CD006181.

Appendix 2

Search Results Using PubMed: "Paediatric", "Cardiac Surgery", "Chylothorax"

1. Day TG, Zannino D, Golshevsky D, d'Udekem Y, Brizard C, Cheyng MMH. Chylothorax following paediatric cardiac surgery: a case-control study. Cardiol Young. 2018;28(2):222–8.
2. Waterhouse SG, Vergales JE, Conaway MR, Lee L. Predictive factors for central line-associated bloodstream infections in pediatric cardiac surgery patients with chylothorax. Pediatr Crit Care Med. 2018; Epub ahead of print.
3. Justice L, Buckely JR, Floh A, Horsley M, Alten J, Anand V, Schwartz SM. Nutrition considerations in the pediatric cardiac intensive care unit patient. World J Pediatr Congenit Heart Surg. 2018;9(3):333–43.
4. Justice LB, Nelson DP, Palumbo J, Sawyer J, Patel MN, Byrnes JW. Efficacy and safety of recombinant tissue plasminogen activator for venous thrombosis after paediatric heart surgery. Cardiol young. 2018;28(2):214–21.
5. Lo Rito M, AlRadi OO, Saedi A, Kotani Y, Ben Sivarajan V, Russell JL, Caldarone CA, Van Arsdell GS, Honjo O. Chylothorax and pleural effusion in contemporary extracardiac fenestrated fontan completion. J Thorac Cardiovasc Surg. 2018;155(5):2069–77.
6. Wu C, Wang Y, Pan X, Wu Y, Wang Q, Li Y, An Y, Li H, Wang G, Dai J. Analysis of the etiology and treatment of chylothorax in 119 pediatric patients in a single clinical center. J Pediatr Surg. 2018. E-pub ahead of print.
7. Weissler JM, Cho EG, Koltz PF, Carney MJ, Itkin M, Laje P, Levin LS, Dori Y, Kanchwala SK, Kovach SJ. Lymphovenous anastomosis for the treatment of chylothorax in infants: A novel microsurgical approach to a devastating problem. Plast Reconstr Surg. 2018;141(6):1502–7.
8. Muniz G, Hidalgo-Capos J, Valdivia-Tapia MDC, Shaikh N, Carreazo NY. Succesfful management of chylothorax with etilefrine: Case report in 2 pediatric patients. Pediatrics. 2018;141(5):e20163309.
9. Ok YK, Kim YH, Park CS. Surgical reconstruction for high-output chylothorax associated with thrombo-occulusion of

superior vena cava and left innominate vein in a neonate. Korean J Thorac Cardiovasc Surg. 2018;51(3):202–4.

10. Winder MM, Eckhauser AW, Delgado-Corcoran C, Smout RJ, Marietta J, Bailly DK. A protocol to decrease postoperative chylous effusion duration in children. Cardiol Young. 2018;28(6):816–25.

References

1. Thoma A, Kaur MN, Farrokhyar F, Waltho D, Levis C, Lovrics P, Goldsmith CH. Users' guide to the surgical literature: how to assess an article about harm. Can J Surg. 2016;59(5):351–7.
2. Song JW, Chung KC. Observational studies: cohort and case-control studies. PRS. 2010;126(5):2234–42.
3. Day TG, Zannino D, Golshevsky D, d'Udekem Y, Brizard C, Cheung MMH. Chylothorax following paediatric cardiac surgery: a case–control study. Cardiol Young. 2018;28(2):222–8.
4. Mery CM, Moffett BS, Khan MS, Zhang W, Guzmán-Pruneda FA, Fraser CD Jr, Cabrera AG. Incidence and treatment of chylothorax after cardiac surgery in children: analysis of a large multi-institution database. J Thorac Cardiovasc Surg. 2014;147(3):678–86.
5. Ismail SR, Kabbani MS, Najm HK, Shaath GA, Jijeh AMZ, Hijazi OM. Impact of chylothorax on the early post operative outcome after pediatric cardiac surgery. J Saudi heart Assoc. 2014;26(2):87–92.
6. Guyatt G, Rennie D, Meade MO, Cook DJ. Users guides to the medical literature: a manual for evidence-based clinical practice. 2nd ed. 2009 JAMA.
7. Hussey P, Anderson GF, Osborn R, Feek C, McLaughlin V, Millar J, Epstein A. How does the quality of care compare in five countries? Health Aff. 2004;23(3):89–99.
8. Yeh J, Brown ER, Kellogg KA, Donohue JE, Yu S, Gaies MG, Fifer CF, Hirsch JC, Aiyagari R. Utility of a clinical practice guideline in treatment of chylothorax in the postoperative congenital heart patient. Ann Thorac Surg. 2013;96:930–7.
9. Chan EH, Russell JL, Williams WF, Van Arsdell GS, Coles JG, McCrindle BW. Postoperative chylothorax after cardiothoracic surgery in children. Ann of Thoracic Surg. 2005;80(5):1864–70.
10. Szumilas M. Explaining Odds Ratios. J Can Acad Child Adolesc Pscyhiatry. 2010;19(3):227–9.
11. Villa-Hincapie CA, Careeno-Jaimes M, Obando-Lopez CE, Camacho-Mackenzie J, Umaña--Mallarino JP, Sandoval-Reyes NF. Risk factors for mortality in reoperations for pediatric and congential heart surgery in a developing country. World J Pediatr Congenit Heart Surg. 2017;8(4):425–9.
12. Jackson R, Ameratunga S, Broad J, Connor J, Lethaby A, Robb G, Wells S, Glasziou P, Heneghan C. The GATE frame: critical appraisal with pictures. Evidence-Based Med. 2006;11(2):35–8.

18 Evaluating Case Series in Surgery

Christopher J. Coroneos and Brian Hyosuk Chin

Introduction

The case series is an observational study design involving a group of similar patients, who share a common exposure, diagnosis, intervention, or outcome [1]. In surgery, they most commonly report rare/unique cases, or the results of novel interventions [2]; several landmark disease classifications, and interventions were first reported in case series [1]. Given the focus on technique and innovation in surgical literature, it is not surprising that the majority of top historical citations and even current publications are case series/case reports [1, 3]. From a methodological perspective, case series represent low-level evidence (Level IV) [4]. With the absence of a control group and commonly retrospective design, they are especially prone to bias [4]. However, the case series remains a design in surgical research for generating hypotheses and feasibility of interventions [5]; patient characteristics and outcomes are often used to plan a higher level study design (e.g., sample size calculation, follow-up timing) [4, 5]. A case series alone is often sufficient to establish diagnostic accuracy or demonstrate safety [4]. Case series can demonstrate "real-world" effectiveness, with high external validity [5, 6]. By design, they remain cheaper, and faster to complete than higher levels of evidence [2]. Given their prevalence in the surgical literature, it is important that every surgeon be familiar with the critical appraisal of case series, with attention to selection bias, recall bias, and information bias.

Clinical Scenario

You are a head and neck reconstructive plastic surgeon at an academic center working in a multidisciplinary team. Your thoracic and general surgery colleagues request you see a patient with an esophageal adenocarcinoma who is awaiting esophagectomy. He is 60 years old, a previous smoker, and has a history of hypertension. The complicating factor is that the adenocarcinoma invaded the stomach requiring a subtotal gastrectomy. This makes a gastric pull-up, the first-choice option for esophageal reconstruction, potentially not viable depending on the remaining stomach. Your colleagues are seeking your reconstructive expertise for this patient.

Having recently attended a conference on advancements in head and neck reconstruction, you recall a presentation on esophageal reconstruction with a "supercharged" jejunal flap,

C. J. Coroneos (✉) · B. H. Chin
Department of Surgery, Division of Plastic Surgery, Faculty of Health Sciences, McMaster University, Hamilton, ON, Canada
e-mail: coronec@mcmaster.ca

B. H. Chin
e-mail: hyosuk.chin@medportal.ca

A. Thoma et al. (eds.), *Evidence-Based Surgery*,
https://doi.org/10.1007/978-3-030-05120-4_18

where the esophagus is replaced with a pedicled jejunal conduit, and the perfusion to the most proximal segment of jejunum is augmented with microsurgical vessel anastomoses. You wonder if the surgeons that presented the work have published their techniques in a peer-reviewed journal.

Literature Search

You visit PubMed.gov and perform a search with the terms: "esophageal" AND "reconstruction" AND "jejunum". The search is limited to human subjects, English language, and a publication date between 2008 and 2018. This yields 116 results and you identify several studies on esophageal reconstruction with free jejunal flaps. There are four case series that interest you. Two of the case series are from Japan with 11 and 24 patients in the study [7, 8]. The third case series is from the United Kingdom with 31 cases [9]. The final case-series published in the *Annals of Surgery* by Poh et al. [10] from MD Anderson Cancer Center (Houston, Texas) includes 51 patients. Given that Poh et al. [10] includes the greatest number of cases, a North American patient population, and is published in a high-profile journal, you select this paper for review. Key characteristics of the case series are listed in Table 18.1.

Appraisal of a Surgical Case Series

The appraisal of case series involves evaluating the validity of the study, interpreting the results, and applying study findings clinically (Box 1).

Table 18.1 Key characteristics of the case series by Poh et al. [10]

Characteristic	Case series
Objective	"To review our experience and technique of the supercharged jejunal flap for total esophageal reconstruction"
Population	n: 51 Esophageal cancer: 38 (75%) Age (mean, min–max): 55 (28–74) Male sex: 36 (71%) Active smoking: 6 (12%) History of smoking: 32 (63%) Hypertension: 22 (43%) Other malignancy: 10 (20%) Coronary artery disease: 7 (14%) Diabetes mellitus: 5 (10%) COPD/asthma: 5 (10%)
Intervention	Supercharged jejunal reconstruction Immediate: 34 (67%) Delayed: 17 (33%) Preoperative chemotherapy: 33 (65%) Preoperative radiation: 34 (67%)
Study design	Retrospective review of prospective database Not explicitly consecutive
Outcomes	30-day mortality: 0 Overall mortality: 2 (4%) Flap re-exploration: 3 (6%) Flap failure: 2 (4%) ICU stay (mean, SD): 9.0 days (11.7) Length of stay (mean, SD): 21.5 days (14.0) Regular diet: 44 (90%) Discontinue tube feeds: 39 (80%) at 103 days (SD 81)
Follow-up	Mean 21.9 months (2–80)
Complications	Overall: 33 (65%) Fistula: 7 (14%) Stricture: 5 (10%)

Box 1. Framework for the appraisal of surgical case-series

I. **Are the results valid?**

i. Is a clear objective stated?
ii. Is the series a prospective study? If not, was data collection prospective?
iii. Was patient recruitment consecutive?
iv. Was outcome assessment appropriate?
v. Is the intervention appropriately described?

II. **What are the results?**

i. Are outcomes appropriately reported?
ii. Are outcomes completely reported?

III. **Will the results change practice?**

i. Are the patients similar to my own?
ii. Is the setting similar to my own?

I. Are the Results Valid?

i. *Is a clear objective stated?*
The case series should have a clear objective, as with any other study design; it can be reported as a stated aim, or more appropriately as a structured research question. The common patient factors (e.g., diagnosis, intervention) and rationale for reporting patients should be defined. The objective should be pertinent and add to the current body of research on the topic. The series by Poh et al. [10] reports an objective "to review our experience and technique of the supercharged jejunal flap for total esophageal reconstruction". There is no structured research question stated. The statement defines the population and intervention but does not incorporate the technical challenges and refinements that are the focus of the paper in optimizing outcomes. These aspects are alluded to in the title, or subsequently discussed in the manuscript.

ii. *Is the series a prospective study? if not, was data collection prospective?*
Prospective study designs demonstrate more rigorous methodology; patient inclusion factors are predefined, baseline characteristics are accurately captured, the intervention is consistent, and outcomes and their timing are established a priori. Patients can be captured at the same time point in their disease process, ideally at initial presentation. This is especially important in studies of exposure; temporal relationships between exposure and acute versus long-term outcomes can be established [11]. A corollary readers must be aware of is information bias, where there is excessive probing into risk factors/outcomes biasing results; data are not collected in a standard manner [12]. Prospective designs are unfortunately more expensive and labor intensive [11].
If the entire case series does not follow a prospective protocol, the data collection element could have been prospective. Data quality is optimized if established a priori [11], with uniform fields for each patient. A common alternative strategy for surgeons is to use their existing prospective patient database if one exists. Retrospective assessment of clinical and administrative records may result in missing outcomes of interest and inconsistent data. Retrospective patient assessment is prone to recall bias, where remembered risk factors or outcomes are inaccurate. Poh et al. [10] report that the series has a retrospective design, but utilizes a prospectively collected database. Given that the series reports results of a surgical

intervention, the reconstructive procedure itself is a consistent time point of reference for all patients. While a prospective study would be ideal, recall and information bias are minimized in this series.

iii. *Was patient recruitment consecutive?*
Inclusion of consecutive patients is the best indication to the reader that selection bias is minimized. In case series where favorable patients are selected or "cherry-picked", results will likely overestimate positive outcomes, namely, the success of a surgical intervention [5]. For example, selecting only American Society of Anesthesiologists (ASA) 1 patients will result in decreased morbidity and mortality. Reporting only ideal patients limits the external validity of the study, and readers cannot be confident the series represents practical effectiveness for all patients in real-world practice [13]. In a special case, for series where an incidence or estimate of risk is reported, it is important that all patients are reported for a given time period, and represent a demographic patient sample. An accurate "denominator" for the patient group must be obtained. For example, a series of all births at a hospital are a demographic sample, and the study can provide the incidence of birth injury for the given patient group. Conversely, a series of cases not resolving with conservative management and subsequently referred to a specialist represents only a portion of all cases, and patient group metrics cannot be calculated.
In case series where consecutive patients are not included, specific inclusion and exclusion criteria should be reported [5]; readers should interpret results accordingly. Further, for case series reporting a high-risk surgical intervention, even consecutive cases will not represent all patients; some discussion of the characteristics for patients who agree to treatment should be included. Poh et al. [10] do not specifically report consecutive, or "all" patients. The series simply reports that patients were identified from a prospective database from 2000 to 2009 with a supercharged jejunal flap within the defined period at MD Anderson Cancer Center (Houston, Texas). There is no discussion pertaining to the percentage of patients agreeing to treatment, though with a cancer diagnosis this procedure is not elective. However, an indication of the proportion of patients "fit" for this procedure should be discussed.

iv. *Was outcome assessment appropriate?*
As with other study designs, the primary outcome of a case series should be specific, clinically relevant, measured at an appropriate time, and be important to patients; these factors are indicative of the series' clinical impact [14]. Readers can consider the modified hierarchy of patient-important outcomes where Class I: mortality, Class II: morbidity, Class III: symptoms/quality of life/functional status, Class IV: surrogate [15, 16]. The highest-class clinically relevant outcome should be reported to have the largest impact on patient care [15, 16]. Class I and II outcomes are considered "hard" outcomes; they are dichotomous, and least subjective (e.g., "life or limb"). For example, a case series on melanoma, or major burn care, can report mortality (Class I), a case series on early laparoscopic cholecystectomy for cholecystitis can measure 30-day major complications (Class II), and a case series on breast reconstruction can report long-term quality of life with BREAST-Q [17] (Class III).
Appropriate timing of outcome assessment is equally important; the reader must consider if sufficient time has accumulated to assess patient survival, the success of a procedure, or quality of life [5]. For example, 30 days may be appropriate for a series assessing survival of acute trauma interventions, whereas 2 years may be necessary for long-term functional outcomes of a nerve reconstruction potentially requiring

multiple procedures or long-term physical therapy. Readers should look for a minimum follow-up period as a criterion for case series inclusion [4]. Finally, possible bias in outcome assessment should be considered. Blinding outcome assessment is frequently feasible in prospective designs [14]. For retrospective designs, "hard" outcomes are the most objective.

Poh et al. [10] report a number of appropriate intra- and postoperative outcomes given the retrospective design. Mortality (Class I) is reported, as are dichotomous Class II outcomes of intensive care admission, reoperation, flap failure, overall major complications (Table 18.1). Finally, Class III outcomes of oral intake, achieving regular diet and discontinuing tube feeds. Mean follow-up time of 22 months is appropriate given the outcomes. The 2–80 month minimum and maximum follow-up interval could include mortality; defining minimum follow-up excluding these cases would improve their methodology and reporting.

v. *Is the intervention appropriately described?*

Most surgical case series describe a procedure; technical details of the intervention and perioperative management should be sufficiently described for readers to appropriately interpret, and possibly reproduce reported results [5]. Beyond the specific description of a surgical procedure, readers should evaluate for operative indications, preoperative workup/care (e.g., imaging investigations, resuscitation protocols), perioperative care (e.g., antibiotics, venous thromboembolism prophylaxis, necessary instruments/disposables, dosages of unique medications), and postoperative care (e.g., physical therapy protocols, imaging surveillance) [1]. Any cointerventions should be described [18] (e.g., comorbid fracture repair with intramedullary nail of lower extremity fractures, abdominoplasty with breast reduction) [5].

Poh et al. [10] comprehensively report the details of a supercharged jejunal flap. The discussion focuses on three important aspects of the reconstruction: "(1) selecting the appropriate jejunal segment, (2) choosing the optimal recipient vessels for microsurgical anastomosis, and (3) creating a suitable conduit passageway." Beyond the meticulous description of the intervention, technical refinements, pitfalls, and the "how" and "why" of these critical steps are rationalized. Further, authors comment on planning the procedure between three teams, with steps that can be performed concurrently between ablative and reconstructive surgeons.

II. **What Are the Results?**

i. *Are outcomes appropriately reported?*

The case series is a descriptive study design, not analytic; no control group is present [4]. As such, "cause and effect" relationships cannot be established. Readers should be cautious that causal inferences between an intervention and outcomes are not reported. Instead, outcomes can be discussed in a descriptive manner, and hypotheses can be generated for testing in a higher level study design [4]. For example, the first case series of breast implant-associated anaplastic large cell lymphomas (BI-ALCL) [19] could not demonstrate causation of silicone breast implants; results suggested an association with silicone implants, and suggested confirmation with higher level studies (e.g., case-control study) . As discussed in *Was patient recruitment consecutive?*, the series also did not include a demographic patient sample, and incidence of BI-ALCL could not be estimated.

Readers should be cautious interpreting statistics beyond simple descriptive statistics, especially if p-values are present; authors should be conservative in reporting case series results [4]. In select cases, authors may report analyses "before and after" a procedure, or compared to historical controls. Any such analyses should have been defined a priori, and have rational sample size calculations. These analyses will detect significant "noise" instead of "signal"; postoperative outcomes are often nonspecific [18]. Patients receiving novel or investigational procedures are likely distinct from the general population, and derive a perceived benefit when assessed [18]. Historical controls are rarely, if ever, an adequate comparison group; patients treated previously were in completely distinct settings, and analyses are thus prone to a number of biases [18].

Poh et al. [10] report essential outcomes (as discussed in *Was outcome assessment appropriate?*), and do so in a cautious manner. Descriptive statistics are reported. Numerators and denominators accompany percentages. Measures of dispersion (e.g., minimum and maximum, SD) are reported. No inappropriate comparisons are present with respect to control groups outside the scope of the case series. No inappropriate analyses or p-values are reported before and after the technical modifications discussed in case series.

ii. *Are outcomes completely reported?*

Complete outcomes, especially beyond those demonstrating benefit, should be reported in a case series. In a prospective series, any loss to follow-up (LTFU) should be reported. Readers can assume patients LTFU have outcomes worse than those completing the study [20]. Patients with poor outcomes or health states do not present for follow-up, and these issues are not accurately captured (e.g., cancer patients not presenting for follow-up with their reconstructive surgeon may mean they are deceased). Further, reporting LTFU is a sign to the reader that a study was completed with higher methodological rigor [21]. For those identified LTFU, some discussion of the tolerability of the intervention, or treatment attrition is appropriate. In retrospective series, readers can similarly assess for missing outcome data; less missing data is a sign that a robust database was used.

In series where mortality or morbidity are not the most clinically important outcomes, reporting harms and potential complications is necessary. Readers should look for conventional reporting of overall major complications, reintervention, readmission, and appropriate intraoperative harms (e.g., blood loss, damage to surrounding structures) [1, 5]. In case series including patients treated over a long period of time, readers should be critical of identifiable and possible unknown changes to the patient population, disease characteristics, and intervention [4]; changes to the surgical procedure over time should be outlined, and rationalized to the reader. Similarly, authors can indicate the presence of a learning curve to the reader [1, 5]. Poh et al. [10] adequately report outcomes. LTFU is not specifically reported, but given the retrospective design of the series and nature of the appropriate outcomes, discussion of LTFU beyond time of follow-up is not of high importance. Poh et al. [10] comprehensively review harm and changes to the intervention over a variety of case series. No major component of missing data is discerned. Poh et al. [10] are appropriately critical of their own results, and interpret early treatment failures in context of an observed learning curve. The length of the learning curve is not specified, it is simply stated that the three flap failures occurred "early" in their experience.

III. Will the Results Change Practice?

i. *Are the patients similar to my own?*

After considering the validity of the case series, and appraising the results, readers must decide if patients are comparable to their own. Case series typically have high external validity [5]. Inclusion and exclusion criteria are not as stringent as in higher level study designs (e.g., RCTs), and results can often be applied to a wider spectrum of patients [4]. Still, readers should consider the comorbidities and characteristics of the patients included in the case series, especially prognostic variables (e.g., age, smoking status, tumor stage) [1].

Poh et al. [10] comprehensively describe their patient population. Table 18.1 describes baseline demographics, with high prevalence of recurrent disease, smoking, major comorbidities, and chemoradiation. These prognostic factors are, however, not surprising given the disease process and intervention described in the case series. The age, sex, comorbidities, and presenting diagnosis of patients in the case series match those of your patient.

ii. *Is the setting similar to my own?*

In applying results, readers must be certain that the care setting is similar to their own. Case series are often single center, however, if outcomes are pooled with a multicenter design, the differences between centers should be defined [5]. Novel and innovative interventions are often introduced by tertiary or even "quaternary" settings, where highly specialized care is delivered to what amounts to a worldwide referral base. While academic centers typically have more resources versus community settings, patients are correspondingly more complicated [5]. Multidisciplinary care is often necessary for increasingly complex interventions, for example, intraoperative anesthesia management, expertise of other surgical specialties, postoperative inpatient monitoring, postoperative imaging surveillance, and functional assessment, and long-term physical therapy.

Poh et al. [10] describe a patient group with high prevalence of recurrent disease and secondary reconstructions after treatment failures at other institutions. Patients similarly have a number of comorbidities. MD Anderson can be classified as a "quaternary" setting, where patients are captured from a global base [22]. Expertise beyond the reconstructive team is necessary, with the series describing a 3-team surgical approach, postoperative ICU and ward management, and subsequent nutrition and barium swallow assessment.

Resolution of Clinical Scenario

You review the case series and discuss it with your colleagues in planning for this challenging case. Given that the stomach will be unavailable for reconstruction, you agree a supercharged jejunal flap is appropriate for reconstruction. The series is appropriately designed, with appropriate outcome assessment for the procedure. You are impressed by the number of technical refinements, the comprehensive description of the surgical steps, and the candid rationale for changes. Your hospital is not a quaternary level center, but it is an academic center with oncologic general surgeons, thoracic surgeons, and microsurgical plastic surgeons who are all fellowship trained, and capable of undertaking the required supercharged jejunum procedure. You have a discussion with your patient regarding the risks of the procedure, the perioperative management, postoperative diet, and expected recovery. Given the complexity of the case, you and your colleagues decide to proceed with a two-stage surgical plan. On the first day of the procedure, the ablative teams will proceed with an esophagectomy, and partial gastrectomy. At the conclusion of the ablative procedure, the patient's remaining stomach will be evaluated, and the teams will decide if reconstruction with a gastric conduit is possible. If this is not possible (as predicted), reconstruction with a supercharged jejunal flap will be performed the following day in a staged manner to minimize operating time. During the procedure, you will incorporate the case series' details in selecting and isolating a jejunal segment of adequate length, creating a pathway through the chest to pass the jejunum, and finally dissecting a recipient artery and vein to perfuse the segment.

Conclusion

Although case series are recognized as Level IV in the hierarchy of evidence, they remain prevalent in the surgical literature. Case series is the most common study design in surgical specialty research and remain predominant in reporting unique patient presentations, and innovative surgical procedures. They are unique in their high external validity, and fast and less costly design. Alone, case series can establish the safety of an intervention, or the diagnostic accuracy of a test [4]. From a methodological standpoint, they are important in demonstrating feasibility, and patient characteristics for higher level study planning. With consideration of the topics discussed in this chapter, surgeons can confidently assess the validity and applicability of a case series relevant to their practice.

References

1. Agha RA, Fowler AJ, Rajmohan S, Barai I, Orgill DP, PROCESS Group. Preferred reporting of case series in surgery; the PROCESS guidelines. Int J Surg [Internet]. 2016;36(Pt A):319–23. Available from: http://www.ncbi.nlm.nih.gov/pubmed/27770639.
2. Chan K, Bhandari M. Three-minute critical appraisal of a case series article. Indian J Orthop [Internet]. 2011;45(2):103–4. Available from: http://www.ncbi.nlm.nih.gov/pubmed/21430861.
3. Joyce KM, Joyce CW, Kelly JC, Kelly JL, Carroll SM. Levels of evidence in the plastic surgery literature: a citation analysis of the top 50 "classic" papers. Arch Plast Surg [Internet]. 2015;42(4):411–8. Available from: http://www.ncbi.nlm.nih.gov/pubmed/26217560.
4. Kooistra B, Dijkman B, Einhorn TA, Bhandari M. How to design a good case series. J Bone Joint Surg Am [Internet]. 2009;91(Suppl 3):21–6. Available from: http://www.ncbi.nlm.nih.gov/pubmed/19411496.
5. Coroneos CJ, Ignacy TA, Thoma A. Designing and reporting case series in plastic surgery. Plast Reconstr Surg [Internet]. 2011;128(4):361e–8e. Available from: http://www.ncbi.nlm.nih.gov/pubmed/21544010.
6. Audigé L, Hanson B, Kopjar B. Issues in the planning and conduct of non-randomised studies. Injury [Internet]. 2006;37(4):340–8. Available from: http://www.ncbi.nlm.nih.gov/pubmed/16483576.
7. Okumura Y, Mori K, Yamagata Y, Fukuda T, Wada I, Shimizu N, et al. Two-stage operation for thoracic esophageal cancer: esophagectomy and subsequent reconstruction by a free jejunal flap. Surg Today [Internet]. 2014;44(2):395–8. Available from: http://www.ncbi.nlm.nih.gov/pubmed/24292600.
8. Takeno S, Takahashi Y, Moroga T, Yamamoto S, Kawahara K, Hirano T, et al. Reconstruction using a free jejunal graft after resection of the cervical esophagus for malignancy. Hepatogastroenterology [Internet]. 2013;60(128):1966–71. Available from: http://www.ncbi.nlm.nih.gov/pubmed/24719936.
9. Laing TA, Van Dam H, Rakshit K, Dilkes M, Ghufoor K, Patel H. Free jejunum reconstruction of upper esophageal defects. Microsurgery [Internet]. 2013;33(1):3–8. Available from: http://www.ncbi.nlm.nih.gov/pubmed/22821641.
10. Poh M, Selber JC, Skoracki R, Walsh GL, Yu P. Technical challenges of total esophageal reconstruction using a supercharged jejunal flap. Ann Surg [Internet]. 2011;253(6):1122–9. Available from: http://www.ncbi.nlm.nih.gov/pubmed/21587114.
11. Bernard T, Armstrong-Wells J, Goldenberg N. The institution-based prospective inception cohort study: design, implementation, and quality assurance in pediatric thrombosis and stroke research. Semin Thromb Hemost [Internet]. 2012;39(1):10–4. Available from: http://www.thieme-connect.de/DOI/DOI?10.1055/s-0032-1329551.
12. Sedgwick P. Prospective cohort studies: advantages and disadvantages. BMJ [Internet]. 2013;347(1):f6726. Available from: http://www.bmj.com/cgi/doi/10.1136/bmj.f6726.
13. Sedgwick P. Bias in observational study designs: prospective cohort studies. BMJ [Internet]. 2014;349(2):g7731. Available from: http://www.bmj.com/cgi/doi/10.1136/bmj.g7731.
14. Voineskos SH, Coroneos CJ, Ziolkowski NI, Kaur MN, Banfield L, Meade MO, et al. A systematic review of surgical randomized controlled trials: part I. Risk of bias and outcomes: common pitfalls plastic surgeons can overcome. Plast Reconstr Surg [Internet]. 2016;137(2):696–706. Available from: http://www.ncbi.nlm.nih.gov/pubmed/26818309.
15. Bala MM, Akl EA, Sun X, Bassler D, Mertz D, Mejza F, et al. Randomized trials published in higher

vs. lower impact journals differ in design, conduct, and analysis. J Clin Epidemiol [Internet]. 2013;66 (3):286–95. Available from: http://www.ncbi.nlm.nih.gov/pubmed/23347852.
16. Lubsen J, Kirwan B-A. Combined endpoints: can we use them? Stat Med [Internet]. 2002;21(19):2959–70. Available from: http://www.ncbi.nlm.nih.gov/pubmed/12325112.
17. Pusic AL, Klassen AF, Scott AM, Klok JA, Cordeiro PG, Cano SJ. Development of a new patient-reported outcome measure for breast surgery: the BREAST-Q. Plast Reconstr Surg [Internet]. 2009;124(2):345–53. Available from: http://www.ncbi.nlm.nih.gov/pubmed/19644246.
18. Carey TS, Boden SD. A critical guide to case series reports. Spine (Phila Pa 1976) [Internet]. 2003;28 (15):1631–4. Available from: http://www.ncbi.nlm.nih.gov/pubmed/12897483.
19. de Jong D, Vasmel WLE, de Boer JP, Verhave G, Barbé E, Casparie MK, et al. Anaplastic large-cell lymphoma in women with breast implants. JAMA [Internet]. 2008;300(17):2030–5. Available from: http://www.ncbi.nlm.nih.gov/pubmed/18984890.
20. Akl EA, Briel M, You JJ, Lamontagne F, Gangji A, Cukierman-Yaffe T, et al. LOST to follow-up Information in Trials (LOST-IT): a protocol on the potential impact. Trials [Internet]. 2009;10:40. Available from: http://www.ncbi.nlm.nih.gov/pubmed/19519891.
21. Schulz KF, Grimes DA, Altman DG, Hayes RJ. Blinding and exclusions after allocation in randomised controlled trials: survey of published parallel group trials in obstetrics and gynaecology. BMJ [Internet]. 1996;312(7033):742–4. Available from: http://www.ncbi.nlm.nih.gov/pubmed/8605459.
22. Van Allen EM, Lui VWY, Egloff AM, Goetz EM, Li H, Johnson JT, et al. Genomic correlate of exceptional erlotinib response in head and neck squamous cell carcinoma. JAMA Oncol [Internet]. 2015;1(2):238–44. Available from: http://www.ncbi.nlm.nih.gov/pubmed/26181029.

19 Quality Improvement and Patient Safety in Surgery

Martin A. Koyle and Jessica H. Hannick

Clinical Scenario

As a new community general urologist on staff, you are asked to see a 5-month-old male in the general pediatric medicine clinic with a unilateral, left non-palpable undescended testis. The right testicle is located in the scrotum and palpably is normal in shape and size. The mother reports to you that the infant's primary care provider had recommended referral to a specialist for correction, if the testis did not spontaneously descend by school age, and had recommended an ultrasound exam be performed in the interim. In your training as a resident, while rotating on pediatric urology, you remember your attending discussing the merits of early orchidopexy while suggesting that ultrasounds not only were rarely necessary in the current approach to the diagnosis and management of cryptorchidism, but could be misleading. As a generalist, rather than pediatric subspecialist, you wish to assure that the recommendations on the assessment and management of the undescended testis are accurate, and hence search your computer for current guidelines to this problem.

Literature Search

The scenario above portrays a situation that is relevant to Quality Improvement and Patient Safety (QIPS). The young surgeon wishes to provide quality care to the patient and feels the current plan of action that the mother has outlined may not be appropriate. Despite being comfortable with a myriad of common adult urological problems, specific pediatric problems are not regularly addressed in his practice setting. He, therefore, pursues a comprehensive search strategy utilizing the Medical Subject Heading (MeSH) terms of 'undescended testis', 'cryptorchidism', 'guidelines', and 'clinical pathways'. He has decided to search only English language papers within the past 5 years to narrow his search. Medline guides him to a recently published critical review of practice guidelines pertaining to the management of the undescended testis [1]. He has not been familiar with the AGREE II tool used in the assessment of several guidelines reviewed in the paper and realizes that he actually knows very little about how guidelines are actually constructed and to whom they are relevant.

M. A. Koyle (✉)
Department of Pediatric Urology, The Hospital for Sick Children, Toronto, ON, Canada
e-mail: martin.koyle@sickkids.ca

J. H. Hannick
Department of Surgery, McMaster University, Hamilton, ON, Canada
e-mail: jhannicklumc@gmail.com

A. Thoma et al. (eds.), *Evidence-Based Surgery*,
https://doi.org/10.1007/978-3-030-05120-4_19

Introduction

The practice of medicine continues to evolve, due to advances, often disruptive in nature, in basic science, pharmaceuticals and technology. However, the ***way*** we practice is also rapidly changing, as a result of the demands and expectations of the environment(s) in which we work (government, private sector, academic, hospital), and newer approaches for whom we care. The paternalistic model of care, where a physician dictated diagnostic and management plans, has become a ***shared decision model***, wherein transparency and joint interaction have become the new norm. Most of us were brought up in an era of volume-based health care delivery. This is now the era of ***evidence-based*** medicine, with ***personalized*** care and ***value*** has become the pivotal goals. Value (V)–based care, will be evaluated based on performance, that is on quality (Q) and cost ($) (V = Q/$) [2]. This approach will likely reimburse or reward providers based on outcomes (quality) rather than on number of cases performed. With skyrocketing healthcare costs, preventable errors have become a target for quality improvement and patient safety (QIPS).

For surgeons, in particular, this constantly changing playing field has to be balanced with patient safety concerns. Yet surgery has so many opportunities to be successful in QIPS initiatives due to the establishment of centrally based registries, standardization when possible, simulation training, and video critiquing of surgeries we perform. To many of us, QIPS is viewed as top-down, where institutions promote measures that we often consider nuisances and hence disregard, that are focused on issues such as hand hygiene, start times, checklists, line, surgical site and catheter-associated urinary tract infections, falls and pressure sores, and ventilator-associated pneumonia. It, therefore, becomes incumbent upon us to define reliable (the right) and meaningful metrics to make QIPS initiatives relevant and to provide evidence that indeed we are delivering quality care.

Background

In essence, surgeons have always pursued the concept of gradual, progressive change leading to ongoing opportunities for improvement. Our surgical results are audited to search for root causes of untoward outcomes caused by errors of omission and commission related to our interventions. At the turn of the twentieth century, Ernest Amory Codman began tracking and reporting his 'end results', a concept that was totally foreign to the established (Harvard) community at Massachusetts General Hospital (MGH). Codman promoted the ***End Result Idea***, through which he would document patient demographics and track their outcomes. He suggested that it was our ethical duty to report each surgeon's results, good or bad, and identify opportunities for improvement His desire to formally assess surgeon competence, rather than promotion based on seniority, led to his dismissal from MGH. Defiantly, he built his own facility, *The End Result Hospital*. There, he could measure efficiency and performance and present it to the public [3, 4]. To the medical community at that time, it was heresy. Ultimately, the concept of frank, scheduled discussion sessions, where analysis of hospital reform and patient outcomes occurs, has led to our now sacrosanct morbidity and mortality (M and M) conferences. He and other leaders of the newly formed American College of Surgeons (ACS), pursued a goal of evaluation and standardization. This culminated in the formation of the Joint Commission on Accreditation, for which Codman is now given much of the credit. Most recently, the ACS has focused on QIPS by developing the National Surgical Quality Improvement Program (NSQIP), which has rapidly expanded beyond North America [5]. NSQIP allows validated risk adjusted outcomes of surgical procedures to be compared between reporting hospitals. Because individual hospitals are often challenged when it comes to analyzing their surgical outcomes, it is difficult to pinpoint areas of concern to improve problem areas. NSQIP provides a tool to allow hospitals to focus on areas where improvement is necessary, where complication rates can be improved.

Quality Improvement and Patient Safety (QIPS) has now become a center of focus in all facets of medicine. It has become a mandated component of every hospital's annual report and a target for a broad variety of stakeholders, including payers and consumers (patients). The Institute of Medicine (IOM) has proposed six principles for improvement: safe, effective, patient-centered, efficient, timely and equitable care [6]. There is even a structure for publishing, the SQUIRE guidelines, as the increasing number of medical journals either entirely devoted, or at least partially devoted to this subject, publish new contributions [7].

What is Quality Improvement?

Although there are many interpretations of what QI is, Batalden and Davidoff have simplistically defined it as '... combined and unceasing efforts of everyone-healthcare professionals, patients and their families, researchers, payers, planners and educators-to make the changes that will lead to better patient outcomes (health), better system performance (care) and better professional development (learning)' [8]. Berwick and colleagues at the Institute for Healthcare Improvement (IHI) developed the triple aim of quality healthcare as that of improving the experience of care, improving the health of populations, and reducing per capita costs of healthcare [9].

Many of the current concepts of continuous process improvement (CPI) are based on the work of W. Edwards Deming, his 'system of profound knowledge' and his 'fourteen points of management' [10]. In QI, the four keys of the system of profound knowledge: appreciating the system, understanding variation, a theory of knowledge (epistemology) and understanding human behaviour/psychology, are pivotal in instituting sustained positive changes. Simplistically, this means viewing an organizational system as a series of interrelated processes not silos where they share a common goal, understanding that variation may be either due to a common or to a special cause, knowing that new knowledge is likely to be present within the organization and that there may be different individual drivers to enhance motivation. A key to Deming's thinking was that robust leaders who could engage stakeholders were mandatory, and that unwanted variation must be reduced. Kilo and IHI adopted the model for improvement in which an aim identifies a change concept to be improved within a defined time period [11]. Through a series of cycles called P-D-S-A (Plan, Do, Study, Act), a concept for change is addressed with an action plan, and an analysis of the effect of that action is then performed to allow further subsequent opportunities. With each ensuing PDSA, or change cycle, small adjustments can be made with hopes of making escalating gains. PDSA reiterates 3 fundamental questions in each cycle: 1. What are we trying to accomplish? 2. How will we know that a change is an improvement? 3. What changes can we make that will result in an improvement? Thus, through CPI, a provider, organization, or system is more likely to improve on an ongoing basis. Other tools such as Lean/Six Sigma may be used in furthering CPI. By reducing waste, one is increasing value for potential stakeholders [12].

Is QI Research?

Both QI and traditional research are based on data. Although it may be folklore as to the originator of the statement, one of the most famous quotations attributed to Deming (and for that matter others) is 'In God we trust, all others must bring data.' Simplistically, research attempts to provide new knowledge while QI takes existing knowledge and seeks improvement. Not that QI lacks rigor, but primarily it is based on rapid cycle tests of change (PDSA). Although statistical methodology can be used in QI, data are best presented visually in real time using run charts or when control limits are required, Shewart (Control) charts. Because of the confusion and inconsistencies regarding the publication of QI Material, the SQUIRE guidelines were introduced in 2008.

Unique to QI reporting in healthcare are the SQUIRE guidelines (**S**tandards for **QU**ality **R**eporting **E**xcellence) [7]. SQUIRE consists of a checklist composed of 19 items/4 categories, that authors should consider when submitting papers describing new QIPs and value knowledge in healthcare. The original descriptions of SQUIRE stressed that these checklist items are common to scientific reporting but with modifications that make them more applicable to the unique aspects of medical QI work. It was acknowledged that it was important to present a system such as this as many peer-reviewed journals and stakeholders were unfamiliar with the design, implementation and reporting of QI projects [13]. In no way are they meant to be exclusive of other guidelines and at times may be synergistic.

Discussion

Healthcare is a dynamic, complex entity that is unpredictable at best. Historically QIPS in healthcare has been driven by external forces (National Health Services (NHS), Centers for Medicare and Medicaid Services (CMS), Joint Commission on Accreditation of Hospital Organizations (JCAHO). As the stakes and emphasis in healthcare change and costs soar, many QIPS initiatives are now central to organizations (ACS), hospitals (Virginia Mason), and providers (Intermountain Healthcare, Kaiser-Permanente). Healthcare has attempted to emulate other highly reliable organizations (HROs) such as aviation and the nuclear agencies, where safety is prioritized and reduced errors are a priority. As value becomes more important, future research and leaders in the field will need to promote our knowledge of QIPS. In 1966, Donabeian identified three approaches in the assessment of quality: structure, process and outcome [14]. To this day, it remains one of the most frequently cited articles in healthcare and is a solid pillar in the evaluation of QI in healthcare [15]. In this seminal paper, structure referred not to the settings but to the qualifications of the providers in those settings and administrative systems within. Process and outcome are more straightforward and related to components of care and fate upon recovery. The Institute of Medicine further promoted QIPS in their 2000 and 2001 publications ***To Err is Human*** and ***Crossing the Quality Chasm*** [5, 16]. The focus of these reports was that systems need to be improved knowing that human fallibility and error are innate. Thus, much harm within healthcare was preventable. With the escalation of healthcare costs, prevention of costly errors, while reducing the onus on human blame, has become a goal as the road towards HROs is travelled.

It has been estimated that approximately half of all hospital complications occur within the operating room itself [17]. Surgery is unique, as it demands the combination of one's surgical skill, knowledge, and the judgment to apply the right operation to the right patient at the right time. Addressing the fact that surgery is a team sport exacerbates this daunting challenge. Although an operating room is as inanimate as a cockpit or an aircraft carrier, the variability in the supporting personnel (resident, fellow nursing, anesthesiologist) are not always as reliably interchangeable as those members of the airline crew or naval vessel. Although it is unlikely that the surgeon him/herself will change during an operation, commonly the other team players will. If anything the value of standardization and checklists should not be underscored. Communication failures have been demonstrated to occur every 7–8 min during an operation [18]. Thus, the longer the operation, with increasing likelihood of greater personnel turnover, the more the opportunity for error increases. Surgical checklists are now a decade old and have been implemented to reduce ***preventable*** surgically related morbidity (and mortality) [19]. Conceptually, this makes sense to assure that indeed it is the right patient who is consented for that scheduled operation, where laterality is confirmed as are issues of allergies and antibiotic administration. Urbach, using a large Canadian provincial database, has appropriately demonstrated that there are indeed potential challenges with checklists when there is non-compliance and inconsistencies with implementation [20, 21]. Although checking boxes per se may not impact the occurrence of adverse events, improved communication amongst operating room personnel, regardless of 'status', is to be encouraged.

Medicine as a whole, but surgery in particular, has housed a culture of ***shame and blame*** where an individual, rather than a system has been held responsible for a given outcome (especially a complication). Lucien Leape, a well known pediatric surgeon who is now at the Harvard School for Public Health, testified before the US Congress in its hearings on health care quality improvement that, 'The single greatest impediment to error prevention in medicine is that we punish people for making mistakes.' As a result of medical error, there is often more than just the patient as a victim, as it is easier to blame an individual than a system. The IOM's ***To Err is*** *Human* [16] focuses on the fundamental issue of human fallibility. In QIPS, James Reason's ***Swiss Cheese Model*** has often been used as an analogy [22]. Reason uses several layers of Swiss cheese with latent and active holes in this model. In an ideal system, errors are trapped between the layers, as the holes do not align. However, given the worst-case scenario, the holes of each layer align, and this creates an opportunity for an untoward event to occur.

Recognizing that human factors play an important role in outcome, it is obvious that an understanding of other elements that either support or hinder an individual's performance. As a core element of QIPS, ***Human Factors Engineering***, often called ergonomic or human engineering uses physical and psychological principles to affect processes and systems, and promote a reduction in errors [23]. In the operating room setting, it has especially been applicable to medical devices, medication safety, and Information Technology.

Clinical Practice Guidelines (CPGs) have increasingly become part of our daily practices in an attempt to enhance the quality of care. To be relevant, CPG's should be based on systematic reviews (SR) of current best evidence regarding a given topic, that has been addressed by an unbiased, multidisciplinary group of experts, so that they can use to assist practitioners and their patients in optimizing patient care. Sackett's description of Evidence-Based Medicine (EBM) of CPG's, 'The conscientious, explicit, and judicious use of current best evidence in making decisions about the care of individual patients', is most apt [24]. Problematically, is that not all CPG's have been based on high-quality evidence which potentially can lead to less than ideal results, and thus has led to scepticism regarding their implementation. CPGs should take voluminous or complex data that is not at our fingertips, and make such data more manageable for that individual patient, who is cared for by that individual physician, at that given time. Hence in no way should CPG's be construed as cookbook medicine or the only option for that specific patient or encounter. Sadly, defensive medicine and 'over testing' are realities of the practice of medicine. This is costly to the system as a whole and impacts the utility of CPGs and other progressive initiatives such as 'Choosing Wisely' [25]. In QIPS, various tools have been developed to construct and to analyze CPGs. GRADE (Grades of Recommendation, Assessment, Development and Evaluation) has been developed as a tool for constructing CPGs that enhances physician evaluation of the quality of medical evidence so that recommendations can be applied most appropriately in patient care [26]. It replaces letter recommendations regarding quality with 'strong' or 'weak/conditional', 'for' or 'against' and avoids 'expert opinion' in the hierarchy of evidence pyramid, while recognizing that even the highest evidence standard, SR, can be flawed. Recommendations using GRADE ideally should be actionable and avoid restating obvious facts and vagaries. The AGREE II tool (Appraisal of Guidelines for Research and Evaluation) has gained acceptance as a standardized technique for the evaluation and comparison of existing CPGs [27]. It consists of 6 quality domains containing 23 items used to quantify each CPG. It requires several appraisers who independently score each domain of each guideline. Importantly each appraiser also assesses the overall quality of the CPGs and makes a recommendation as to whether that guideline should be used. CPGs should be used judiciously, remembering that medical judgment and experience remain essential components of our fostering shared decision making and optimal care. CPGs will increasingly be available to us. As such, practitioners must understand how they are developed and what their qualities and their relevance are [28]. Electronic Health Records likely will improve their availability, as well as be an adjunct in improving compliance with their utilization.

Resolution of the Clinical Scenario

After reading this single aforementioned article, the surgeon found that five major guidelines all recommended that referral of an infant with presumed cryptorchidism should occur by 6 months of age [1]. The guidelines agreed that palpation under anesthesia followed by laparoscopic evaluation if the testis remained non-palpable should be the next step of care. All of these modern guidelines were in concordance, with rare exceptions, supporting that ultrasound and other diagnostic imaging were not recommended as an adjuvant is assessment, as imaging rarely improve diagnostic accuracy, and does not impact management. Given this information in hand, the surgeon suggests that as the boy, who is approaching 6 months of age, should be scheduled for exam under anesthesia and laparoscopy with potential orchidopexy as indicated, under the care of a pediatric urologist or pediatric surgeon, who performs cases such as this on a routine basis. Therefore, the ultrasound is deemed unnecessary and is cancelled.

Conclusion

QIPS is more than checklists and evidence-based guidelines. There are many tools that can be used in QI that are applicable to promote a culture of change and safety, eliminate silos, understand the basic problem(s) at hand, test changes, with continuous study of outcomes and performance, and to report pertinent findings to sustain change(s) to allow for opportunities to improve further [29]. The environment of the operating room is complex and each patient is unique. As such the opportunity for error is heightened, as are opportunities to reduce, or ideally, prevent such occurrences.

References

1. Kim JK, Chua ME, Ming JM, Dos Santos J, Zani-Ruttenstock E, Marson A, et al. A critical review of recent clinical practice guidelines on management of cryptorchidism. J Pediatr Surg. 2017. [Epub ahead of print].
2. Institute of Medicine, Committee on Redesigning Health Insurance Performance Measures, Payment, and Performance Improvement Programs. Rewarding provider performance: aligning incentives in medicare. Washington, DC: National Academies Press; 2016.
3. Berwick DMEA. Codman and the rhetoric of battle: a commentary. Milbank Q. 1989;67(2):262–7.
4. Donabedian A. The end results of health care: Ernest Codman's contribution to quality assessment and beyond. Milbank Q. 1989;67(2):233–56.
5. Birkmeyer JD, Shahian DM, Dimick JB, Finlayson SR, Flum DR, Ko CY, et al. Blueprint for a new American College of Surgeons: National Surgical Quality Improvement Program. J Am Coll Surg. 2008;207(5):777–82.
6. Institute of Medicine, Committee on Quality of Health Care in America. Crossing the quality chasm: a new health system for the 21st century. Washington, DC: National Academies Press; 2001.
7. Davidoff F, Batalden P, Stevens D, Ogrinc G, Mooney S, SQUIRE Development Group. Publication guidelines for quality improvement in health care: evolution of the SQUIRE project. Qual Saf Health Care. 2008;17(Suppl 1):3–9.
8. Batalden P, Davidoff F. What is "quality improvement" and how can it transform healthcare? Qual Saf Health Care. 2007;16:2–3.
9. Berwick DM, Nolan TW, Whittington J. The triple aim: care, health, and cost. Health Aff. 2008;27(3): 759–69.
10. Walton M. The Deming management method. New York: Perigee Books; 1986.
11. Kilo CM. A framework for collaborative improvement: lessons from the Institute of Healthcare Improvement's breakthrough series. Qual Manag Health Care. 1998;6(4):1–13.
12. Cima RR, Brown MJ, Hebl JR, Moore R, Rogers JC, Kollengode A, et al. Use of lean and six sigma methodology to improve operating room efficiency in a high volume tertiary-care academic medical center. J Am Coll Surg. 2011;213(1):83–92.

13. Davidoff F, Batalden P. Toward stronger evidence on quality improvement. Draft publication guidelines: the beginning of a consensus project. Qual Saf Health Care. 2005;14:319–25.
14. Donabedian A. Evaluating quality of medical care. Milbank Q. 1966;44:166–206.
15. Ayanian JZ, Markel H. Donabedian's lasting framework for health care quality. New Eng J Med. 2016;375:205–7.
16. Kohn LT, Corrigan J, Donaldson MS. To err is human: building a safer health system. Washington, DC: National Academies Press; 2000.
17. Gawande AA, Thomas EJ, Zinner MJ, Brennan TA. The incidence and nature of surgical adverse events in Colorado and Utah in 1992. Surgery. 1999;126(1): 66–75.
18. Hu YY, Arriaga AF, Peyre SE, Corso KA, Roth EM, Greenberg CC. Deconstructing intraoperative communication failures. J Surg Res. 2012;177(1):37–42.
19. Haynes AB, Weiser TG, Berry WR, Lipsitz SR, Breizat AH, Dellinger EP, et al. A surgical safety checklist to reduce morbidity and mortality in a global population. N Engl J Med. 2009;360(5):491–9.
20. Urbach DR, Govindarajan A, Saskin R, Wilton AS, Baxter NN. Introduction of surgical safety checklists in Ontario, Canada. N Engl J Med. 2014;370(11): 1029–38.
21. Leape LL. The checklist conundrum. N Engl J Med. 2014;370(11):1063–4.
22. Reason J. Human error models and management. Br Med J. 2000;320:768–70.
23. Vosper H, Hignett S, Bowie P. Twelve steps for embedding human factors and ergonomics principles in healthcare education. Med Teach. 2018;40(4): 357–63.
24. Sackett DL, Rosenberg WM, Gray JA, Haynes RB, Richardson WS. Evidence based medicine: what it is and what it isn't. BMJ. 1996;312:71–2.
25. Welk B, Winick-Ng J, McClure JA, Lorenzo AJ, Kulkarni G, Ordon M. The impact of the choosing wisely campaign in urology. Urology. 2018 Mar 20. [Epub ahead of print].
26. Guyatt GH, Oxman AD, Vist G, Kunz R, Falck-Ytter Y, Alonso-Coello P, et al. GRADE: an emerging consensus on rating quality of evidence and strength of recommendations. BMJ. 2008;336:924–6.
27. Brouwers MC, Kho ME, Browman GP, Burgers JS, Cluzeau F, Fedar G, et al. AGREE II: advancing guideline development, reporting, and evaluation in health care. CMAJ. 2010;182:839–42.
28. Koyle MA. Truth and consequences—the issue with standards and guidelines. Can Urol Assoc J. 2018; 12(4):79–80.
29. Koyle MA, Koyle LCC, Baker, GR. Quality improvement and patient safety: reality and responsibility from Codman to today. J Pediatr Urol. 2018:14(1):16–9.

Diagnostic Studies in Surgery

20

Stuart Archibald, Jessica Murphy, Achilles Thoma and Charles H. Goldsmith

Introduction

Surgeons are challenged every day in clinical practice to make a diagnosis. A correct diagnosis is foundational to recommending the proper approach, whether that is to perform a procedure or to refrain from such. The present climate, in which patients often come primed with internet-derived 'expertise', can add social complexity and time to the consultation process. Furthermore, patients have continually rising expectations for certainty in the diagnosis before making their decision on the treatment recommendations that they get, often unaware that certainty in diagnosis is elusive.

As surgeons, we follow the time-honoured process of starting with the history and physical examination to arrive at an initial differential diagnosis. Then, by applying diagnostic tests, often in a sequential multistep process, we narrow the diagnostic possibilities. In this chapter, using a clinical scenario of an informed patient who has typical expectations, we will demonstrate how to use the best evidence to find, evaluate and apply diagnostic tests.

Clinical Scenario

A 42-year-old woman is referred to you with an asymptomatic thyroid nodule found on ultrasound (US), which was done for vague swallowing symptoms. She had no history of previous thyroid disease or head and neck radiation exposure. However, she is alarmed with the identification of the nodule because her grandmother died years ago of a thyroid cancer. She is 'surgery averse', and only wants an operation 'if it is necessary'. Accordingly, she went on the Internet and found that there is a molecular test, ThyroSeq ver3, which, it is claimed, will determine if her lesion is malignant and what kind of

S. Archibald (✉)
Department of Surgery, Division of Head and Neck Surgery, McMaster University, Hamilton, ON, Canada
e-mail: archibs@mcmaster.ca

J. Murphy · A. Thoma
Department of Surgery, Division of Plastic Surgery, McMaster University, Hamilton, ON, Canada
e-mail: murphj11@mcmaster.ca

A. Thoma
e-mail: athoma@mcmaster.ca

A. Thoma · C. H. Goldsmith
Department of Health Research Methods, Evidence and Impact, McMaster University, Hamilton, ON, Canada
e-mail: cgoldsmi@sfu.ca

C. H. Goldsmith
Faculty of Health Sciences, Simon Fraser University, Burnaby, BC, Canada

C. H. Goldsmith
Department of Occupational Science and Occupational Therapy, Faculty of Medicine, The University of British Columbia, Vancouver, BC, Canada

A. Thoma et al. (eds.), *Evidence-Based Surgery*,
https://doi.org/10.1007/978-3-030-05120-4_20

malignancy it is. Before looking at her printed handout, you examine her; the examination discloses only that there is a fullness to her right lower neck in the thyroid compartment, without any well-defined mass. No neck adenopathy could be palpated. Laryngoscopy showed that her vocal cords moved normally. The remainder of the examination is non-contributory. This negative history and non-palpable nodule cannot influence the probability of this patient having cancer, thus the baseline prevalence of thyroid cancer in the general population remains. You know that the prevalence of thyroid nodules and thyroid cancer has increased in recent years, with most of this increase considered to be due to the widespread use of US examinations [1, 2]. This constitutes 'detection bias' , where the event of interest (thyroid nodules and thyroid cancer) is observed more frequently in the group which has a more sensitive detection method, in this case US, applied to it than is applied to the other group; this may lead to the mistaken interpretation that nodules and cancers are truly increasing [3]. You believe that this patient falls into this category.

Nodules may be found in 70% of the population when US is used [4], and about 5% of thyroid nodules are malignant [5, 6], thus a reasonable estimate for the prevalence of thyroid cancer is 3%. On review of this patient's US report, unfortunately, there is very little additional information on the characteristics of the nodule aside from its dimensions. In your own institution, US reports are given in the TIRADS (Thyroid Imaging Reporting and Data System) format, which, provides more information than was given in this patient's study. You decide to search the literature to find out what are the current recommendations for diagnostic tests on thyroid nodules, their sequence, and the role of TIRADS.

Literature Search

As outlined in Chap. 3, the first step to solving a clinical dilemma is to form your research question using the PICOT format (Box 1).

Box 1. The PICOT Format Applied to the Current Clinical Scenario

Population	Patient with **thyroid nodules**
Intervention	TIRADS (Thyroid Imaging Reporting and Data System)
Comparative intervention	NA
Outcome	Risk classification for cancer diagnosis
Time horizon	NA

Using the following search terms, you perform a literature search using Cochrane Library: 'Thyroid Nodules' AND 'TIRADS' AND 'Risk Classification'. Your search yields one article and a conference publication for the same article (see Appendix 1), however, neither of these articles are ideal as the studies are performed in Korea, and therefore may not be generalizable to your patient. You decide to perform a literature search using the same terms in PubMed, and this time your search yields 18 articles. By restricting your search to publications in 2017 and 2018, your search results decrease to 12 (Appendix 2). Out of these 12 publications, you choose a 2017 paper by Horvath et al. [7]; you choose this study as it was a prospective study by the authors who first proposed TIRADS.

Brief Study Summary

It is clear that the most commonly recommended initial test of a thyroid nodule is US of the thyroid. Although there are several ways that the US is reported, the use of TIRADS categories has become dominant. In this study, the investigators used total thyroidectomy specimens for surgical pathology on all nodules as the standard against which TIRADS was tested, and they provided Likelihood Ratios (LR). Other studies have used Fine-Needle Aspiration Biopsy (FNAB) against which TIRADS was tested, but since FNAB includes an 'indeterminate' category where only some nodules come to surgery, the actual status of those nodules which were not resected remains uncertain, thus those studies do not have a consistently applied 'gold standard' against which TIRADS was compared. In the recent study by Horvath et al. [7], consecutive eligible patients underwent US for nodule pattern and TIRADS categorization of the dominant nodule, as well as of any additional nodules which were considered likely to be identifiable on gross examination of the surgical specimen. A subset of US images were used to determine inter-observer agreement. US-guided FNAB's of nodules in TIRADS categories 4 (including 4A, 4B and 4C) and 5 were then carried out. FNAB was not done on TIRADS 2 and 3 because the likelihood of cancer is 0 and <5%, respectively (Table 1 in the Horvath et al. [7] article). However, in the total thyroidectomy specimens done for dominant nodules classified as TIRADS 4 or 5, other non-dominant nodules were studied with histopathology, and this includes some TIRADS 2 and 3 lesions, even though they may not have had FNAB. In this way, some TIRADS 2 and 3 incidentally found nodules were studied with pathology. The radiologists who performed the US and FNAB test were all highly experienced. A single experienced pathologist who performed the surgical pathology studies was blinded to the US and TIRADS results. In total, 210 patients, and 520 nodules were studied, Fig. 20.1 outlines the study design by Horvath et al. [7].

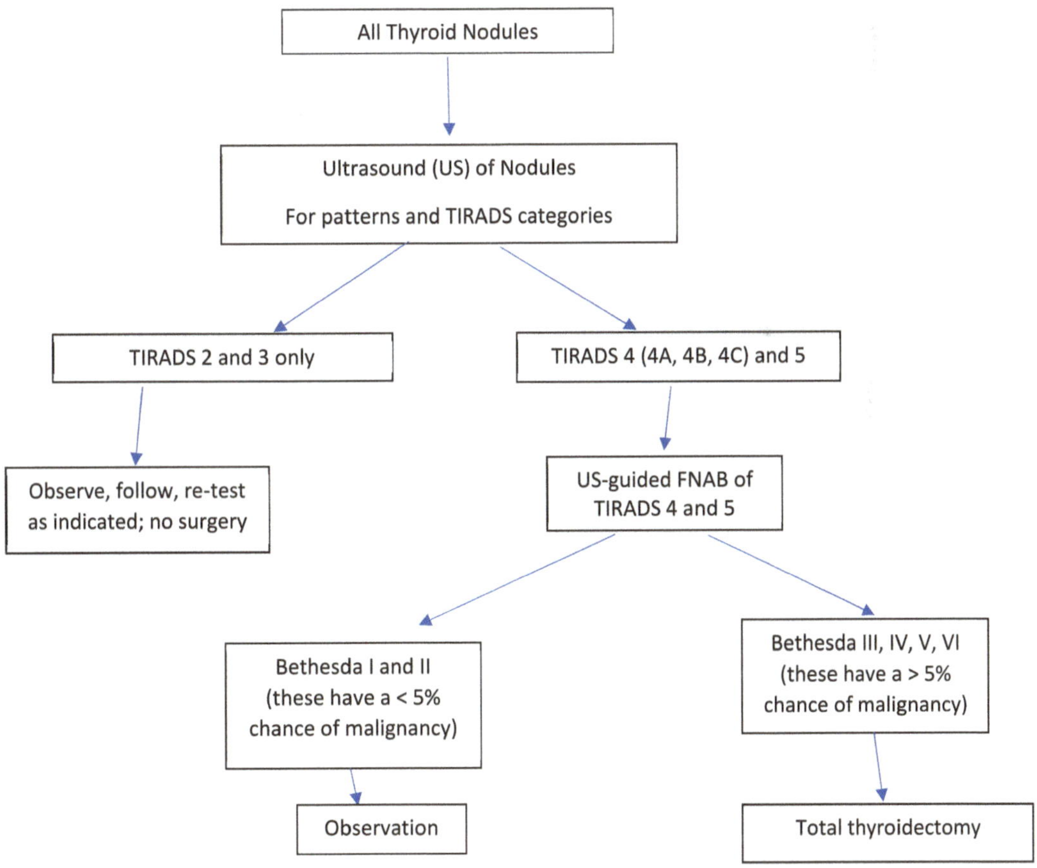

Fig. 20.1 Flow chart of study design. Created using information from Horvath et al. [7]

Important Aspects of Diagnostic Studies

The first step in successfully understanding and appraising a diagnostic study is to understand the terms commonly used in this area of research. These terms are summarized in Box 2. As also seen in Chap. 29, diagnostic studies use the terms 'True Positive' (TP), 'False Positive' (FP), 'True Negative' (TN) and 'False Negative' (FN). True Positive, refers to when the test correctly diagnoses the presence of a disease, whereas False Positive, incorrectly diagnoses an individual with a disease when they do not have the disease. Similarly, a True Negative, is when a test correctly determines that a disease is not present, and a False Negative refers to when a diagnostic test determines a patient does not have a disease, when in fact they do. These terms, which describe how useful test is, are outlined in terms of cancer diagnosis in Table 20.1.

Box 2. Important Terms for Understanding Diagnostic Tests

- **True Positive (a)**
  The test indicates a positive result AND the reference standard indicates a positive result
- **True Negative (d)**
  The test indicates a negative result AND the reference standard indicates a negative result
- **False Positive (b)**
  The test indicates a positive result BUT the reference standard indicates a negative result
- **False Negative (c)**
  The test indicates a negative result BUT the reference standard indicates a positive result
- **Positive Predictive Value (PPV): a/(a + b)**
  The proportion of positive tests that is correct
- **Negative Predictive Value (NPV): d/(c + d)**
  The proportion of negative tests that is correct
- **Sensitivity: a/(a + c)**
  The proportion of patients with disease that is correctly identified by the test
  Synonyms: True-Positive Rate or Positivity in Disease
- **Specificity: d/(b + d)**
  The proportion of patients without the disease correctly identified by the test
  Synonyms: True-Negative Rate or Negativity in Health
- **Likelihood Ratio (LR):**
  Ratio of the probability that a test result is correct to the probability that the test result is not correct
- **Likelihood Ratio of a Positive Test (LR+)**
  The equivalent of dividing the true-positive rate by the false positive rate, or $\frac{\text{Sensitivity}}{1\text{–Specificity}}$ *
- **Likelihood Ratio of a Negative Test (LR−)**
  The equivalent of dividing the false negative rate by the true-negative rate, or $\frac{1\text{–Sensitivity}}{\text{Specificity}}$ *
- **'Accuracy' (best avoided) = (a + d)/(a + b + c + d)**

	Reference standard/ disease is positive/present	Reference standard/disease is negative/absent	Total
Test is positive	*a*	*b*	*a* + *b*
Test is negative	*c*	*d*	*c* + *d*
	a + *c*	*b* + *d*	*a* + *b* + *c* + *d*

**For two-level tests*

When a clinician is making a diagnosis (Box 3), the direction of reasoning moves from a test result to the probability of disease. The Likelihood Ratio (LR), a computation not commonly used by surgeons (although it should be),

Table 20.1 Diagnostic testing and true results in cancer diagnosis

	Cancer Present	Cancer Absent
Test Positive for Cancer	True Positives (TP)* a**	False Positives (FP) b
Test Negative for Cancer	False Negatives (FN) c	True Negatives d
Totals	(TP + FN) (a + c)	(FP + TN) (b+d)

* 'TP', 'FP', 'FN' and 'TN' are used to designate the cell

** '*a*', '*b*', '*c*' and '*d*' are used to designate the numerical values in a cell

does this. It can be either 'LR+' or 'LR−' depending on whether or not one is considering a positive test or a negative test with exactly two levels. An LR+ test answers the question: 'What is the probability that this positive test is found in a patient with the disease compared to the chance that this same positive test is found in a patient without the disease?' Referring to Table 20.1, where the data are displayed in a 2 × 2 table,

$$\text{LR+ is calculated as : LR+} = \frac{\text{Probability of a positive test in those with cancer}}{\text{Probability of a positive test in those without cancer}} = \frac{\text{sensitivity}}{(1-\text{specificity})}$$

LRl− answers the question: 'What is the probability that this negative test will be found in a patient with the disease compared to the probability that this negative test will be found in a patient without the disease?'

$$\text{LR− is calculated as :} = \frac{\text{Probability of a negative test in those with cancer}}{\text{probability of a negative test in those without cancer}} = \frac{(1-\text{sensitivity})}{\text{specificity}}.$$

The above is applied to the results from Horvath et al. [7], as follows:

$$\begin{aligned}\text{LR+} &= \{a/(a+c)\}/\{b/(b+d)\}\\ &= (270/272)/(43/230) = 5.31\end{aligned}$$

This is how Horvath et al. [7] used the data, which meant reducing it to two levels to get a 'pooled LR' .

$$\begin{aligned}\text{LR}- &= \{c/(a+c)\}/\{d/(b+d)\}\\ &= (2/272)/(187/230) = 0.01\end{aligned}$$

LR also can be applied to a single level out of a multilevel data set, avoiding the need to collapse the data into a 2 × 2 table which results in a loss of information. The data from Horvath et al. [7] is shown for each level in Table 20.2.

When an LR is 1.0, the pre-test probability (prevalence), and post-test probability are unchanged. When an LR is greater than 1.0, then the post-test probability of the diagnosis has been increased from the pre-test probability (prevalence), and conversely when an LR is less than 1.0, then the post-chance probability of the diagnosis has been decreased from the pre-test probability (prevalence). Generally, LRs greater than 10 indicate large and likely conclusive changes in the pre-test probabilities and 'rule in' the condition of interest, whereas LRs less than 0.1 indicate large and likely conclusive changes in the pre-test probabilities and 'rule out' the

Table 20.2 Results as reported by Horvath et al. [7] showing LR for each category

Test result *(TIRADS categories)*	Cancer (shown by surgical pathology)	No cancer (shown by surgical pathology)	Totals	LR
5	86	1	87	72.7
4C	135	13	148	8.8
4B	49	29	78	1.4
4A	1	16	17	0.05
3	1	55	56	0.02
2	0	116	116	0.00
Totals	272	230	502	

condition of interest. LRs between 2 and 5, or between 0.5 and 0.2 indicate modest but possibly important changes in the pre-test probabilities. LRs between 1 and 2, or between 0.5 and 1.0 indicate small and not usually conclusive changes in pre-test probabilities [8]. The additional advantages of LRs are that the value is not influenced by prevalence of the condition. LRs can be used sequentially in several tests, which follows the pattern of use in clinical practice. Thus, the pre-test probability and LR can give the post-test probability of the first test, which serves as the pre-test probability with the LR to give the post-test probability on the second test, and so on. This can be done using mathematical formulae for each test, or more simply by applying a nomogram to visually give the results [9]. This nomogram, shown in Fig. 20.2, makes it easy to use cascading tests in this manner [8]. By placing a ruler on the pre-test probability and aligning it with the calculated LR we can obtain on the far right of the nomogram the post-test probability of the disease. As TIRADS has multiple categories various cut-off points may be selected for determining sensitivity, specificity, positive predictive value, negative predictive value, and likelihood ratios. The cut-off point shown in Table 20.3 in the Horvath et al. [7] article is at 4B; thus TIRADS 2, 3, and 4A are considered 'negative' for cancer, and TIRADS 4B, 4C and 5 are considered 'positive' for cancer.

Sensitivity and specificity are commonly stated measures of a diagnostic test, even though they reverse the process used clinically by using the known disease categories to get test performance measures. The term 'sensitivity' describes the proportion of diseased individuals in the population that are classified as having the disease using the test. In other words, sensitivity describes the probability that the test is able to correctly diagnose a disease. Sensitivity is calculated using the formula below:

$$\text{Sensitivity} = \frac{a}{(a+c)}$$

Specificity is the term used to describe the proportion of those people without the disease who were correctly identified by a negative test as non-diseased. Specificity is calculated using the formula below:

$$\text{Specificity} = \frac{d}{(b+d)}.$$

Using results from the Horvath et al. [7] study (Table 20.3), sensitivity and specificity would be calculated as:

$$\text{Sensitivity} = \frac{270}{(270+2)} = \frac{270}{272} = 0.993 \text{ or } 99.3\%$$

and

$$\text{Specificity} = \frac{187}{(187+43)} = \frac{187}{230} = 0.813 \text{ or } 81.3\%$$

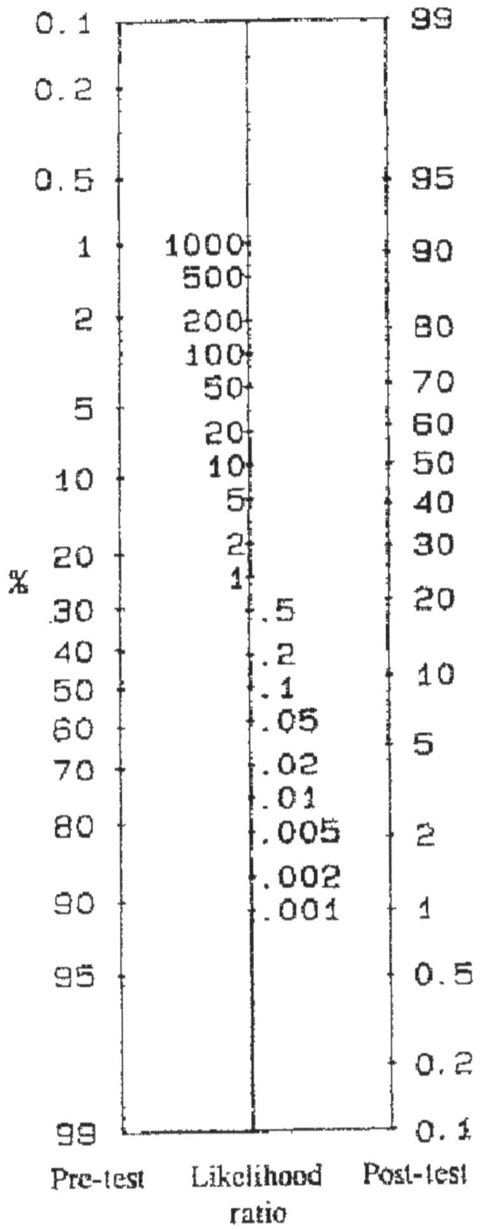

Fig. 20.2 Nomogram for interpreting diagnostic test result

While sensitivity and specificity are useful in characterizing diagnostic tests and are commonly reported, they have major limitations when applied to 'real-life' practice [10]. For instance, as noted above, in using sensitivity and specificity, the clinician's reasoning must move from the disease to the test result. But the presence or absence of the disease is precisely what is being sought in a diagnostic quest, where the clinical reasoning moves from the test result to whether the disease is present or not. Furthermore, sensitivity and specificity do not allow sequential use in tests, and thus are limited in refining the diagnosis. Sensitivity and specificity, are developed from binary data, and are not amenable to being used on a single level in a multilevel data set, without reducing the data to a 2 × 2 table, thereby losing information. Finally, as explained by Parikh et al. [10], in the early stages of a disease it is difficult to determine the presence of health or illness and so the sensitivity may decrease; on the other hand, in cases of severe disease, the sensitivity may increase. Despite this, for most diagnostic tests in common situations, the sensitivity and specificity are considered to be stable. For all of these reasons, the most useful test for a clinician is the LR. The reported Positive Predictive Value (PPV) and Negative Predictive Value (NPV) also answer a relevant question when making a diagnosis, but they are computed using prevalence of disease in the data set, which may not be the prevalence of disease in your clinical setting [10]. In the study by Horvath et al. [7], the prevalence is $(a + c)/(a + b + c + d) = 272/502 = 0.54$ or 54%. This makes the PPV and NPV really only useful at around 50% prevalence. You need to ask, 'Is this true for my clinical setting?'.

You decide to review the article by Horvath et al. [7] and a subsequent systematic review article by Kwak et al. [11] to see how the TIRADS system was developed and how it has evolved. You discover that the TIRADS system, as first proposed by Horvath et al. [12] in 2009, used diagnostic ultrasonography to stratify the risk of cancer into six levels. The original proposal by Horvath et al. [12] had 10 ultrasound patterns to define the levels of cancer risk, and it has been validated by using surgical pathology as the 'gold standard' [7]. However, while the concept of a model stratifying cancer risk remained attractive, this TIRADS system has proven too cumbersome for most investigators, and some nodules do not fit the patterns [11]. Thus, modifications to simplify the system have

Table 20.3 Results as reported by Horvath et al. [7] grouping TIRADS categories. Pooled LR = 5.31

Test Result (TIRADS Categories)	Cancer (shown by surgical pathology)	No Cancer (shown by surgical pathology)	Totals
"Positive": 4B, 4C, 5 (cancer prob > 5%)	270 <u>TP</u> *a*	43 <u>FP</u> *b*	313 *a*+*b*
"Negative": 2, 3, 4A (cancer prob < 5%)	*c* <u>FN</u> 2	*d* <u>TN</u> 187	*c*+*d* 189
Total	*a* + *c* 272	*b* + *d* 230	502

**TP, True Positive; FP, False Positive, FN; False Negative, and TN; True Negative, denote the "cell names".*
**"a", "b", "c", "d" refer to the numerical values of those cells: 270, 43, 2, 187, respectively*

been made. The first suggestion was to de-emphasize the criteria designed to characterize specific benign conditions because with most thyroid nodules, the main goal is to identify those nodules which are malignant. The second was to reduce the number of ultrasound characteristics of the nodule to the five considered relevant for determining risk of cancer: composition (solid, cystic, mixed), echogenicity (hyper, hypo, marked hypo), adverse margins (yes/no), adverse calcifications (yes/no), and adverse shape (yes/no). These suggested modifications were used to define levels 4A, 4B, 4C and 5, where 4A has one of the US characteristics present, 4B has two, and 4C has three or four [11]. The risk of malignancy associated with each category is shown in Table 20.4. The effect of these modifications has been to simplify the TIRADS system and so making it easier to apply. An additional result is that 'TIRADS' may mean slightly different things depending on whether one is using Horvath's model [12], or one of the others.

For instance, using the modified system by Kwak et al. [11], the probabilities of malignancy for each level are similar to, but not exactly the same, as the probabilities quoted by Horvath et al. [7]. The use of different criteria for the levels is a weakness of the present status of TIRADS. In any TIRADS system, the expertise of the US operator is important. The US operators in published studies are usually the most expert available, and this level of expertise may affect the generalizability of the results.

Once an US, using the TIRADS categories, has been found to warrant FNAB (generally considered for 4B and higher), then the patient is usually sent for an US-guided FNAB, as was done in the 2017 paper by Horvath et al. [7], and the results of this test are reported using the commonly accepted Bethesda System for Reporting Thyroid Cytopathology [13]. The Bethesda System uses 'diagnostic categories' designated by Roman numerals, rather than Arabic numerals as with TIRADS levels. A meta-analysis of the Bethesda System by Bongiovanni et al. [14] presents data that allow LRs to be calculated for the various Diagnostic Categories. Thus, the diagnostic tests of US with TIRADS Levels can be followed by FNAB with Bethesda Diagnostic Categories, and by using LRs in each test in the sequence, the probabilities

Table 20.4 Risk of malignancy associated with each category

Level	Risk of cancer (%)
5	87.5
4C	44.4–72.4
4B	9.2
4A	3.3
3	1.7
1 and 2	0

Created using information from Kwak et al. [11]

Table 20.5 Bethesda diagnostic categories showing probabilities of cancer and likelihood ratios

Diagnostic category[a]	Risk of cancer (%)	Likelihood ratio (LR)
VI	99.0	592
V	75.0	18.2
IV	30.0	2.6
III	14.0	1.1

Created using information from Bongiovanni et al. [14]
[a]Diagnostic categories I and II are not shown as the risk of cancer is <5% [14]. None of these LRs can be used to 'rule out', but V and VI clearly exceed 10, so could be used to 'rule in' cancer

of cancer may be refined. The LRs for the Bethesda Diagnostic Categories calculated from data in the Bongiovanni et al. [14] study are displayed in Table 20.5.

Evaluating the Literature on a Diagnostic Test

Three key steps must be taken to assess a diagnostic test, and this can be done by answering the three main questions outlined in Box 3.

Box 3. Questions to Appraise the Literature on a Diagnostic Test

1. Are the results valid?
   Primary guides
   (a) Is there an independent, blind comparison with a reference standard?
   (b) Does the patient sample include an appropriate spectrum of patients whom the diagnostic test will be applied in clinical practice?
   Secondary guides
   (a) Do the results of the test being evaluated influence the decision to perform the reference standard?
   (b) Are the methods for performing the test described in sufficient detail to permit replication?
2. What are the results?
   (a) Are likelihood ratios of the test being evaluated? Or, are the data necessary for their calculation provided?
3. Will the results help me in caring for my patients?

(a) Will the reproducibility of the test result and its interpretation be satisfactory in my setting?
(b) Are the results applicable to my patient?
(c) Will the results change my management?
(d) Will patients be better off as a result of the test?

Created using information from Jaeschke et al. [15]

Are the Results of the Study Valid?
The answer to this question is critical because it determines whether the results can be trusted. You need to know if the test was compared to an appropriate reference standard, and what the characteristics of the study population are.

Primary guide #1(a): Is there an independent blind comparison with a reference standard?
In the study by Horvath et al. [7] all eligible patients' thyroids underwent US and TIRADS categorization, and those nodules categorized as TIRADS 4 and 5 underwent FNAB, and those found to be Bethesda Diagnostic Categories III–VI went on to surgery. The pathologist was blinded to the TIRADS readings.

Primary guide #1(b): Does the patient sample include an appropriate spectrum of patients to whom the diagnostic test will be applied in clinical practice?
Given that the centre reporting is a tertiary referral centre [7], the spectrum of disease might at first be thought to be of advanced disease. However, the size of the nodules indicates that many small and therefore early nodules are included, so the spectrum seems to be applicable more broadly.

Any dominant TIRADS 2 and 3 nodules were eliminated from surgery, and thus the gold standard was not applied to them. Some information was obtained from other TIRADS 2 and 3 nodules found in the total thyroidectomy specimens taken out for a dominant TIRADS 4 or 5 nodule, but the full spectrum of benign nodules was not studied. Such a limitation may not be clinically important when the goal of diagnosis is to determine malignancy, but it does affect the study of benign nodules. All TIRADS 4 and 5 nodules which were Bethesda III–VI on FNAB went on to surgery. We are not told in how many cases there was a discrepancy where high levels of TIRADS were not matched by high categories of Bethesda, that is, where TIRADS 4 and 5 which have a high probability of malignancy were only Bethesda I or II, which have a less than 3% chance of malignancy, although the number is likely very few. Properties of a test can change with different degrees of disease severity. Likelihood ratios tend to increase when patients with the target disease all have severe disease and tend to decrease towards 1 when the subjects all have mild disease. Knowing the study population will help you decide if the results are applicable to your practice.

Given that the data came from a single tertiary centre known for its interest in thyroid cancers, the prevalence of malignant disease in the population from which the study sample was drawn will be high. This, plus the elimination of probably many TIRADS 2 and 3 nodules likely accounts for the high (54%) percentage of remaining nodules that are malignant. The stage and cell type of cancers are not specified. However, given the small size of the nodules (median size 7 mm), it is likely that most of the disease is early stage, with some more advanced lesions, as the largest was 6 cm. It seems therefore that an appropriate sample of cancer patients was studied.

Once validity has been confirmed, and the subjects characterized, two more questions need to be answered.

Secondary guide #1(a): Do the results of the test being evaluated (in this case TIRADS) influence the decision to perform the reference standard test(s) (in this case, FNAB and surgery)?
In this study, the TIRADS level did affect whether or not the FNAB and surgery were

performed. This is unavoidable for ethical reasons because to do otherwise would require that all patients have the reference standard performed knowing that those with TIRADS Levels 2 and 3 have a very low probability of malignancy. A sensitivity analysis using confidence intervals could be used for those Levels.

Secondary guide #1(b): Are methods for performing the test described in sufficient detail to permit replication?

The performance of all of the tests, TIRADS, and FNAB, are well-described with examples of each of the ten US levels in the case of TIRADS, the equipment (US machine) for TIRADS, and laboratory process for FNAB to get the Bethesda Classification specified [7].

What Are the Results?

Given the above considerations, you are becoming more confident that the study's results will be believable. We have presented LRs as the most versatile and applicable way to use tests to refine the diagnosis. LRs answer the relevant question, use the same pattern of reasoning as does a diagnostician (unlike sensitivity and specificity), are not affected by prevalence, (unlike PPV and NPV), can be applied to multilevel data without loss of information (unlike sensitivity and specificity), and can be used on sequential tests to narrow the diagnostic probabilities.

Are likelihood ratios for the test results presented, or are the data necessary for their calculation available?

Sufficient data are presented to allow LRs to be calculated. Referring to the previous calculations, and the Horvath et al. [7] paper, the data give a pooled LR of 5.31 (Table 20.3). Consider this option 1, which accepts that only some of the TIRADS 2 and 3 (and likely a minority, although we do not know) are included, thus not fully evaluating the TIRADS system. What if other ways of studying TIRADS are considered? A full evaluation of TIRADS (consider this Option 2) would require all of the TIRADS 2 and 3 be studied in the same way as TIRADS 4 and 5, operating on those patients knowing that the diagnosis of cancer is very low; this is not ethical. TIRADS 4 and 5 alone are considered in the data by Horvath et al. [7] (Option 3), the LRs are different as seen in Table 20.6. 4C is less likely to change the pre-test probability than was the case in option 1, because LR is now 2.3 instead of 8.8, and 4B is reduced to 0.37 from 1.4.

Which should be chosen? Option 2 is not feasible. Option 3 discards the information on TIRADS 2 and 3, even though that is incomplete, and lowers the LRs. We are left, then, with option 1. See Table 20.3.

The article by Horvath et al. [7] used FNAB and the Bethesda Classification to confirm the malignant potential of TIRADS 4 and 5, leading to surgery, but the data from the cytology is not otherwise discussed. Acknowledgement is given that TIRADS was used to select patients for FNAB, and the FNAB results lead to treatment recommendation.

Will the Results Help Me in Caring for My Patient?

3(a) Will the reproducibility of the test result and its interpretation be satisfactory in my setting?

Your centre already uses the TIRADS and Bethesda Systems, so application of this test will

Table 20.6 Calculated LR's for each category of TIRADS 4 and 5 when TIRADS 2 and 3 are discarded (Option 3)

TIRADS level	Cancer	No cancer	Totals	LR
5	86	1	87	18.7
4C	135	13	148	2.3
4B	49	29	78	0.37
4A	1	16	17	0.01
	271	59	330	

Created with data from Horvath et al. [7]

be straightforward, unlike situations where neither of these systems are currently used.

3(b) Are the results applicable to my patient?
We have assessed the validity of the Horvath et al. article [7] and its results, and now want to know if it helps us in caring for the patient. The pre-test probability of cancer is estimated at 3%, and for TIRADS 4B application of the LR of 5.31 gives a post-test probability of about 22% (see Nomogram in Fig. 20.2). This is not enough to exceed the patient's threshold for surgery, although it would be high enough for most surgeons.

You decide, therefore, to obtain an US-guided FNAB and apply LR from that test [14]. The result was read as Bethesda Level IV. Taking the pre-test probability as 22%, and applying the LR of 1.7, on the Fagan nomogram the post-test probability becomes about 33%. The patient is impressed that so much more information could be obtained from minimally invasive tests, but she remains unconvinced that surgery is necessary. She wants to know how the new test, ThyroSeq ver3 might affect the probabilities.

3(c) Will the results change my management?
The data on ThyroSeq ver3 presented at the American Thyroid Association 2017 meeting by Stewart et al. [16] allows calculation of the diagnostic test variables. Seeing that multiple diagnostic categories of Bethesda Classification are reported is reassuring that the article is comprehensive. Two of the categories, III and IV, are shown here, with calculation of LRs (Tables 20.7 and 20.8).

$$\begin{aligned} LR- &= [c/(a+c)]/[d/(b+d)] \\ &= (3/35)/(101/119) = 0.1 \end{aligned}$$

This does not exceed 10, so it indicates a modest change in probabilities from pre-test to post-test.

$$\begin{aligned} LR- &= [c/(a+c)]/[d/(b+d)] \\ &= (3/35)/(101/119) = 0.1 \end{aligned}$$

At 0.1, this rules out the diagnosis of malignancy

$$\text{Sensitivity} = 0.91$$

$$\text{Specificity} = 0.8$$

$$\text{PPV} = 0.64 \text{ or } 64\%$$

$$\text{NPV} = 0.97 \text{ or } 97\%$$

$$LR+ = 3.52$$

$$LR- = 0.04$$

$$\text{Sensitivity} = 0.97$$

Table 20.7 ThyroSeq version 3: performed on thyroid nodules subjected to FNAB, and read as 'Bethesda III' (follicular neoplasm or suspicious for a follicular neoplasm, probability of cancer 5–15%)

Test Result	Cancer Present	Cancer Not Present	Totals
Positive	32 **a**	18 **b**	50
Negative	**c** 3	**d** 101	104
	35	119	154

Table 20.8 ThyroSeq version 3: Performed on thyroid nodules subjected to FNAB, and read as 'Bethesdal IV' (follicular neoplasm or suspicious for a follicular neoplasm, probability of cancer 15–3%)

Test result	Cancer present	Cancer not present	Totals
Positive	34	16	50
Negative	1	42	43
	35	58	93

$$\text{Specificity} = 0.72$$

$$\text{PPV} = 0.68 \text{ or } 68\%$$

$$\text{NPV} = 0.98 \text{ or } 98\%$$

Although insufficient information is provided for you to carry out the full assessment of a diagnostic test as was done for Horvath's paper, there is enough data to determine, for a Bethesda IV sample the LR+ is 3.5, and the LR− is 0.04. You can tell the patient that if the test were applied, and she 'fit' the study sample of patients, then using the Fagan nomogram a positive test would change her pre-test probability of cancer from 33% to a post-test probability of 68%, and if the test is negative, the pre-test probability would change from 33% to a post-test probability of 1.3%.

You also point out that if the ThyroSeq ver3 test had been applied initially without first doing the US-TIRADS and the FNAB in sequence as was done, given a pre-test probability of 3% and an LR + of 3.5 then the post-test probability would be about 10%, not high enough for her to choose surgery, although a negative test with LR− of 0.04 would have ruled out cancer, with a post-test probability of less than 0.1%.

3(d) Will patients be better off as a result of the test?

The use of sequential tests for which the LRs are known or can be calculated as shown in this example to be very helpful. It is important to use all levels available in the data for LR. With multiple levels, there is a greater chance to find the LR > 10, which is sufficient to move almost any pre-test probability of disease to the post-test 'rule in' disease threshold (Fig. 20.3). Now that you have worked this out for this clinical problem, and you have the LRs already calculated, and the nomogram available, future patients with the same problem can be approached with confidence and efficiency.

Caution should be used when applying the latest new 'wonder test' to try to gain the requisite information all at once, as these tests need to be subjected to the same rigorous scrutiny as was demonstrated for TIRADS to be considered valid and applicable to a particular situation.

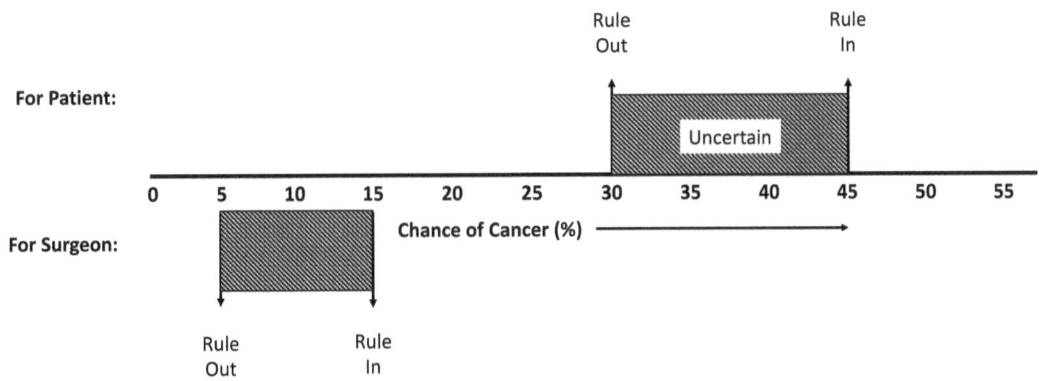

Fig. 20.3 Rule in, rule out line

Appendix 1: Results of Cochrane Literature Review

1. Ha EJ, Mood W-J, Na DG, Lee YH, Choi N, Kim SJ, et al. A multicenter prospective validation study for the Korean thyroid imaging reporting and data system in patients with thyroid nodules. Korean J Radiol. 2016;17(5):811.
2. Ju Ha E, Mood W-J, Na D, Lee YH, Choi N, Kim JK. A multicenter, prospective validation study for the Korean thyroid imaging reporting and data system in patients with thyroid nodules (K-TIRADS). European Thyroid Journal. In: 29th conference on annual meeting of the European thyroid association. Denmark; 2016.

Appendix 2: Results from PubMed Literature Search

1. Nguyen QT, Lee EJ, Huang MG, Park YI, Khullar, Plodkowski RA. Diagnosis and treatment of patietns with thyroid cancer. Am Health Drug Benefits. 2015;8(1): 30–40.
2. Parikh R, Parikh S, Arun E, Thomas R. Likelihood ratios: clinical application in day-to-day practice. Indian J Ophthalml. 2009;57(3): 217–21.
3. Archibald S, Bhandari M, Thoma A. For the evidence-based surgery working group. Users' guides to the surgical literature: how to use an article about a diagnostic test. CJS. 2001;44(1): 17–23.
4. Zhuang Y, Lic C, Hua Z, Chen K, Lin JL. A novel TIRADS of US classification. Biomed Eng Online. 2018;17(82):1–17
5. Ching CL, Tan HC, Too CW, Lim WY, Chiam PPS, Chu L, et al. Diagnostic performance of ATA, BTA and TIRADs sonographic patterns in the predication of malignancy in histologically proven thyroid nodules. Singapore Med J. 2018. [EPub Ahead of Print]. https://doi.org/10.11622/smedj.2018062.
6. Schenke S, Zimny M. Combination of sonoelastography and TIRADS for the diagnostic assessment of thyroid nodules. Ultrasound Med Biol. 2018;44(3):575–83.
7. Migda B, Migda, Migda MS, Slapa RZ. Use of the Kwak Thyroid Image Reporting and Data System (K-TIRADS) in differential diagnosis of thyroid nodules: systematic review and meta-analysis. Eur Radiol. 2018;28(6):2380–88.
8. Middleton WD, Teefey SA, Reading CC, Langer JE, Beland MD, Szabunio MM, et al. Multiinstitutional analysis of thyroid nodule risk stratification using the American College of Radiology Thryoid Imaging Reporting and Data System. AJR Am J Roentgenol. 2018;208(6): 1331–41.
9. Vargas-Uricoechea H, Meza-Barera I, Herrera Chaparro J. Concordance between the TIRADS ultrasound criteria and the BETHESDA cytology criteria on nontoxic thyroid nodule. Thyroid Res. 2018;10(1). eCollection 2017. https://doi.org/10.1186//s13044-017-0037-2.
10. Trimboli P, Fulciniti F, Zilioli V, Ceriani L, Giovanella L. Accuracy of international ultrasound risk stratification systems in thyroid lesions cytologically classified as indeterminate. Diagn Cytopathol. 2017;45(2): 113–7.
11. Horvath E, Silva CF, Majlis SM Rodriguez I, Skoknic V, Castro A, et al. Prospective validation of the ultrasound based TIRADS (Thyroid Imaging Reporting And Data System) classification: results in surgically resected thyroid nodules. Eur Radiol. 2017;27(6): 2619–28.
12. Dhyani M, Faquin W, Lubitz CC, Daniels GH, Samir AE. How to interpret thyroid fine-needle aspiration biopsy reports: a guide for the busy radiologist in the era of the Bethesda Classification System. *AJF* 2013;201(6):1335–39.

References

1. Davies L, Welch HG. Current thyroid cancer trends in the United States. JAMA Otolaryngol Head Neck Surg. 2014;140(4):317–22.
2. Topstad D, Dickinson JA. Thyroid cancer incidence in Canada: a national cancer registry analysis. CMAJ Open. 2017;5(3):E612–6.
3. Altman DG. Practical statistics for medical research. London: Chapman and Hall; 1991. p. 95.
4. Corso C, Gomez X, Sanabria A, Vega V, Dominguez LC, Osorio C. Total thyroidectomy versus hemithyroidectomy for patients with follicular neoplasm. A cost-utility analysis. Int J Surg. 2014;12:837–42.
5. Cooper DS, Doherty GM, Haugen BR, et al. For the American Thyroid Association (ATA) guidelines taskforce on thyroid nodules and differentiated thyroid cancer. Revised American thyroid association management guidelines for patients with thyroid nodules and differentiated thyroid cancer: the American Thyroid Association (ATA) guidelines taskforce on thyroid nodules and differentiated thyroid cancer. Thyroid. 2009;19:1167–214. Errata in: Thyroid. 2010;20:674–5; Thyroid. 2010;20:942.
6. Welker MJ, Orlov D. Thyroid nodules. Am Fam Phys. 2003;67:559–66.
7. Horvath E, Silva CF, Majlis SM, Rodriguez I, Skoknic V, Castro A, et al. Prospective validation of the ultrasound based TIRADS (Thyroid Imaging Reporting And Data System) classification: results in surgically resected thyroid nodules. Eur Radiol. 2017;27(6):2619–28.
8. Archibald S, Bhandari M, Thoma A. For the evidence-based surgery working group. Users' guides to the surgical literature: how to use an article about a diagnostic test. CJS. 2001;44(1): 17–23.
9. Fagan TJ. A nomogram for applying likelihood ratios [letter]. NEJM. 1975;293:257.
10. Parikh R, Parikh S, Arun E, Thomas R. Likelihood ratios: clinical application in day-to-day practice. Indian J Ophthalml. 2009;57(3):217–21.
11. Kwak JY, Han KH, Yoon JH, Moon HJ, Son EJ, Park SH, et al. Thyroid imaging reporting and data system for US features of nodules: a step in establishing better stratification of cancer risk. Radiology. 2011;260(3):892–9.
12. Horvath E, Majlis S, Rossi R, Franco C, Niedmann JP, Castro A, et al. An ultrasonogram reporting system for thyroid nodules stratifying cancer risk. J Clin Endocrinol Metab. 2009;94:1748–51.
13. Dhyani M, Faquin W, Lubitz CC, Daniels GH, Samir AE. How to interpret thyroid fine-needle aspiration biopsy reports: a guide for the busy radiologist in the era of the Bethesda Classification system. AJF. 2013;201(6):1335–9.
14. Bongiovanni M, Spitale A, Faquin WC, Mazzucchelli L, Baloch ZW. The Bethesda system for reporting thyroid cytopathology: a meta-analysis. Acta Cytol. 2012;56:333–9.
15. Jaeschke R, Guyatt G, Sackett DL. The evidence-based medicine working group. Users' guides to the medical literature. III. How to use an article about a diagnostic test. A: are the results of the study valid? JAMA. 1994;271(9):703–7.
16. Stewart D, Carty S, Sippel R, Yang P, Sosa J, Sipos J, et al. Clinical validation of THYROSEQ V3 performance in thyroid nodules with indeterminate cytology: a prospective blinded multi-institutional validation study. Thyroid. 2017;27(Suppl1):A-167.

How to Assess a Prognostic Study

21

Saurabh Gupta, Kevin Kim, Emilie Belley-Côté and Richard P. Whitlock

Clinical Scenario

You are a cardiac surgeon consulting on a 63-year-old man with severe aortic stenosis. He has a bicuspid aortic valve, followed by his cardiologist for years, and is becoming increasingly dyspneic. He also describes an episode of pre-syncope. On physical examination, he weighs 100 kg (220 lbs) and is 183 cm (6 ft) tall, and you auscultate a 3/6 systolic ejection murmur. His echocardiogram shows a calcified aortic valve with a mean gradient of 60 mm Hg and a valve area of 0.8 cm^2. You discuss aortic valve replacement with a bioprosthetic prosthesis. You review the risks and benefits of the surgery. He asks you two questions: "How long will the bioprosthetic valve last?" and "What are the possible operative and long-term complications?" You ask your senior resident to check for prognostic studies around bioprosthetic valves to discuss during the patient's next appointment.

How and Why We Measure Prognosis?

As surgeons, we aim for interventions that do more benefit than harm and intend for better outcomes than the natural course of the pathology. Prognostic studies examine the effect of variables, like surgical interventions, on disease progression [1]. Understanding prognosis can help us better advise our patients on treatment options and natural disease progression. Further, knowledge of expected outcomes after a given procedure informs us, and our patients, in the decision-making process [2].

Providing accurate estimates of patient prognosis requires a study that reports outcomes in patients with a similar clinical presentation [3]. For example, a surgeon looking to determine

S. Gupta
Department of Surgery, Division of Cardiac Surgery, Department of Health Research Methods, Evidence, and Impact, McMaster University, Hamilton, ON, Canada
e-mail: Saurabh.gupta@medportal.ca

K. Kim
Department of Health Research Methods, Evidence and Impact, Hamilton Health Sciences, Hamilton General Hospital, Hamilton, ON, Canada
e-mail: kevinskim94@gmail.com

E. Belley-Côté
Department of Health Research Methods, Evidence, and Impact, Department of Medicine, Division of Cardiology & Critical Care, Population Health Research Institute, McMaster University, Hamilton, ON, Canada
e-mail: emilie.belley-cote@phri.ca

R. P. Whitlock (✉)
Department of Surgery, Division of Cardiac Surgery, Department of Health Research Methods, Evidence, and Impact, McMaster University, Population Health Research Institute, Hamilton, ON, Canada
e-mail: Richard.whitlock@phri.ca

A. Thoma et al. (eds.), *Evidence-Based Surgery*,
https://doi.org/10.1007/978-3-030-05120-4_21

in-hospital mortality after replacing the ascending aorta and aortic valve in a patient with Marfan syndrome would need studies that report outcomes in other Marfan patients. Such patient data are referred to as prognostic factors; clinical characteristics that are objectively measured and can help predict patient outcomes [4].

In the remainder of this chapter, we will focus on identifying trustworthy prognostic information and using the results in patient care.

Study Designs for Prognostic Studies

Before undertaking a literature search, it is important to understand what study designs best answer our clinical question. When determining the effectiveness of treatment, we consider randomized controlled trials (RCTs) as high quality evidence and observational studies as lower quality [5]. When determining prognosis, however, we might place more confidence in estimates of prognosis from observational studies than RCTs [6]. This is because RCTs include filters in their eligibility criteria (e.g., age restriction, comorbidity, drug intolerance, etc) that exclude patients relevant to the broader prognostic question of interest. Eligible patients may decline to participate in an RCT due to reasons related to their prognosis. One exception to this rule is large, simple, pragmatic trials with broad eligibility criteria. For example, Stassano et al. [7] randomized 310 patients to receive a mechanical or bioprosthetic aortic valve. If our patient wanted to compare the effectiveness of one valve type over the other, "Aortic valve replacement: a prospective randomized evaluation of mechanical versus biological valves in patients ages 55–70 years" by Stassano et al. [7] might be a good study to use. However, our patient wants to know his prognosis specifically after receiving a bioprosthetic valve. As such, a cohort of study is ideal in identifying associations between our prognostic factors of interest and outcomes [8].

In cohort studies (a type of observational study), patients receive the intervention (i.e., they are not randomized) and are observed over a period of time. Furthermore, cohort studies can be conducted prospectively—forward in time—or retrospectively—data are collected on patients who received the intervention some time ago, and we want to know their outcome [9]. Both approaches have advantages and disadvantages. Prospective designs are powerful for assessing incidence and investigating potential causes. They measure the stage of disease prior to treatment, preventing the true effect from being influenced by the knowledge of the outcome. Most importantly, investigators using a prospective cohort design can measure outcomes more completely and accurately than a retrospective design [10]. The disadvantages are high cost and inefficiency when studying rare outcomes. Alternatively, a retrospective study design is less costly and time-intensive. A retrospective cohort study fundamentally has the same methodology as a prospective study, except that it looks back in time. Subjects already had their exposure to the variable of interest, had baseline measurements recorded, and follow-up period completed. The main disadvantage of a retrospective study is that biases may affect the selection of patients and recall of information. Further, we must use the data available, which may be incomplete, inaccurate, or measured in ways not suited to answer our question [11]. The 2017 study by Goldstone et al. [12], which we chose to help answer our patient's questions, is a retrospective cohort study. The authors identified patients who underwent surgical aortic valve replacement from 1996 through 2013 and evaluated their outcomes [12].

Investigators can also use a "case-control" design to study prognosis. They evaluate patients who have experienced an outcome of interest (cases) and compare them to those without the outcome (controls) [13]. Investigators are then able to assess the relative frequency of prognostic factors among both study groups. For example, Sleder et al. [14] retrospectively evaluated socioeconomic and racial disparities among severe aortic stenosis (AS) patients receiving transcatheter aortic valve replacement (TAVR) in a case-control study. They compared 67 patients with severe AS who underwent TAVR (cases) to patients with severe AS who were not offered TAVR (controls). They noted a statistically significant income disparity between the "cases" and "controls" [14]. By definition, case-control studies are retrospective and share the limitations of retrospective cohort studies. In addition, case-control studies provide relative odds of outcomes, but not absolute risks. Case-control studies are particularly useful when the outcome of interest is rare or requires lengthy time to occur—beyond what would be feasible for a prospective study design [15].

Literature Search

To identify relevant literature to our patient with aortic stenosis, we entered relevant key words into an established database of publications (Please see Chap. 4: How to Perform a Literature Search). In our scenario, entering the keywords "biologic" AND "aortic valve" AND "replacement", along with activating filters for human, full texts, and published within the last 2 years identified 27 articles in PubMed. If an initial search does not produce articles of interest, we could employ other strategies such as querying multiple databases (EMBASE and MEDLINE). We can also review references of relevant publications and recent textbooks (hand-searching) or reach out to field experts for guidance. Scanning through the most recent publications, we did not identify any relevant RCTs or prospective cohort study. Ten studies were excluded for focusing on basic science, two were excluded because they were case studies, and four studies excluded for evaluating outcomes with specific repair types in comparison to valve replacement. The search revealed one promising article: "Mechanical or Biological Prostheses for Aortic-Valve and Mitral-Valve Replacement" by Goldstone et al. [12]. This is a retrospective cohort study that identified patients who underwent surgical aortic valve replacement from 1996 through 2013 and evaluated their outcomes. This study seems promising in answering our patient's questions. The steps in appraising a surgical study that deals with prognosis are shown in Table 21.1.

Table 21.1 User's guide to surgical literature: guide to an article about prognosis [16]

I. Guide for validity (study methodology)
Step 1:
• Is the sample representative?
– Were patients homogeneous with respect to their prognostic risk? Are they at a similar point in the course of the disease?
– If subgroups were identified, did investigators provide estimates for clinically relevant subgroups and adjust for important prognostic factors?
Step 2:
• Was follow-up sufficiently long and complete?
• Were assessed outcomes objective and unbiased?
II. Understanding the results
Step 3: How likely are the outcomes to occur over time?
Step 4: How precise are the estimates of likelihood?
III. Using the results to determine patient care (applying the results to your patients)
Step 5: Can I apply the results to my practice or patient?

Appraising the Surgical Literature on Prognosis

Before applying the study results to our patient, we must critically appraise the Goldstone et al. [12] publication. Key questions to ask are (1) Is the sample representative of my patient? (2) Was the follow-up sufficiently long and complete? (3) Were the assessed outcomes objective and unbiased? (4) How likely are the outcomes to occur over time? (5) How precise are the estimates of likelihood? (6) Can I apply the results to my practice or patient? Table 21.1 outlines these questions, and more, that are important when interpreting and using prognostic studies [16].

Is the Sample Representative?

Ideally, we would like to determine prognosis by studying an affected population from the onset of exposure to the end. However, we cannot study entire populations and must instead determine the prognosis of a sample. As such, evaluating a representative sample of the entire population is crucial for generalizable results [17]. If a sample population is systematically different from the population of interest, it is not representative and may be biased. Biased prognostic studies can result in over- or underestimating event rates. A common way to identify an unrepresentative sample is to look for any systematic processes that patients passed through before entering the study, which may introduce bias; for example, patients with more complex or severe forms of the disease are more likely to be referred for tertiary care [3]. As a consequence, the prognosis in a tertiary center sample may differ from the prognosis of the disease in general due to referral bias. To determine whether a sample is a representative, look for a description of inclusion and exclusion criteria as well as a recruitment strategy. In addition, the authors should report objective criteria for sample selection and disease diagnosis. Unclear or inadequate definition of patients within a study increases the risk that the sample will not be representative, and its results biased. This is achieved through precise and consistent inclusion criteria [18]. For instance, we want studies reporting outcomes in a study group with similar baseline characteristics as our patient from the clinical scenario (63-year-old male with severe, symptomatic aortic stenosis). If a study included a diverse spectrum of patients undergoing aortic valve replacement (a wide age range, for example), a subgroup analysis of study participants similar to our patients would suffice. In addition to similar disease severity, other prognostic factors such as age, smoking history, diabetes, among others, should be considered. It is important to consider these prognostic factors in relation to each other to avoid making false conclusions.

In situations where a patient characteristic impacts prognosis, a stratified analysis may be used. In a stratified analysis, participants are separated into groups (i.e., strata) by prognostic factors [19]. When a large number of variables predict prognosis, stratified analyses are impractical and statistical methods, like regression, adjust for multiple variables, and determine the strongest prognostic factors [20].

When evaluating the sample in the Goldstone et al. [12] study, we see that the authors obtained all patient records from the California Office of Statewide Health Planning and Development (OSHPD) Patient Discharge, Emergency Department, and Ambulatory Surgery Center in the Patient Discharge, Emergency Department, and Ambulatory Surgery Centre datasets [12]. This database includes all patients treated across California in different centers and regions [12]. The authors use the ICD-9-CM codes—objective criteria—to define the inclusion of patients undergoing, "primary aortic valve replacement, or mitral valve with biologic prosthesis or mechanical prosthesis". They also state clear exclusion criteria: not residing in California during initial surgery, previous cardiac surgery, multiple valve replacements, aortic valve repair, mitral valve repair, and thoracic aortic surgery. They included a diverse group of patients and stratified them by age. Mortality outcomes were also analyzed in these strata and reported. We can confidently say that Goldstone et al. [12] included a representative sample, with characteristics similar to our patient's.

Was Follow-up Sufficiently Long and Complete?

Investigators should follow their patients for an adequate length of time to capture all patient-important outcomes. This is especially important in determining long-term outcomes, where the risk of loss to follow-up is increased [21]. A study reporting follow-up results of patients at 5 years after surgery may be helpful, but not adequate for our patient who is expected to live for another 10–15 years after his surgery.

Losing participants to follow-up threatens the validity of prognostic studies and increases the risk of bias as outcomes in those lost to follow-up may differ from those who remain in the study [21]. For example, anticoagulation therapy is a lifelong commitment for patients receiving a mechanical aortic valve [22]. In a study reporting the survival of patients after valve replacement surgery, those lost to follow-up may not be deceased but may have moved or followed up by another physician. The patients surviving and not lost to follow-up are no longer representative of the sample or even the entire study group. The threat to study validity is greatest when outcomes of interest are infrequent, and/or many participants are lost to follow-up. Let us consider the example of mechanical valve thrombosis. In a study by Cannegeiter et al. [23], the incidence of mechanical valve thrombosis in patients receiving appropriate anticoagulant therapy was 0.2 per 100 patient-years. If data for 10 participants were lost to follow-up, and they all experienced valve thrombosis, the true incidence of mechanical valve thrombosis would be higher than reported. This carries important clinical implications, suggesting that valve thrombosis was underreported due to loss of follow-up. One of the weaknesses in the Goldstone et al. [12] study is that while they report that the median follow-up for patients receiving bioprosthetic aortic valve replacement was 5 years, they do not report number lost to follow-up at 10 and 15 years. In consequence, we cannot exclude the possibility of differential loss to follow-up—when the dropout rate differs between treatment groups—potentially introducing bias into the results. Therefore, we must view their data on long-term mortality with caution as the authors do not report completeness of follow-up [24].

Were Objective and Unbiased Outcome Criteria Used?

Outcomes can be objective (e.g., mortality), require adjudication (e.g., myocardial infarction), or subjective (e.g., quality of life). Whenever possible, investigators should specify outcomes based on a consensus definitions [25]. For instance, a patient's heart failure symptoms can be measured using the New York Heart Association Functional Classification, whereas the general quality of life is measured by validated instruments [26]. In the study by Goldstone et al. [12], the authors present mortality as the primary outcome, but also discuss stroke, bleeding, and reoperation. While mortality and reoperation are objective outcomes, stroke and bleeding require definitions. The authors appropriately define stroke, bleeding, and reoperation by ICD-9 codes in table S4 of the supplementary appendix of their article.

How Likely are the Outcomes to Occur Over Time?

Results from prognostic studies help determine the risk of events occurring over time [8]. If our patient wanted to understand his 5-year survival after receiving a prosthetic valve, we would look for a study that reports outcomes of patients 5 years after their initial surgery. Goldstone et al. demonstrate that in patients between ages 55 and 64 years, the probability of mortality at 5 years is approximately 0.1 [12]. If our patient asked about changes in his chances of survival over time, we would show him a survival curve, which illustrates the incidence of events over time. To create a survival curve, events must be discrete (death, reoperation, hospitalizations), and the precise time at which they occur must be recorded [27]. According to Goldstone et al. [12], probability of mortality at 15 years is approximately 0.4 [12], suggesting a fourfold increase in risk between 5 years and 15 years after the valve replacement.

How Precise are the Estimates of Likelihood?

The more precise a prognostic estimate, the closer to certainty and useful it is. Usually, risks of adverse outcomes are reported with their associated 95% confidence interval, (CI) which define the interval within which the true risk likely lies [28]. For example, in a prospective cohort of 196 patients who received bioprosthetic aortic valve replacement, Messe et al. [29] reported clinical strokes in 34 patients (17, 95% CI [12–23%]). That is, assuming the study is valid, there is a 95% chance that the population risk for stroke after the surgery lies between 12 and 23%. Put another way, if the study were repeated 100 times, the incidence of stroke would be between 12 and 23%, approximately 95 of those 100 times. In the Goldstone et al. [12] paper, the authors report 15-year mortality as 36.1% for patients 55–64 years of age, but do not report a confidence interval around this. As such, we cannot estimate precision. However, they did report hazard ratios with mechanical valve patients as a reference point (1.04, 95% CI [0.91–1.18]) [12]. This implies that for patients between the ages of 55 and 64, risk of mortality at 15 years among patients with biological valves or mechanical valves is not statistically significantly different, and likely not important clinically either, because the 95% CI includes 1.0. For more information on confidence intervals please see Chap. 28.

Can I Apply the Results to my Practice or Patient?

The authors should describe patient characteristics and demographics in enough detail that we can compare to our own patients and determine applicability. Further, surgical interventions change and evolve over time [30]. The surgical procedure and risks involved with aortic valve replacement in 1975 are not the same in 2018. With evolving valve types and cardiopulmonary bypass technology, outcomes have improved dramatically [31]. Therefore, it is prudent that the study we review be current, and applicable to current practice. Goldstone et al. [12] recognized the differences in surgical techniques and preferences over time. They reported patient enrollment by study period; of the 3854 patients receiving bioprosthetic aortic valve replacement, 51.7% were enrolled from 2008 to 2013. 69.6% of the patients were male, and over 80% were white [12]. These characteristics of the study sample, along with stratification of outcomes by age, make the study applicable to our patient.

Resolution of Clinical Scenario

Goldstone et al. [12] reported an unbiased assessment of risk in their cohort. The authors provided long-term mortality estimates in patients resembling our patient. There were some limitations related to study design and loss to follow-up, but we can apply the results to our patient and answer his question about long-term prognosis. Since the study included multiple surgeons' outcomes, the long-term data reported can be compared with your surgical skills and capability.

Therefore, we can confidently tell our patient that his risk of mortality is approximately 36% at 15 years after a bioprosthetic valve replacement. Based on the information provided to him, the patient opted to undergo a surgical aortic valve replacement with a biological valve.

References

1. Moons KGM, Vergouwe Y, Grobbee DE, Altman DG. Prognosis and prognostic research: what, why, and how? BMJ. 2009;338:375.
2. Mack JW, Joffe S. Communicating about prognosis: ethical responsibilities of pediatricians and parents. Pediatrics. 2014;133(Suppl 1):S24–30.
3. Randolph AG, Guyatt GH, Richardson WS. Prognosis in the intensive care unit: finding accurate and useful estimates for counseling patients. Crit Care Med. 1998;26:767–72.
4. Italiano A. Prognostic or predictive? It's time to get back to definitions! J Clin Oncol. 2011;29:4718; author reply 4718–9.
5. Barton S. Which clinical studies provide the best evidence? The best RCT still trumps the best observational study. BMJ. 2000;321:255–6.
6. Iorio A SF, Falavigna M. Use of GRADE for assessment of evidence about prognosis: rating confidence in estimates of event rates in broad categories of patients. BMJ. 2015;350.
7. Stassano P, Di Tommaso L, Monaco M, Iorio F, Pepino P, Spampinato N, et al. Aortic valve replacement: a prospective randomized evaluation of mechanical versus biological valves in patients ages 55 to 70 years. J Am Coll Cardiol. 2009;54:1862–8.
8. Hansebout RR, Cornacchi SD, Haines T, Goldsmith CH. How to use an article about prognosis. Can J Surg. 2009;52:328–36.

9. Gamble JM. An introduction to the fundamentals of cohort and case-control studies. Can J Hosp Pharm. 2014;67:366–72.
10. Berger ML, Dreyer N, Anderson F, Towse A, Sedrakyan A, Normand SL. Prospective observational studies to assess comparative effectiveness: the ISPOR good research practices task force report. Value Health. 2012;15:217–30.
11. Thiese MS. Observational and interventional study design types; an overview. Biochem Med (Zagreb). 2014;24:199–210.
12. Goldstone AB, Chiu P, Baiocchi M, Lingala B, Patrick WL, Fischbein MP, et al. Mechanical or biologic prostheses for aortic-valve and mitral-valve replacement. N Engl J Med. 2017;377:1847–57.
13. Mihailovic A, Bell CM, Urbach DR. Users' guide to the surgical literature. Case-control studies in surgical journals. Can J Surg. 2005;48:148–51.
14. Sleder A, Tackett S, Cerasale M, Mittal C, Isseh I, Radjef R, et al. Socioeconomic and racial disparities: a case-control study of patients receiving transcatheter aortic valve replacement for severe aortic stenosis. J Racial Ethn Health Disparities. 2017;4:1189–94.
15. Song JW, Chung KC. Observational studies: cohort and case-control studies. Plast Reconstr Surg. 2010;126:2234–42.
16. Hansebout RR, Cornacchi SD, Haines T, Goldsmith CH. User's guide to the surgical literature: how to use an article about prognosis. Can J Surg. 2009;52(4):328–36.
17. Banerjee A, Chaudhury S. Statistics without tears: populations and samples. Ind Psychiatry J. 2010;19:60–5.
18. Randolph AG CD, Guyatt G. Prognosis. In: Guyatt G, Rennie D, Meade MO, Cook DJ, editors. Users' guides to the medical literature: a manual for evidence-based clinical practice. New York, NY: McGraw-Hill, 2018.
19. Farrokhyar F, Bajammal S, Kahnamoui K, Bhandari M. Practical tips for surgical research. Ensuring balanced groups in surgical trials. Can J Surg. 2010;53:418–23.
20. Christenfeld NJ, Sloan RP, Carroll D, Greenland S. Risk factors, confounding, and the illusion of statistical control. Psychosom Med. 2004;66:868–75.
21. Akl EA, Briel M, You JJ, Sun X, Johnston BC, Busse JW, et al. Potential impact on estimated treatment effects of information lost to follow-up in randomised controlled trials (LOST-IT): systematic review. BMJ. 2012;344:e2809.
22. Jaffer IH, Whitlock RP. A mechanical heart valve is the best choice. Heart Asia. 2016;8:62–4.
23. Cannegieter SC, Rosendaal FR, Wintzen AR, van der Meer FJ, Vandenbroucke JP, Briet E. Optimal oral anticoagulant therapy in patients with mechanical heart valves. N Engl J Med. 1995;333:11–7.
24. Carlson MD, Morrison RS. Study design, precision, and validity in observational studies. J Palliat Med. 2009;12:77–82.
25. Walton MK, Powers JH 3rd, Hobart J, Patric D, Marquis P, Vamvakas S, et al. Clinical outcome assessments: conceptual foundation-report of the ISPOR clinical outcomes assessment—emerging good practices for outcomes research task force. Value Health. 2015;18:741–52.
26. Russell SD, Saval MA, Robbins JL, Ellestad MH, Gottlieb SS, Handberg EM, et al. New York heart association functional class predicts exercise parameters in the current era. Am Heart J. 2009;158:S24–30.
27. Rich JT, Neely JG, Paniello RC, Voelker CC, Nussenbaum B, Wang EW. A practical guide to understanding Kaplan-Meier curves. Otolaryngol Head Neck Surg. 2010;143:331–6.
28. du Prel JB, Hommel G, Rohrig B, Blettner M. Confidence interval or p-value?: part 4 of a series on evaluation of scientific publications. Dtsch Arztebl Int. 2009;106:335–9.
29. Messe SR, Acker MA, Kasner SE, et al. Stroke after aortic valve surgery: results from a prospective cohort. Circulation. 2014;129:2253–61.
30. Gawande A. Two hundred years of surgery. N Engl J Med. 2012;366:1716–23.
31. Maganti M, Rao V, Brister S, Ivanov J. Decreasing mortality for coronary artery bypass surgery in octogenarians. Can J Cardiol. 2009;25:e32–5.

22 Decision Analysis and Surgery

Gloria M. Rockwell and Jessica Murphy

Clinical Scenario

A junior plastic surgery resident assesses a 50-year-old male patient who presents to the clinic with worsening paresthesia in the ulnar nerve distribution of the hand without important weakness. The patient was seen by neurology three months previously and confirmed to have moderate ulnar neuropathy at the elbow, advised to modify activity and wear an extension splint at the elbow. He has done this but without any improvement in his symptoms. The junior resident discusses the case with the chief resident, anticipating that a surgical intervention would be required. The chief resident explains the pathophysiology of ulnar neuropathy at the elbow, and the four different types of surgery they have seen performed for this problem. The junior resident asks the chief resident how to decide which technique is the best to perform for this patient, and in general. The chief resident is unsure and both residents decide to do a literature search.

G. M. Rockwell (✉)
Department of Surgery, Division of Plastic Surgery, University of Ottawa, Ottawa, ON, Canada
e-mail: grockwell@toh.ca

J. Murphy
Department of Surgery, Division of Plastic Surgery, McMaster University, Hamilton, ON, Canada
e-mail: murphjl1@mcmaster.ca

A. Thoma et al. (eds.), *Evidence-Based Surgery*,
https://doi.org/10.1007/978-3-030-05120-4_22

Literature Search

Using PubMed, the residents performed a literature search (see Chap. 4) using the following search terms: "Ulnar Nerve" AND "Surgical Treatment" and "Systematic Review", and a filter of years (2015–2018); this search yielded over 300 articles. To make the task manageable the chief resident suggested they narrow the search strategy and consider using an article with a decision analytic approach. They keep the same criteria for year, but change their search terms to "Ulnar Nerve" AND "Surgical Treatment" AND "Decision Analysis" ; this search yields 10 articles (Appendix 1). The residents screen the titles and abstracts of the articles; three of the articles (Article numbers 5, 7, and 8) have the term decision analysis in the title. Of those three articles, one is in children (Article 5) and is therefore not appropriate. The second article (Article 7) was an individual decision analysis. The third article (Article 8) by Brauer and Graham [1] was a proper decision analysis using evidence from the literature, and the one likely to provide the answer for them.

Background on Decision Analysis in Surgery

Clinical decision-making involves weighing the risks and benefits associated with the various treatment alternatives available for the management of a clinical scenario. Clinicians are guided in their decisions by personal experience, and by their ability to critically appraise the evidence in the literature. Decision-making becomes more difficult when there are multiple variables that can influence the outcome, when evidence in the literature is conflicting, inadequate, poorly designed or absent, and when clinical scenarios differ from the conditions of available studies. Under these circumstances of uncertainty, a formal decision analysis can help in addressing the clinical problem [2–6].

Decision analysis is the translation of a complex clinical scenario and its component parts into a manageable model. Competing management strategies are quantitatively compared despite the presence of clinical uncertainty. All possible therapeutic options and potential outcomes associated with each strategy are identified and assigned a value [7].

Decision analysis starts with a clinical question that must have a defined population, intervention, and outcome. Decision models use clinical experience and the literature to design the decision tree with all possible treatment outcomes for a given strategy. The probability that a specific outcome will occur is established from the literature. The strength of the literature for these outcomes is best achieved through high-quality randomized control trials or systematic reviews combining studies in a meta-analysis to determine the "base case" probabilities with confidence intervals. Base case is the best estimate of the probabilities for each variable; in other words it is the value closest to the truth in the author's estimation [6]. The base case is determined through combining all the known estimates of outcomes, by using a meta-analysis [6]. A sensitivity analysis is used to determine the robustness of the base case and can be performed by repeating the analysis in a one-way- or multi-way fashion to determine reasonable alternatives to the outcomes as determined by confidence intervals or other intervals of values for the various outcome states [2–4, 8].

Components of Decision Analysis

Decision Tree

Decision analysis is composed of several stages in the model design. The first is accumulating outcome possibilities, probabilities and utilities that are integrated into a decision tree. Utilities are defined as a health state with 0 (zero) representing death, and 1 (one) representing perfect health, with possible negative values. The decision tree incorporates the elements of the clinical problem in a schematic format that represents all the clinical options, becoming more complex if multiple decisions are required to reach the final outcome for each strategy. The details behind the design and construction of a decision tree can be found in various references [3, 4, 8–10].

A decision tree is a standardized graphical display that is oriented from left to right. The decision that is to be made is placed on the left and marked with a square node (the decision node) [9]; the clinical outcomes are displayed to the right. The lines (branches) originating from the decision node represent the different clinical strategies that are being compared. The circle nodes represent chance nodes, or chance events; outcomes are illustrated as triangles or rectangles [9]. Numbers can be present on decision trees, when these numbers are on the lines, they represent probabilities; when they are near the triangles, they represent utilities [9]. Figure 22.1 illustrates a simple decision tree, and its parts. Figure 22.2 illustrates an example of a decision tree that could be used in the decision analysis by Brauer and Graham [1] for surgical treatment of ulnar neuropathy at the elbow.

In the current example of ulnar nerve decompression at the elbow; clinical outcomes were determined from the perspective of the patient with chance nodes of good or bad outcomes. Bad outcomes were assumed to require secondary surgery in the form of a submuscular transposition. A good outcome was the complete resolution of sensory neuropathy at 2 years. Complications for each good or bad outcome

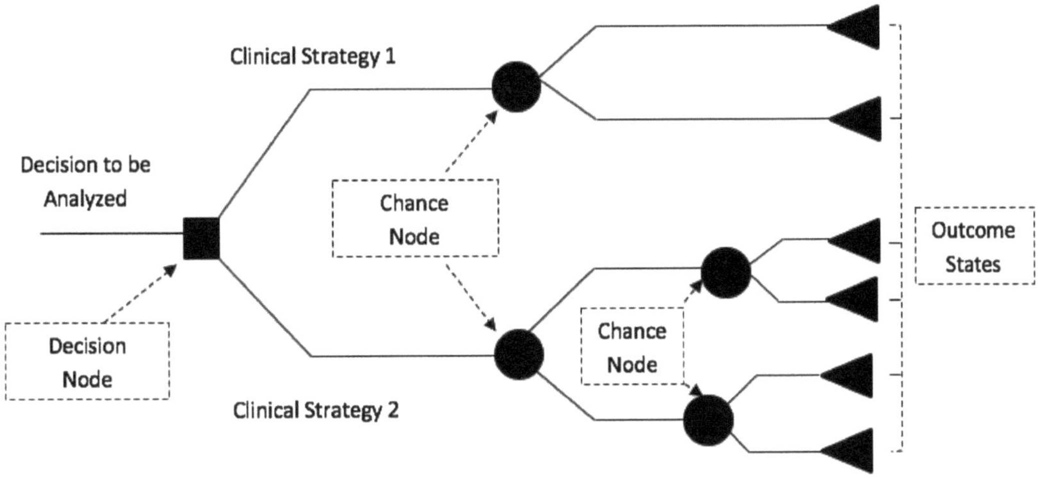

Fig. 22.1 Parts of a decision tree. Created using information from Richardson and Detsky [9]

were also included as chance nodes in the decision tree. Figure 22.2 demonstrates a pictorial schematic of the decision tree for the ulnar nerve at the elbow treatment surgical treatment modalities. The four surgical choices included in the decision analysis are shown in Table 22.1.

The value of the given outcomes can be expressed in terms of utilities. The techniques to measure utilities for different health states can involve time trade-off, standard gamble, visual analog scales measured directly from experts and patients, or indirectly interpreted from similar clinical scenarios with previously published health utilities [4].

Disutility represents a transient health state that can downgrade quality of life temporarily and, for surgical interventions, could involve peri-operative discomforts, inconvenience from hospitalization and immobilization. Disutilities can be measured for short-term complications occurring in each health state. Disutilities are subtracted from the utilities of that health state to give an overall utility value for each specific outcome [4]. Permanent undesirable consequences decrease utility associated with a health state and can be converted to Quality-Adjusted Life Years (QALY) for comparison to other health states, interventions, and even used in further economic evaluations such as cost-effectiveness analyses (see Chap. 23).

When the decision tree is folded back on itself the expected outcomes (utility, cost, QALY, etc.) can be calculated for each decision pathway by multiplying the probability of each branch in the tree with the final outcome for that pathway [4].

The Outcomes

All clinically relevant outcomes for the available management options must be identified, analyzed, and incorporated into the decision tree for the tree to be an accurate representation of a clinical scenario. Uncertainties (confidence intervals or other intervals) are identified during the literature systematic review. The sensitivity analysis of the tree is repeated by varying either one variable or multiple variables, throughout their plausible intervals, to determine the robustness of the decisions derived from the decision analysis [6]. Conclusions are not as strong if they change during the sensitivity analysis within the plausible interval of a variable. Extreme values can be used in the sensitivity analysis to debug the decision tree and help refine the design for obvious areas that give illogical results [4, 5, 14, 15].

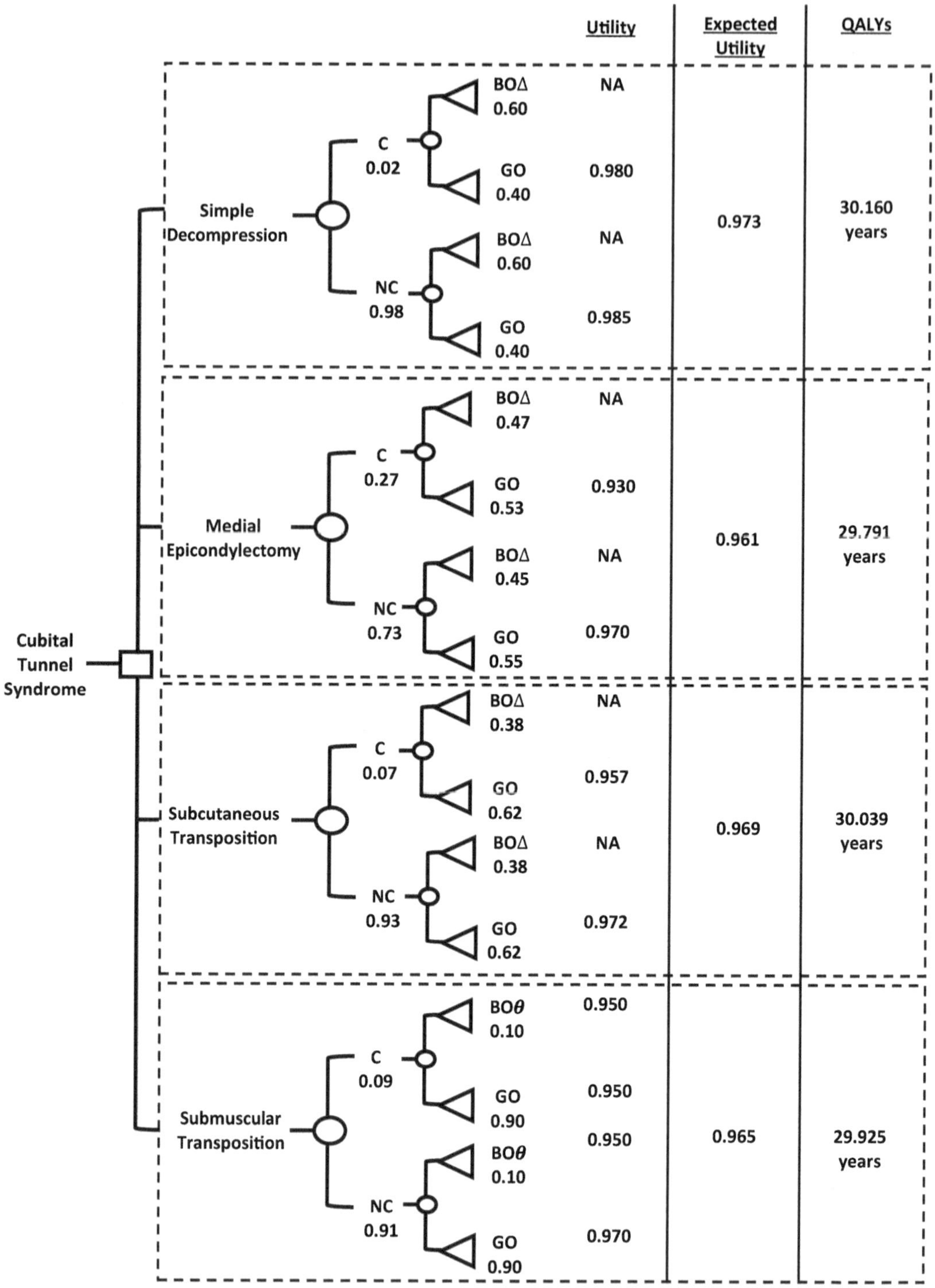

Fig. 22.2 Note *C* Complication, *NC* No complication, *BO* Bad outcome, *GO* Good outcome, *QALYs* Quality-adjusted life years, *BOθ* Was considered an endpoint, *BOΔ* Resulted in revision submuscular transposition surgery, *Circle nodes* Chance event, *Square nodes* Decision to be made, *Triangle nodes* Outcome

Table 22.1 The four surgical treatment modalities

Treatment	Expected utilities
Simple decompression	0.973
Medial epicondylectomy	0.961
Subcutaneous transposition	0.969
Submuscular transposition	0.965

Adapted from Brauer and Graham [1]

Clinical Application

When applying a decision analysis clinicians must carefully consider the generalizability of the model to their own specific patient's characteristics. The value of utilities a patient may apply to the various outcomes could vary and need to be considered when applying the decision tree.

Users' Guide: A Framework

Using the principles of decision analysis theory stated above and a previously devised methodological framework for use in interpreting the literature, we can now critically appraise the Brauer and Graham [1] article using the questions found in Box 1.

Box 1. Questions to Appraise Decision Analysis Literature

1. Are the Results Valid?

   (a) Were all the important strategies and outcomes included?
   (b) Was an explicit and sensible process used to identify, select and combine the evidence into probabilities?
   (c) Were the utilities obtained in an explicit and sensible way from the credible sources?
   (d) Was the potential impact of any uncertainty in the evidence determined?

2. What are the Results?

   (a) In the baseline analysis, does one strategy result in a clinically important gain for patients? If not,
   (b) Is the result a toss-up?
   (c) Is the Difference Between the Strategies Clinically Important?
   (d) How strong is the evidence used in the analysis?
   (e) Could the uncertainty in the evidence change the result?

3. Will the Results Help Me in Caring for My Patients?

   (a) Do the probability estimates fit my patients' clinical features?
   (b) Do the utilities reflect how my patients would value the outcomes of the decision?

Created using information from Refs. [6, 9, 10].

In their study, Brauer and Graham [1] review the literature surrounding the diagnosis and surgical therapy for moderate to severe ulnar neuropathy at the elbow that has failed nonsurgical management. They expressed the advantages and disadvantages of each of the four most common surgical treatment options. The authors described their design of the decision analysis and decision tree including the outcomes in terms of utilities and probabilities for each outcome state. The choice of the various outcomes was determined through a previous review of the literature by Brauer and Graham [1]. The authors describe how they determine the various probabilities and utilities related to their "base case" and summarize their findings (see Fig. 22.2 and Table 22.2). They have given a detailed description of how they chose utilities and disutilities from previously published utility values for different health states including upper extremity arthritis and wrist arthroplasty, which is a more demanding

Table 22.2 Probabilities, disabilities and utilities by variable

Probabilities		Probability value
Complications	Simple Decompression	0.02
	Medial Epicondylectomy	0.27
	Anterior Subcutaneous Transposition	0.07
	Anterior Submuscular Transposition	0.09
Bad outcomes	Simple Decompression/Complication	0.60
	Medial Epicondylectomy/Complication	0.47
	Anterior Subcutaneous Transposition/Complication	0.38
	Anterior Submuscular Transposition/Complication	0.10
	Simple Decompression/No Complication	0.60
	Medial Epicondylectomy/No Complication	0.45
	Anterior Subcutaneous Transposition/No Complication	0.38
	Anterior Submuscular Transposition/No Complication	0.10
Utilities		Utility value
Bad outcomes	Anterior Submuscular Transposition	0.95
Good outcomes	Simple Decompression	0.99
	Medial Epicondylectomy	0.98
	Anterior Subcutaneous Transposition	0.98
	Anterior Submuscular Transposition	0.98
Disutilities		Disutility value
Procedures	Simple Decompression	0.005
	Medial Epicondylectomy	0.008
	Anterior Subcutaneous Transposition	0.01
	Anterior Submuscular Transposition	0.01
Complications	Simple Decompression	0.005
	Medial Epicondylectomy	0.04
	Anterior Subcutaneous Transposition	0.015
	Anterior Submuscular Transposition	0.02

Adapted from Brauer and Graham [1]

surgery with a longer recovery and potential for chronic disability (see Table 22.3) [11–13].

Table 22.3 Utility by health status

Health state	Utility
Menopause symptom	0.99
Anti-hypertensive treatment side effects	0.95–0.99
Wrist arthrodesis	0.95
Kidney transplant	0.84
Hospital dialysis	0.57
Severe angina	0.50

Adapted from [11–13]

Are the Results Valid?

Before applying the decision analysis to the patient in question, it is important to determine if the decision analytic model the authors formulated is applicable to the clinical scenario. This means examining the methodology of the model's design, as to how the authors determined the outcomes, the methods used to combine the evidence, the sources and credibility of the utilities chosen, as well as the potential impact of uncertainty.

Were All the Important Strategies and Outcomes Included?

The first step in appraising a decision analysis is determining whether the authors have included all clinically relevant treatment strategies and outcomes. The decision analysis by Brauer and Graham [1] reviews the literature of the four most common surgical interventions for ulnar nerve entrapment at the elbow. Brauer and Graham [1] tabulate the advantages and disadvantages of each surgical intervention as well as the peri-operative and postoperative care. They provide a table of the variables determined from their review of various randomized controlled trials comparing several of each of the operative interventions. They clearly state the limitations of the available studies, but do not explicitly describe the search criteria, nor provide tabulated or confidence intervals or other intervals for each variable. The authors constructed a decision model to fit the clinical scenario usually encountered in clinical practice; in this case, the four different operative interventions (Table 22.1). The failure of an initial surgery either a direct release, or subcutaneous transposition, or medial epicondylectomy, would result in the secondary surgical treatment of submuscular transposition. Failure of submuscular transposition was equated as the endpoint.

How well the structure of the model fits with our clinical scenario depends on reviewing the decision tree. Figure 22.2 is the complete decision tree for their surgical management of ulnar neuropathy at the elbow. There are four clinically important surgical options each with good outcome (GO) or bad outcome (BO). The objective for the study was to establish a general policy for recommendations of treatment recognizing that this policy may not fit all situations. The outcomes of the decision analysis are labeled as health states. In this decision analysis, a good outcome was defined as complete relief of all sensory symptoms for greater than 2 years and all other results were considered bad outcomes.

Was an Explicit and Sensible Process Used to Identify, Select, and Combine the Evidence into Probabilities?

The methods used to combine the evidence in a decision analysis are predictive of the clinical value of the final result. Providing the proper methodological steps is necessary to determine applicability to a given patient and also to minimize the introduction of bias. Brauer and Graham [1] state that they performed a literature review and that they were guided by results from various clinical trials and guidelines [2–5]. They described the reasoning for defining the outcomes as good outcome versus bad, and also data limitations and assumptions used in the model. Unfortunately, their tabulated base case data for probabilities, utilities and disutilities as well as the sensitivity analysis and threshold values, did not include confidence intervals or other intervals to more easily allow the reader to analyze the model and compare to their clinical case. Brauer and Graham [1] report the use of SMLTREE (JP Hollenberg, Roslyn, NY, USA) software to construct the decision tree. Figure 22.2 showing the basic tree design moving from right to left, demonstrates that after each decision node for the four various surgical options there was then a chance node of complication (C) or no complication (NC), with a further chance node of bad outcome or good outcome as the final pathway state. They did summarize the risks from the literature to establish an overall rate but without the intervals being given. The papers analyzed by Brauer and Graham [1] were explicitly given in their appendix. The authors chose base case failure rates of 10% for submuscular transposition (3–50%), 38% (10–73%) for anterior subcutaneous transposition, 60% for subcutaneous decompression and 45% for medial epicondylectomy [1]. Their model base case is biased towards a better outcome, by choosing a lower initial base case complication rate of 10% within an interval of 3–50% from their literature review for submuscular transposition and 38% from a range of 10–73% for anterior subcutaneous transposition; with a poorer outcome with simple decompression (60%) or medial epicondylectomy (45%) [1]. Further analysis with a one-way sensitivity analysis was performed to determine threshold values (Table 22.2).

They assume the outcomes would not change with minor complications, except in the pathway for medial epicondylectomy, which could result in medial instability or ectopic bone formation and therefore the probability of a failure with complications was slightly higher than with no complications. They considered most complications for the various surgical treatments to be transient and to have little effect on the failure of a treatment and therefore the probabilities of a good or poor outcome were unchanged with complications or no complications. This is an assumption that may not necessarily be true for all patient groups but they have explicitly described this. Outcome estimates were transformed into quantitative estimates, or probabilities with zero being impossible and one being certain. The authors do highlight the data limitations and assumptions used.

Were the Utilities Obtained in an Explicit and Sensible Way from Credible Sources?

The authors used a simple decision analysis with two possible outcomes "good outcome (complete resolution of all sensory deficits at 2 years)" or "bad outcome." In this model, utilities were determined in comparison to similar disabilities in the upper extremity, and other disease states (Table 22.3) [11–13]. Several methods are available to measure utilities directly; different methods use different scales with zero equaling death and one equaling perfect health. These authors report sources of utilities directly from standardized health states [25–27]. Patient specific utilities can be measured directly from the patient. Clinical policy utilities can be measured directly from large groups of patients with the disorder; from published studies of quality of life ratings by patients; and from large groups of people representing the general population.

In the decision analysis by Brauer and Graham [1], they used indirect measures of published utilities from the quality of life outcomes in upper extremity and hand disorders from patients with osteoarthritis of the wrist, as well as from the American Medical Association Guides to the Evaluation of Permanent Impairment [11–13]. They stated their chosen utilities of 0.99 for a small scar without pain, 0.98 for a large scar, and 0.954 for chronic mild sensory or motor disturbances [1]. They assumed the utility would be unchanged despite a minor temporary complication. The effect of most complications was measured through disutilities also taken from the literature and varying from 0.005 to 0.01 [1]. Disutilities would occur for either hospitalization, discomfort associated with the intervention, length of postoperative immobilization and need for rehabilitation postoperatively (Table 22.2).

The indirect values chosen may not represent those of either patients or the general public. By comparison, a Cost-Utility Analysis study by Song et al. [14] directly measured utility values, from family members and paticnts undergoing surgical interventions for ulnar neuropathy, using time trade-off techniques. Despite the differences in either indirect calculations of utilities versus direct measurement, Brauer and Graham [1] and Song et al. [14] had found similar expected utilities for direct decompression and anterior subcutaneous transposition (0.98 and 0.98 for Song et al. [14] versus 0.973 and 0.969 for Brauer and Graham [1], respectively. Medial epicondylectomy and submuscular transposition had a statistically significant difference between the two authors (Brauer and Graham [1]: 0.961 and 0.965, vs. Song et al. [14] 0.88 and 0.82 respectively). When compared to standardized health state utility measurements (Table 22.3) a utility of 0.84 is that of a kidney transplant. Thus despite direct measurements from patients and family, undergoing the specific surgery for ulnar neuropathy, and measured with time trade off, utilities measure by Song et al. [14] appear lower than expected. Utilities by Brauer and Graham [1] seem more logical when compared to those of other health states, though indirectly measured.

Was the Potential Impact of Any Uncertainty in the Evidence Determined?

Uncertainty in the evidence, and poor model design can lead to miscalculation of both the utilities assigned to outcomes and the probabilities of each health state. As in any critical appraisal of the literature, the highest quality of evidence comes from well designed, adequately powered randomized controlled trials (RCTs), and meta-analysis derived from such RCTs. Authors should acknowledge the quality of the literature in their review. Much of the uncertainty in decision-making arises from a lack of valid evidence in the literature. Even when present, published evidence is often imprecise with wide intervals of estimates. Brauer and Graham [1] report some of the limitations in the quality of the studies in their review, with wide intervals of success and failure. The less valid the methods or less precise the estimates from the literature the wider the intervals that must be included in the sensitivity analysis to determine when a threshold level is reached. Threshold levels occur when a change in a variable results in a change in the outcome conclusions would occur (Table 22.4).

Sensitivity analysis is the systematic exploration of uncertainty in the data to see what effect varying estimates or probabilities for risks, benefits and utilities have on the expected outcome and change of a clinical strategy. Performing a sensitivity analysis is akin to exploring the best and worst case scenario. In this case, the authors used a wide sensitivity analysis to determine threshold values between the two highest rated

Table 22.4 Results of one-way sensitivity analysis comparing simple decompression and subcutaneous transposition

Variable		Base value probability (Threshold)
Complication rate	Simple Decompression	0.02 (NT)
	Medial Epicondylectomy	0.27 (NT)
	Anterior Subcutaneous Transposition	0.07 (NT)
	Anterior Submuscular Transposition	0.09 (NT)
Probability of a bad outcome	Simple Decompression/Complication	0.60 (0.82)
	Medial Epicondylectomy/Complication	0.47 (NT)
	Anterior Subcutaneous Transposition/Complication	0.38 (NT)
	Anterior Submuscular Transposition/Complication	0.10 (NT)
	Simple Decompression/No Complication	0.60 (NT)
	Medial Epicondylectomy/No Complication	0.45 (NT)
	Anterior Subcutaneous Transposition/No Complication	0.38 (NT)
	Anterior Submuscular Transposition/No Complication	0.10 (0.82)
Disutility of individual procedures	Simple Decompression	0.005 (0.0158)
	Medial Epicondylectomy	0.01 (NT)
	Anterior Subcutaneous Transposition	0.008 (0.001)
	Anterior Submuscular Transposition	0.01 (0.0296)

NT no threshold
Adapted from Brauer and Graham [1]

procedures, simple decompression, and subcutaneous transposition. The threshold, in this case, refers to the value beyond which the preferred strategy shifted from simple decompression to subcutaneous transposition.

What are the Results?

In the baseline analysis does one strategy results in a clinically important gain for the patient? If not is the result a toss-up?

The choice between various outcomes strategies is based on the outcome with the highest value of expected utility. One calculates this by folding back the decision tree probabilities from right to left for each outcome. The decision analyst chooses the scale on which to measure the expected utilities to fit the clinical problem: Quality of life, reduction of mortality or other gains in remaining life expectancy. Quality of life and quantity of life can both be combined in calculating the QALYs or healthy year equivalents. The authors chose to present their outcomes in a table of expected utilities for each procedure (Fig. 22.2).

Is the Difference Between the Strategies Clinically Important?

A difference means that any given patient may gain more or less than others and this is where using a policy decision analysis loses the specificity for an individual patient. A gain in QALYs greater than 2–3 months is considered an important gain as published by Naimark et al. [12] and Tsevat et al. [13]. In the study by Brauer and Graham [1] they display expected utilities, which, can be converted to QALYs assuming a 50-year-old man with 31 years of remaining life as determined from the literature where the mean age of a patient with ulnar nerve neuropathy is 52.5 years. This would give a net gain for the base case of 1.45, 2.94, and 4.43 months comparing subcutaneous decompression, to anterior subcutaneous transposition, submuscular transposition with medial epicondylectomy, respectively. Of note, this is based on the base case where there was bias for better outcomes with submuscular transposition and worse with direct decompression. The gain would be much more if a more realistic base case was calculated. This decision analysis model has very small differences in outcome indirect utilities and perhaps may be an over-simplification because transient complications were not used in the outcomes.

How Strong is the Evidence in the Analysis?

The strength of evidence used in creating a decision analysis depends on the quality of the studies from which the probabilities and utilities were estimated. Ideally, every probability at each node in the decision tree is supported by precise estimates from primary RCT data or meta-analysis of high methodological quality. Good decision analysis can still be performed with some imprecise or ambiguous data as long as most of the data are good and the analysts explain any limitations and plan for sensitivity analysis accordingly. The weaker the evidence is used in the analysis the weaker the overall inference one to make from the results [3].

The strength of the evidence cited by Brauer and Graham [1] is good; this is reflected by their systematic review of the data from three randomized controlled studies, one meta-analysis, and various other studies totaling 24 studies. A Cochrane database systematic review of ulnar neuropathy at the elbow updated in 2016 and initially published in 2010 with a second update in 2012 tabulated all available studies which showed that most trials had fewer than 60 participants and nine randomized control trials with a total of only 587 participants [15]. Their meta-analysis concluded that there was at best moderate quality of evidence. It should be remembered that this study was a deterministic analysis based on secondary data collected from the literature, rather than randomized controlled trial comparing all four surgical options under consideration. Deterministic data uses indirect information and requires a wider sensitivity analysis to test the robustness of conclusions. High quality directly measured data from RCTs or meta-analysis of RCTs provide the strongest evidence on which clinical decisions can be based. However, in such circumstances, where strong data are readily available, the use of decision analytic modeling may not be necessary, unless residual uncertainty exists.

Could the Uncertainty in the Evidence Change the Results?

After interpreting the results in the base case analysis, it is critical to test how vulnerable the results are to the variation in probabilities and key outcome measures. If minor changes in the probability or effectiveness measures affect the outcome in a way that would be clinically important to the patient in question, then the decision model may have errors in design and should be reconsidered. A sensitivity analysis is considered robust if changing the variables throughout its possible intervals do not change the strategy or conclusion.

In the Brauer and Graham [1] article, the authors explored the strength of their model with a wide sensitivity analysis. The robustness of their conclusions is demonstrated by the clinically unlikely probability requiring the failure of direct decompression to be greater than 82% before subcutaneous transposition would be the preferred treatment. The authors also found stable conclusions unless submuscular transposition had a bad outcome greater than 82% (eight times their base case of 10%) The sensitivity analysis recommending direct decompression as the treatment of choice was also stable and robust unless the disutility tripled to greater than that for subcutaneous transposition and submuscular transposition which they stated would be clinically unlikely. Threshold levels were also encountered if the disutility of submuscular transposition was greater than a factor of two times, which, would be similar to that of a complex wrist reconstruction with scaphoid excision and metacarpal arthrodesis which is likely more chronically disabling than an ulnar nerve submuscular transposition at the elbow.

Will the Results Help me in Caring for My Patient?

Can the Results be Generalized to This Patient?

The perspective, design, and assumptions used in creating a decision analysis become critical in determining the generalizability of the model, and in particular its relevance to the target population. The model must be based on clinical scenarios that are similar, predictive and helpful to the actual reality of the clinical question at hand. Probabilities and utilities must reflect the values and risks present in the decision-makers' environment.

The applicability of a decision analysis for policy, group, or patient-specific interventions depends on the clinical characteristics of patients for whom the analysis is intended. The analysis should have a description of the patients' conditions to allow for generalizability. If the authors do not describe the samples used in the studies you can search inclusion and exclusion criteria in the original references to see how similar the characteristics are to your patient. If the analysis is designed for patients with differing characteristics than yours, you can assess the sensitivity analysis for the variable used, and intervals, to see where your patient may fall in this current model.

In the decision analysis by Brauer and Graham [1] the authors state their objective is to create a general policy for recommended surgical treatment for moderate, sensory only ulnar neuropathy at the elbow. They outline the advantages and disadvantages of the four procedures as well as the assumptions used in this decision model. The clinical features match that of your patient as he does not have any motor loss or other comorbidities.

Do the Probability Estimates fit my Patient's Clinical Features?

Every decision analysis should contain pertinent positive and negative characteristics for the patient population to which it is applied. Reviewing the sensitivity analysis in the article will permit the gauging of similarities with the patient in question. In this article, the authors clearly state the target population has moderate sensory ulnar neuropathy at the elbow, no motor weakness, and unresponsive to conservative interventions. The generalizability of this decision analysis is therefore limited to this group of patients.

Do the Utilities Reflect How my Patients will Value the Decision Outcomes?

Quality of life, despite having universally accepted quantitative values, is strongly influenced by individual values and social context. Surgeon comfort, experience, and discussion of potential risks for various interventions can all influence patients' choices. In this decision analysis all bad outcomes were treated with an additional surgery in the form of a revision submuscular transposition. This may not be representative of the reality in any given clinical scenario and may impact on decision nodes and thereby the validity of the model. If the decision analysis is designed for an individual patient then the utilities should be measured directly from that patient. If utilities are based on a large group of patients or members of the public, then the utility values may include those of your patient, but the intervals of values must be very broad. One-way or two-way sensitivity analysis can further see if the value of your patient will affect the final decision.

In this example, utilities were decided on by experts from published guidelines in the field of upper extremity and hand surgery compared to standard known utilities for wrist fusion reconstruction and normal patients. Elsewhere, utilities were 0.95 for chronic sensorimotor disturbance mild in nature, 0.99 for small scar with no pain, 0.98 for large scar no pain. The effect of complications was measured by disutilities also measured from the literature. The authors describe explicitly their postoperative routine, the complications, and advantages and disadvantages associated with each procedure to determine the disutilities measured. The authors do emphasize the threshold and robustness of their models from their one-way sensitivity analysis.

This decision analysis has limited generalizability to our current patient due to the indirect calculation of utilities determined from similar disease states in the literature, which are neither patient nor procedure specific. However, the broad sensitivity analysis demonstrated robustness of their conclusions, despite a bias against the direct decompression.

A more recent study with directly measured utilities for ulnar nerve at the elbow from family and patients with ulnar nerve entrapment using time trade-off techniques demonstrated similar utilities for direct decompression and anterior subcutaneous transposition at 0.98 but much lower utilities 0.82 for anterior submuscular transposition and 0.88 for medial epicondylectomy. Despite the more elaborate time trade-off and direct measurement of utilities from patients with the disease process in the study by Song et al. [14], the overall conclusion on the choice of direct decompression being the preferred treatment option for primary cubital tunnel release was the same as the simpler decision analysis by Brauer and Graham [1].

Resolution of the Scenario

After working through the above steps, the residents had a much clearer understanding of the approach to surgical management of moderate sensory ulnar neuropathy at the elbow. Despite the absence of a well-powered randomized control trial comparing the four most common surgical treatment strategies for ulnar nerve decompression at the elbow, the decision analysis by Brauer and Graham [1], demonstrated fairly robustly that simple decompression is the preferred surgical treatment for ulnar neuropathy at the elbow. The residents felt happy to discuss this management plan with their patient.

Appendix 1. Articles Located During Literature Search

1. Wali AR, Park CC, Brown JM, Mandeville R. Analyzing cost-effectiveness of ulnar and median nerve transfers to regain forearm flexion. Neurosurg Focus. 2017;42(3):E11.
2. Park SE, Bachman DR, O'Discoll SQ. The safety of using proximal anteromedial portals in elbow arthroscopy with prior ulnar nerve transposition. Arthroscopy. 2016;32(6): 1003–9.
3. Nagi SS, Mahns DA. Mechanical allodynia in human glaborous skin mediated by low-threshold cutaneous mechanoreceptors with unmyelinated fibres. Exp Brain Res. 2013;231(2):139–51.
4. Page MH, O'Connor D, Pitt V, Massy-Westropp N. Exercise and mobilisation interventions for carpal tunnel syndrome. Cochrane Database Syst Rev. 2012;13(6): CD009899.
5. Lee KM, Chung CY, Gwon DK, Sung KH, Kim TW, Choi IH, et al. Medial and lateral crossed pinning versus lateral pinning for supracondylar fractures of the humerus in children: decision analysis. J Pediatr Orthop. 2012;32(2):131–8.
6. Koscielniak-Nielsen ZJ, Frederiksen BS, Rasmussen H, Hesselbjerg L. A comparison of ultrasound-guided supraclavicular and infraclavicular blocks for upper extremity surgery. Acta Anaesthesiol Scan. 2009;53 (5):620–6.
7. Gasco J. Surgical options for ulnar nerve entrapment: an example of individualized decision analysis. Hand (NY). 2009;4 (4):350–6
8. Brauer CA, Graham B. The surgical treatment of cubital tunnel syndrome: a decision analysis. J Hand Surg Eur Vol. 2008;32(6):654–62
9. Bartels RH. Ulnar neuropathy at the elbow: follow-up and prognostic factors determining outcome. Neurology. 2005;64(9):1664–5. (author reply 1664–5).
10. Prpa B, Huddleston PM, An KN, Wood MB. Revascularization of nerve grafts: a qualitative and quantitative study of the soft-tissue bed contributions to blood flow in canine nerve grafts. J Hand Surg Am. 2002;27 (6):1041–7.

References

1. Brauer CA, Graham B. The surgical treatment of cubital tunnel syndrome: a decision analysis. J Hand Surg (Eur Vol). 2007;6(32E):654–62.
2. Detsky AS, Naglie G, Krahn MD, Naimark D, Redelmeier DA. Primer on medical decision analysis: part I—getting started. Med Decis Making. 1997;17:123–5.
3. Detsky AS, Naglie G, Krahn MD, Redelmeier DA, Naimark D. Primer on medical decision analysis: part 2—building a tree. Med Decis Making. 1997;17:126–35.
4. Naglie G, Krahn MD, Naimark D, Redelmeier DA, Detsky AS. Primer on medical decision analysis: part 3—estimating probabilities and utilities. Med Decis Making. 1997;17:136–41.
5. Naimark D, Krahn MD, Naglie G, Redelmeier DA, Detsky AS. Primer on medical decision analysis: part 5—working with Markow process. Med Decis Making. 1997;17:152–9.
6. Mastracci TM, Thoma A, Farrokhyar F, Tandan VR, Cina CS. User's guide to the surgical literature: how to use a decision analysis. Can J Surg. 2007;50 (5):403–9.
7. Davis Sears E, Chung KE. Decision analysis in plastic surgery: a primer. Am Soc Plast Surg. 2010;126(4):1373–80.
8. Krahn MD, Naglie G, Naimark D, Redelmeier DA, Detsky AS. Primer on medical decision analysis: part 4—analyzing the model and interpreting the results. Med Decis Making. 1997;17:142–51.
9. Richardson WS, Detsky AS. User's guides to the medical literature. VII. How to use a clinical decision analysis. A. Are the results of the study valid? Evidence-Based Medicine Working Group. JAMA. 1995;273:1292–5.
10. Richardson WS, Detsky AS. User's guides to the medical literature. VII. How to use a clinical decision analysis B. What are the results and will they help me in caring for my patients? JAMA. 1995;273:1610–3.

11. Torrance GW. Utility approach to measuring health related quality of life. J Chronic Dis. 1987;40:593–600.
12. Naimark DM, Naglie G, Detsky AS. The meaning of life expectancy: what is a clinically significant gain? J Gen Intern Med. 1994;9:702–7.
13. Tsevat J, Weinstein MC, Williams L, Tosteson AN, Goldman L. Expected gains in life expectancy for various coronary heart disease risk factor modifications. Circulation. 1991;83:1194–201.
14. Song JW, Chung KC, Prosser LA. Treatment of ulnar neuropathy at the elbow: cost-utility analysis. J Hand Surg. 2012;37A:1617–29.
15. Caliandro P, La Torre G, Padue R, Giannini F, Padua L. Treatment for ulnar neuropathy at the elbow. Cochrane Database Syst Rev. 2016;15: CD006839.

23 Economic Evaluations in Surgery

Achilles Thoma, Feng Xie, Jenny Santos and Charles H. Goldsmith

Surgeons of all specialties are constantly introduced to new surgical techniques or approaches to solve surgical problems. These innovations are disseminated via conferences, workshops, or publications in specialty journals. The typical surgeon faces difficulty in deciding whether to adopt a new surgical innovation when conflicting opinions by experts are presented. A surgeon needs to consider the opportunity cost when adopting a novel surgical intervention and abandoning one that they usually use. Opportunity cost is defined as "the value of the forgone benefits" because the resource is not available for its alternative use [1].

New innovations in surgery are often touted by their proponents as being cost-effective with the recommendation to adopt them in our practice and patients. Unfortunately, the term cost-effective is more often than not misused in the surgical literature. For example, Ziolkowski et al. [2] found that most economic evaluations published in plastic surgery and touted to be cost-effectiveness studies were simply cost comparisons.

A surgical technique or surgical approach to be considered as "cost-effective" must have integrated the costs and effectiveness [3, 4]. Economic analysis is a set of formal, quantitative methods used to compare alternative strategies with respect to their resource use and their expected outcomes [4]. Economic evaluation is a unique study design just as randomized controlled trial and case-control studies are. As most surgeons do not have background training in health economics, one can understand how important terminology such as "cost-effective", is misused. This misuse, however, may have direct consequences if surgeons adopt new techniques or surgical approaches, which are touted "cost-effective", when in truth they are not; inefficient use of scarce healthcare resources is one consequence. OECD data estimate that 20% of health expenditure worldwide is wasted, resulting in minimal-if any-improvement of health outcomes [5]. Although we do not have specific breakdown figures for surgery, we have

A. Thoma (✉) · J. Santos
Department of Surgery, Division of Plastic Surgery, McMaster University, Hamilton, ON, Canada
e-mail: athoma@mcmaster.ca

J. Santos
e-mail: santosj8@mcmaster.ca

F. Xie
Faculty of Health Sciences, McMaster University, Hamilton, ON, Canada
e-mail: fengxie@mcmaster.ca

A. Thoma · F. Xie · C. H. Goldsmith
Department of Health Research Methods, Evidence, and Impact, McMaster University, Hamilton, ON, Canada

C. H. Goldsmith
Faculty of Health Sciences, Simon Fraser University, Burnaby, BC, Canada

C. H. Goldsmith
Department of Occupational Science and Occupational Therapy, Faculty of Medicine, The University of British Columbia, Vancouver, BC, Canada

A. Thoma et al. (eds.), *Evidence-Based Surgery*,
https://doi.org/10.1007/978-3-030-05120-4_23

no reason to believe that surgery is immune to wasteful practices.

This chapter has three objectives. First, it will introduce surgeons to the terminology used in the economic evaluations and demystify this important study design. Second and most importantly, it will help the reader appraise and understand an article that purports to be an economic evaluation in surgery. Third, it will hopefully stimulate surgeons to consider "piggy-backing" economic evaluations to their effectiveness studies. We believe that an economic evaluation alongside a robust randomized control trial that compares a novel surgical technique to a standard technique provides the best level of evidence to adopt or reject a novel surgical intervention. We will attempt to keep the mathematics to the bare minimum and make the chapter understandable and hopefully fun to read.

Explanation of the Types of Economic Evaluations and Terminology Used

There are four types of health economic evaluations; Cost analysis (CA): this is cost comparison study and usually not considered a full economic evaluation, it is often called a partial economic evaluation, Cost-Effectiveness analysis (CEA), Cost–Utility Analysis (CUA), and Cost–Benefit Analysis (CBA) [4]. The main difference in these analyses is how the outcome or consequences of the treatments under comparison are measured. The distinguishing features of these four economic evaluations have been summarized in Table 23.1.

There are two main types of methodologies used in economic evaluations. The first type is the model-based and the second is trial-based economic evaluations. In the first, the model-based evaluation (also known as *Deterministic Analysis* or probabilistic analysis), a model is built which in its simpler form is the decision tree which is explained in Chap. 22 of this book. Primary data are usually derived from the literature, for example, by pooling the evidence (preferably through a systematic review of the literature). From these pooled data, one derives probabilities of complications or positive health outcomes labeled as "health states". These health states are then entered into a decision analysis tree, which in its most basic form will look like the one illustrated in Fig. 23.1a.

Clinical investigators then proceed to estimate the expected costs and expected benefits of the "health states" of the interventions under study

Table 23.1 Distinguishing features of the four types of economic evaluations

Type of analysis	Valuation of costs	Identification of outcomes (Consequences)	Metric used in the analysis
Cost analysis (CA)	Monetary units (i.e., \$, £, €)	None	None. This analysis is only a comparison of costs
Cost-effectiveness analysis (CEA)	Monetary units (i.e., \$, £, €)	Common effect of interest. Common outcomes to the competing surgical interventions but with different probability of success (i.e., lives saved, successful hernia repairs, viable flaps, viable replants, sick days averted, hospital days averted)	\$ per natural unit (i.e., \$ per successful replant, \$ per life saved, \$ per hospital day averted)
Cost–utility analysis (CUA)	Monetary units (i.e., \$, £, €)	Single or multiple effects that are not necessarily common to both interventions. Outcomes are measured in health utilities that are used to calculate Quality-Adjusted Life Years (QALYs)	\$, £, or € spent per QALY
Cost–benefit analysis (CBA)	Monetary units (i.e., \$, £, €)	Single or multiple effects not necessarily common to both surgical procedures and are calculated in \$, £, or €	Monetary units (i.e., \$, £, €)

by multiplying the costs and consequences (outcomes) by their probability of occurrence. The decision analysis tree model becomes more complex as we add more branches to the main pathways. This type of analysis is based on modeling. An example of a more complex model is shown in Fig. 23.1b, representing the cost and utility associated with various complications of a Deep Inferior Epigastric Perforator (DIEP) flap in postmastectomy breast reconstruction [6]. A similar analytic tree was also constructed for the other intervention for breast reconstruction being studied; the free Transverse Rectus Abdominis Myocutaneous (TRAM) flap.

The second type, the trial-based economic evaluation (also known as *Stochastic Analysis*), derives data directly from the patients in the trial. It incorporates sampling uncertainty that is inherent probabilistic by nature. Parallel to a prospective, and preferably, a randomized controlled trial the researchers capture not only clinical outcome data but also direct and indirect costs related to the comparative interventions.

Formulas Used in Economic Evaluations that Inform Adoption of Novel Surgical Interventions

For Cost Analysis

$$\begin{aligned}\text{Cost Analysis} &= \text{Mean Cost}_{\text{novel surgical intervention}} \\ &\quad - \text{Mean Cost}_{\text{comparative surgical intervnetion}}\end{aligned}$$

(This is a partial economic evaluation. It assumes that the outcomes are the same, which may not be correct unless one measures them and finds them to be so).

If the outcome is similar, we adopt the novel intervention if it is found to be less costly.

For Cost-Effectiveness Analysis

Here we calculate the Incremental Cost-Effectiveness Ratio (ICER)

$$\text{ICER} = \frac{\Delta C}{\Delta E} = \frac{\begin{pmatrix}\text{Mean Cost}_{\text{novel surgical intervention}} \\ -\text{Mean Cost}_{\text{comparative surgical intervention}}\end{pmatrix}}{\begin{pmatrix}\text{Mean Effectiveness}_{\text{novel surgical intervention}} \\ -\text{Mean Effectiveness}_{\text{comparative surgical intervention}}\end{pmatrix}}$$

The adoption of a novel surgical intervention will be based on some threshold, which is arbitrarily set by clinical investigators or health economists based on consensus or in the case of CBA on showing a Net Social Benefit [4].

An important outcome that unfortunately is not commonly used in surgical comparative studies is Quality-Adjusted Life Years (QALYs) [7]. This is an outcome that captures both quality of life and quantity of life in a single measure. It can be measured with preference-based instruments, such as the EuroQOL 5-Dimension (EQ-5D) and the Health Utilities Index [7].

(Although a full economic evaluation, because the outcomes are measured differently, it cannot be used across disparate surgical interventions that measure outcomes differently).

The main limitation of this type of analysis is that it is difficult to compare disparate surgical interventions. Imagine the hypothetical scenario where two specialties, plastic surgery and orthopedic surgery, present each to a third-party payer a CEA and ask that their novel surgeries be funded but there is funding for only one. If the ICER submitted by each specialty were as follows:

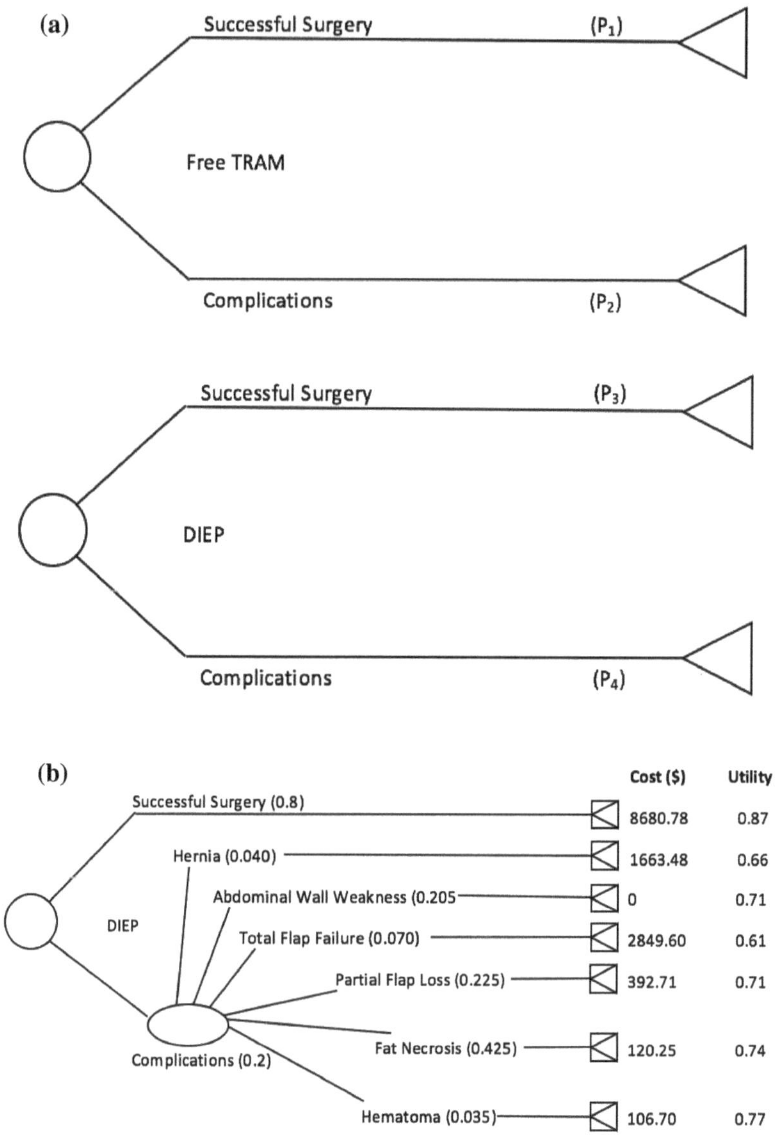

Fig. 23.1 **a** Decision analytic tree illustrating possible health state (pathway) probabilities for free TRAM versus DIEP. **b**. DIEP flap in postmastectomy breast reconstruction. *P* probability of each pathway; figure from Thoma et al. [6]

- ICER = $40,000/successful breast reconstruction after mastectomy
- ICER = $50, 00/successful knee replacement

How should the third-party payer decide? This is akin to comparing apples and oranges. This dilemma is obviated by the CUA where a common outcome (QALYs) is used by both specialties and the decision is easier to make.

For Cost–Utility Analysis

This is a full economic evaluation, recommended to be used to inform reimbursement policy making [3, 4]. Here, we calculate the Incremental Cost–Utility Ratio (ICUR).

$$\mathrm{ICUR} = \frac{\Delta C}{\Delta U} = \frac{\left(\begin{array}{c}\text{Mean Cost}_{\text{novel surgical intervention}} \\ -\text{Mean Cost}_{\text{comparative surgical intervention}}\end{array}\right)}{\left(\begin{array}{c}\text{Mean QALY}_{\text{novel surgical intervention}} \\ -\text{Mean QALY}_{\text{Comparative intervention}}\end{array}\right)}$$

(If the ICUR < $50,000/QALY, this is a strong indication that the novel intervention should be adopted [8]). As a general guidance, it is probably better to use a Willingness-to-Pay (WTP) threshold as the $50,000 figure has no theoretical basis and it is mostly used in the USA.

For Cost–Benefit Analysis

In this type of analysis, we attach a monetary value to the consequence of an intervention using a Willingness-to-Pay (WTP) approach.

$$\mathrm{NSB}_i = \sum_{t=1}^{n} \frac{b_i(t) - c_i(\mathrm{t})}{(1+r)^{t-1}}$$

where NSB = Net Social Benefit, t = year, $b_i(t)$ = benefits derived in year t, $c_i(t)$ = costs derived in year t and r = discount rate, n = lifetime of study.

(This type of economic evaluation is not used much in health care as it attaches a monetary value to the effectiveness of a health state, which health economists believe discriminates against the poor) [4].

Sensitivity Analysis

In clinical effectiveness studies, the results are reported by a point estimate such as a mean and a validity estimate such as a standard deviation. Hypothesis testing is done via the p-value. In economic evaluations, one performs a sensitivity analysis to determine how robust the conclusions are [4]. After the main analysis is performed based on the point estimate, the investigators redo the analysis based on one or two standard deviations around the point estimate of the costs or effectiveness or both, to see whether or not the conclusions of the study change. Probabilistic analyses with nonparametric "bootstrapping" with replacement are used in more advanced economic analyses [4, 9]. The conclusions are reported as robust if all calculations, main analysis, and sensitivity analyses favor the novel surgical intervention.

Now that you have mastered the important terminology and principles, we will help you understand how to appraise and understand a published economic evaluation report, by taking you through the following clinical scenario.

Clinical Scenario

At the hospital orthopedic rounds, a young surgeon asks his chief of service for an additional OR room for arthroscopic knee surgery. He claims there is an increasing demand for this useful procedure. His chief is skeptical because what he read that the benefits of arthroscopic surgery is controversial. He doubts he can persuade the hospital administration to invest money in this endeavor and asks his junior colleague to present supporting evidence that arthroscopic surgery is cost-effective compared to just physical therapy from the patient's point of view.

Finding the Evidence

To identify the best evidence and inform his colleagues, the surgeon begins by conducting a literature search, as described in Chap. 3, in this book and according to the "Users" guide to the surgical literature: how to perform a high-quality literature search" [10].

The effectiveness of a surgical intervention can be found in a high-quality Randomized Controlled Trial (RCT) or a meta-analysis of number of RCTs. In this case, an RCT that compares arthroscopic surgery to optimal non-operative therapy, in which the investigators coupled an economic evaluation, would provide the best evidence of cost-effectiveness. The surgeon follows the PICOT format, as described in Chap. 4, for the identification of important key words used in the search process:

Population: Patients with knee arthritis
Intervention: Arthroscopic surgery
Comparison: Physical Therapy (Physiotherapy or Optimal nonsurgical therapy)
Outcome: Cost-effectiveness
Time horizon: At least a year follow-up

We performed a literature search by choosing the filtered database, COCHRANE reviews and an unfiltered database, PubMed. With the PICOT format in mind, we used the search strategy: "osteoarthritis (P) AND arthroscopic surgery (I) AND physical therapy (C) AND cost-effectiveness analysis (O)". Between COCHRANE and PubMed, we identified 7 articles. We excluded articles because they did not include cost-effectiveness analyses, if they were not recent (last 10 years), or if they did not measure QALY.

One by Marsh et al. [11], which was listed in both databases, caught our attention. We read the abstract and we found it relevant to our purpose. This article includes both costs and effectiveness measured in QALYs and it is a full economic evaluation. It compares arthroscopic knee surgery and nonoperative methods. Now, we proceed to appraise the economic evaluation to determine whether the results are valid and whether they are relevant to our practice.

Are the Results Valid?

Did the Analysis Provide a Full Economic Comparison of Healthcare Strategies?

An economic analysis compares two or more healthcare interventions; in our case two surgical interventions to a surgical problem. Specifically, it compares the costs and the consequences (outcomes) of these interventions. The Marsh et al. [11] article is a full economic evaluation as they compared the costs in dollars and the effectiveness of the interventions, arthroscopy and a nonoperative method, using the Western Ontario McMaster Ostearthritis Index (WOMAC) and Quality-Adjusted Life Years (QALYs). It seems this is a full economic evaluation and we proceed to the next question.

Were Relevant Viewpoints Considered?

In an economic evaluation, there are a few possible perspectives (viewpoints). By this, we mean who bears the costs associated with the use of the new surgical procedures. In appraising an economic evaluation specifically, we ask who is benefiting from this study? Is it the patient, the hospital, the third-party payer or the society or others? There are occasions where a novel intervention may be found to be cost-effective from one perspective (i.e., the hospital) but not necessarily from another (i.e., the patient). For example, the hospital may save money by discharging patients earlier after a surgical intervention compared to an older program when the patients are hospitalized for a longer period but from the patient's point of view, this may be more costly if the patient's spouse has to take time off work to care for them during recovery at home.

In the Marsh et al. [11] study, we are told that the investigators conducted the cost-effectiveness analysis from the perspective of the Canadian healthcare payer and the societal perspectives. These perspectives are legitimate; however, we were concerned that they did not mention the patient's perspective. As the societal perspective also includes any out of pocket costs to the patient such as physical therapy, medications or assistive devices not covered by the provincial insurance plan and indirect costs such as time off employment, we wonder why they did not include explicitly the patient perspective. Their claim of taking a societal perspective may be incomplete, as other aspects, such as childcare and other familial obligations, could be different for the patient between the two interventions.

The perspective taken in an economic evaluation may depend on the question asked. The panel in cost-effectiveness in health strongly recommended that the societal perspective is the most important and should be considered, if possible [3]. Marsh and colleagues did this but as mentioned above, there may be some limitations to it [11].

Were All Relevant Clinical Strategies Compared?

When conducting an economic evaluation, it important that the investigators compare all relevant strategies for the condition under investigation. For example, the investigators should be comparing a novel procedure to a standard one and not one that is rarely used. In addition, investigators should be considering patients of different baseline risks. For example, if a general surgeon is performing a CEA on a novel hernia repair in the military population, this may not be generalizable to a retirement community population. If a CEA is performed comparing two approaches to hand surgery, one should consider both the Workers Compensation Benefit (WCB) patient and the non-WCB patient population, as the WCB patients are considered high-risk patients.

This is accomplished by doing a literature review of the population at risk. It seems that Marsh et al. considered different baseline risks as they performed a subgroup analysis [11]. This included patients with less severe radiographic disease (KL grade 2) and patients reporting mechanical symptoms of catching or locking. The clinical strategies they considered, arthroscopic versus nonoperative seems appropriate.

Were the Costs and Outcomes Properly Measured and Valued?

Was Clinical Effectiveness Established?

As mentioned in the introduction, there are two methodologically distinct types of economic evaluations, the model-based (deterministic) method, and the trial-based (stochastic) method. The preferred method is trial-based. In this type, patient-derived data are extracted from a well-executed RCT, in which the investigators collect costs from various perspectives parallel to the RCT. This type of economic evaluation provides high internal validity but at the expense of external validity as the subjects in the study may not be typical of community patients. If multiple RCTs exist, one can then pool the results in meta-analysis thus increasing generalizability because the pooled estimate of the effectiveness is derived from a wider spectrum of patients. To improve generalizability, one may relax the inclusion criteria in the RCT thus including patients that represent the whole population thus making this a pragmatic RCT and pragmatic economic evaluation.

The clinical effectiveness in the Marsh et al. article was measured by the WOMAC scale, which is a validated osteoarthritis instrument with total scores varying from 0 to 2400, higher scores indicating more pain and stiffness and reduced physical function [12–14].

Marsh et al. [11] also uses QALYs for performing a cost–utility analysis, the preferred type of economic evaluation by policy makers. To use QALYs, health utilities (such as HRQL or weights) are required [4, 7, 15]. Marsh et al. [11] used the Standard Gamble Technique to estimate health utilities. A health utility score is anchored at 0 (death) and 1 (perfect health). The other measure taken into account to measure QALYs is the duration of the corresponding health state. We believe that the investigators measured the effectiveness of the competing interventions appropriately.

Were Costs Measured Accurately?

How the cost of the interventions is reported depends on the perspective taken, as certain aspects such as costs of physiotherapy will not be relevant if comparing a hospital perspective, as these services is usually provided outside the hospital. Reporting healthcare resource use in natural units and unit costs separately allows for appraisal and replication by others.

As mentioned previously, Marsh et al. [11] include two perspectives, the Canadian healthcare payer perspective and the societal perspective, in which they breakdown further considering both short-term and long-term costs (physical therapy vs. time off employment) directly or indirectly associated with the two treatments.

For the operative intervention, Marsh et al. [11] took the average procedure costs from the Ontario Case Costing Initiative, which includes things such as medical tests, operating room costs, equipment, and laboratory testing. For surgeon billing fee for each procedure, Marsh et al. [11] used the Ontario Schedule of Benefits. The investigators did not mention about anesthesia costs here, which we consider an important component of the procedure cost.

Direct medical cost estimates of the nonoperative intervention used information such as the number of physical therapy sessions attended by each patient, as well as medication (pain medication, anti-inflammatory medications, and hyaluronic injections) and device use (cost per unit obtained from the Ontario Drug Benefit Formulary) were considered [11].

Patient out of pocket costs include medications or devices that are not covered by any type of insurance program, Indirect costs cover items such as time off employment and caregiving activities. The indirect costs and out of pocket costs combined are included in the "societal perspective". The out of pocket costs fall into the patient perspective, so we are perplexed as to why Marsh et al. [11] were not explicit on using the patient perspective separately.

Were Data on Costs and Outcomes Appropriately Integrated?

Studies that claim to be full economic evaluations often compare direct medical costs to each other, which does not necessarily mean that whichever one is the least costly is the most cost effective. Another common mistake is to take a ratio of cost and effect of the novel intervention and compare it to that of the comparative intervention.

To determine whether a novel surgical treatment is cost-effective, one needs to calculate an incremental cost–utility ratio (ICUR). This integrates the costs and effectiveness of the competing interventions, telling us what the extra unit of benefit is for each extra unit of cost. This is precisely what the investigators in the Marsh et al. study did. They calculated the marginal cost per marginal unit of utility [11]. This measure divides the difference in the mean cost of the novel and comparative treatment by the difference in the mean effectiveness, which in this case is QALY.

The investigators also report an Incremental Cost-Effectiveness Ratio (ICER), to look at the other outcome, WOMAC. This equation is identical to the one used for ICUR (described above) other than the denominator:

$$\text{ICER} = \frac{\begin{pmatrix}\text{Differences in costs between} \\ \text{Intervention 1 and Intervention 2}\end{pmatrix}}{\begin{pmatrix}\text{Differences in health effects between} \\ \text{Intervention 1 and Intervention 2}\end{pmatrix}}$$

These measures are critical because they represent the treatment which has the greatest incremental cost per unit gained in either QALY or pain and mobility measures from the WOMAC index. In other words, the higher the value of ICER/ICUR, the greater the cost to improve the outcome (patient health). Acceptance or rejection of novel surgical technologies is based on this. It also depends on the patient and the circumstances at hand, such as frequency of the intervention and ability of the healthcare system to support it. Ultimately, some type of threshold of acceptability will be decided upon by a consensus of experts.

In the Marsh et al. [11] study, there was also an estimate of the total cost for each patient over the 2-year follow-up, therefore discounting (accounting for the difference in cost presently versus the cost in the future) was not necessary [11]. Therefore, it seems that costs and outcomes were appropriately integrated.

Was Appropriate Allowance Made for Uncertainties in the Analysis?

It is imperative to determine whether the ICER/ICUR values actually represent cost-effectiveness, as there are many values that can fall around the mean. This can be accomplished by recalculating the ICER/ICUR using both the best- and worst-case scenarios, referred to as a sensitivity analysis. If the conclusion on cost-effectiveness stays the same, it can be decided with more confidence that the treatment is truly cost-effective. Marsh et al. included a sensitivity analysis, in which they used either extreme of their 95% CI surrounding the mean differences in WOMAC scores and QALY. They estimated ICER and ICUR values that assumed the highest possible treatment effect observed in their sample, favoring either added arthroscopy or nonoperative treatments only, followed by Cost-Effectiveness Acceptability Curves (CEAC). We believe they satisfied this criterion.

The economic evaluation by Marsh et al. also includes the CEACs, which indicate the probabilities of an intervention being cost-effective at various Willingness-to-Pay (WTP) values [11]. WTP values represent the amount one is willing to spend per one unit increase in WOMAC or QALY value [16]. Marsh et al. [11] performed a Net Benefit Regression model (NBR) for each outcome (WOMAC and QALY), by WTP (up to the clinically relevant threshold of $100,000 per unit gained), and stratified by perspective (Health care and Societal).

Are Estimates of Costs and Outcomes Related to the Baseline Risk in the Treatment Population?

As patients who are considered "high risk" are generally more likely to benefit from a treatment than those who are considered "low risk" , it is imperative to divide the population to reflect these groups to determine if there is in fact a difference in cost and benefit between groups.

Marsh et al. [11] included a table outlining the baseline characteristics of the population by intervention group (operative vs. nonoperative) and they were very similar between groups. However, the investigators could have categorized the continuous variables (i.e., age and BMI). This would provide a better sense of the different baseline risks or benefits of one treatment over the other for older individuals or those considered "over-weight" or "obese". Those who have less severe disease (KL grade 2) and patients reporting mechanical symptoms of catching or locking may not be the only groups to consider [11].

What Are the Results?

What Were the Incremental Costs and Outcomes Between the Two Strategies?

Marsh et al. [11] found a statistically significant difference in mean cost between groups, health-care payer perspective and societal perspective (Table 23.2). In terms of outcomes, there were differences in both outcomes WOMAC (favoring surgery) and QALY (favoring nonoperative) between intervention groups. However, these were not statistically significant ($p = 0.87$ and $p = 0.72$, respectively; Table 23.2).

The net benefit regression models (WOMAC and QALY) did not indicate arthroscopic surgery

Table 23.2 Cost and effect of outcomes (WOMAC and QALY)

	Surgery[a]	Nonoperative[a]	Incremental difference[b]
WOMAC			
Baseline	1222.91 (478.16)	1355.26 (548.92)	−132.35 (−24.58 to 289.29), 0.10
24-month	1526.45 (623.83)	1510.77 (570.21)	15.69 (−198.35 to 166.98), 0.87
Utility			
Baseline	0.79 (0.22)	0.80 (0.21)	0.01 (−0.06 to 0.07), 0.85
24-month	0.84 (0.23)	0.86 (0.16)	0.02 (−0.04 to 0.08), 0.47
QALY	1.64 (0.40)	1.66 (0.30)	−0.02 (−0.09 to 0.13), 0.72
Cost[c]			
Healthcare payer perspective	2633.25 (574.43)	737.40 (542.93)	1895.85 (1716.13–2075.57), <0.01
Societal perspective	3825.60 (1443.48)	1614.22 (1784.94)	2211.38 (1716.04–2706.51), <0.01

Note Table 23.2 was taken directly from Marsh et al. [11]
QALY quality-adjusted life yearn, *WOMAC* Western Ontario and McMaster Universities Osteoarthritis Index
[a]Mean (SD)
[b]Mean difference between groups (95% CI), p value
[c]2014 Canadian dollars

as a cost-effective alternative to nonoperative methods from either perspective at all levels of WTP (Table 23.3).

Do Incremental Costs and Outcomes Differ Among Subgroups?

In terms of cost and outcomes in the subgroup analysis, surgery was also not cost-effective in terms of either WOMAC or QALY. This was seen in both subgroups chosen by the investigators (patients with less severe disease and patients reporting mechanical symptoms of catching or locking) at all the levels of WTP.

How Much Does Allowance for Uncertainty Change the Results?

Marsh et al. stated that the ICER value was $140.94 from the societal perspective and $120.83 from the healthcare payer perspective, per one-point improvement on the 2400 point WOMAC total score, translating to $28,188 (societal) and $24,166 (payer) for a clinically important improvement (200 points). Additionally, the ICUR was −$110,569 from the societal perspective and −$94,792.50 from the healthcare payer perspective per QALY gained, where the negative value indicates paying more and not getting a better outcome (surgery costs more but is less effective than nonoperative care). As reporting of economic evaluations with negative values is not intuitive, health economists prefer to use terms such as “dominant strategy”, “win-win “scenario, “lose-lose” scenario. In the Marsh et al. [11] study, the ICUR from the societal perspective should have been reported as a “lose-lose” strategy as surgery was more costly and less effective (Figs. 23.2 and 23.3).

When we compare a novel surgical intervention to a prevailing technology, there are nine possibilities, which are illustrated in Fig. 23.2. The novel intervention may be more, same or less effective than the prevailing intervention illustrated on the horizontal axis of Fig. 23.2. The vertical axis illustrates whether the novel intervention is more, same or less costly than the prevailing intervention. If a novel intervention falls in *cell 1*, we adopt the new surgical technology, as it is more effective and less costly. Using the same reasoning, if it falls in cell 2, we reject it, as it is less effective and more costly. Most novel interventions fall in cell 7, where new technologies are more

Table 23.3 Net-benefit regression analysis results

(a) WOMAC

WTP[a]	Healthcare payer[b]		Societal[b]	
	Incremental net benefit	95% CI. *p*-value	Incremental net benefit	95% CI. *p*-value
0	−1179.20 (386.56)	−1942.58 to −415.82, <0.01	−1670.507 (66.18)	−2978.30 to −362.71, 0.01
1500	−352,418.73 (332804.27)	−1,009,643.31 to 304,805.85, 029	−369,151.74 (334,686.56)	−1,030,156.42 to 291,852.95, 0.27
2000	−469,498.57 (443753.31)	−1,345,826.20 to 406,829.05, 0.29	−491,645.48 (446,248.44)	−1,372,984.45 to 389,693.49. 0.27
2500	−586,578.42 (554702.36)	−1,682,009.13 to 508,852.29, 029	−614,139.22 (557,810.37)	−1715812.60 to 487534.16, 0.27
5000	−1,171,977.63 (1109447.72)	−3,362,923.98 to 1,018,968.72, 0.29	−1,226,607.94 (1,115,620.38)	−3,429,953.97 to 976,738.10, 0.27
10,000	−2,342,776.07 (2218938.56)	−6,724,753.89 to 2,039,201.76, 0.29	−2,451,545.36 (2,231,240.70)	−6,858,237.29 to 1,955,146.56, 0.27
20,000	−4,684,372.93 (4437920.28)	−13,448,413.80 to 4,079,667.94, 0.29	−4,901,420.22 (4,462,481.46)	−13,714,804.20 to 3,911,963.77, 0.27
30,000	−7,025,969.80 (6656902.01)	−2,0172,073.70 to 6,120,134.15, 0.29	−7,351,295.06 (6,693,722.26)	−20571371.20 to 5,868,871.04, 0.27
40,000	−9,367,566.66 (8875883.74)	−26,895,733.70 to 8,160,600.36, 0.29	−9,801,169.94 (8,924,963.07)	−27,427,938.20 to 7,825,598 33, 0.27
50,000	−11,709,163.50 (11094865.47	−33,619,393.60 to 10,201,066.58, 0.29	−12,251,044.80 (11,156,203.89)	−3,428,450,520 to 9,782,415.63. 0.27
60,000	−14,050,760.40 (13313847.20)	−40,343,053.60 to 12,241,532.79, 0.29	−14,700,919.70 (13,387,444.70)	−41,141,072.20 to 11,739,232.93, 0.27
70,000	−16,392,357.30 (15532828.94	−47,066,713.50 to 14,281,999.01, 0.29	−17,150,794.50 (15,618,685.51)	−47,997,639.20 to 13,696,050.23, 0.27
80,000	−18,733,954.10 (17751810.67)	−53,790,373.50 to 16,322,465.23, 0.29	−19,600,669.40 (17,849,926.33)	−54,854,206.30 to 15,652,867.53, 0.27
90,000	−21,075,551.00 (19970792.40)	−60,514,033.40 to 18,362,931.44, 0.29	−22,050,544.20 (20,081,167.14)	−61,710,773.30 to 17,609,684.84, 0.27
100,000	−23,417,147.90 (22189774.14)	−67,237,693.40 to 20,403,397.66, 0.29	−24,500,419.10 (22,312,407.96)	−68,567,340.30 to 19,566,502.14, 0.27

(b) QALY

WTP[c]	Healthcare payer[b]		Societal[b]	
	Incremental net benefit	95% CI. *p*-value	Incremental net benefit	95% CI, *p*-value
0	−2020.18 (558.61)	−3123.38 to −916.98, <0.01	−2048.89 (946.17)	−3917.66 to −180.11, 0.03
1500	−2226.59 (608.74)	−3427.75 to −1023 38, <0.01	−2250.38 (1006.93)	−4239.15 to −261.59, 0.03
2000	−2294.02 (645.94)	−3569.69 to −1018.34, <0.01	−2317.54 (1039.73)	−4371.10 to −263.98, 0.03
2500	−2362.48 (691.03)	−3727.19 to −997.77, <0.01	−2384.70 (1077.94)	−4513.73 to −255.67, 0.03
5000	−2704.77 (991.35)	−4662.60 to −746.96, 0.01	−272052 (1331.67)	−5350.69 to −90.34, 0.04
10,000	−3389.38 (1735.70)	−6817.21 to 38.45, 0.05	−339214 (2007.52)	−7357.19 to 572 91, 0.09
20,000	−4758.57 (3339.13)	−11,353.01 to 1835.87, 0.16	−4735.40 (3560.87)	−11768.45 to 2297.66, 0.18
30,000	−6127.77 (4972.26)	−15,947.50 to 3691.96, 0.22	−6078.65 (5181.15)	−16311.90 to 4154.60, 0.24

(continued)

Table 23.3 (continued)

(b) QALY				
WTP[c]	Healthcare payer[b]		Societal[b]	
	Incremental net benefit	95% CI. *p*-value	Incremental net benefit	95% CI, *p*-value
40,000	−7496.98 (6613.14)	−20,557.26 to 5563.32, 0.26	−7452.72 (6820.82)	−20,893.66 to 6049.85, 0.28
50,000	−8866.17 (8257.13)	−25,173.19 to 7440.86, 0.29	−8765.16 (8468.63)	−25,491.49 to 7961.16, 0.30
60,000	−10,235.27 (9902.70)	−29,792.22 to 9321.50, 0.30	−10,108.42 (10,120.60)	−30,097.54 to 9880.70, 0.32
70,000	−11,604.56 (11549.16)	−34,413.03 to 11,203.90, 0.32	−11,451.68 (11,774.98)	−34,708.34 to 11,804.99, 0.33
80,000	−12,973.76 (13196.19)	−39,034.94 to 13,087.42, 0.33	−12,794.93 (13,430.88)	−39,322.15 to 13,732.30, 0.34
90,000	−14,342.96 (14,843.59)	−43,657.60 to 14,971.67, 0.34	−14,138.19 (15,087.81)	−43,937.98 to 15,661.62, 0.35
100,000	−15,712.16 (16,491.26)	−48,280.77 to 16,856.45, 0.34	−15,481.44 (16,745.45)	−48,555.23 to 17,592.53, 0.36

Note Table 23.3 was taken directly from Marsh et al. [11]

QALY quality-adjusted life year, *WOMAC* Western Ontario and McMaster Universities Osteoarthritis Index, *WTP* willingness-to-pay

[a]WTP for a one-point improvement on the WOMAC total score

[b]Incremental net benefit (SD)

[c]WTP for an additional QALY

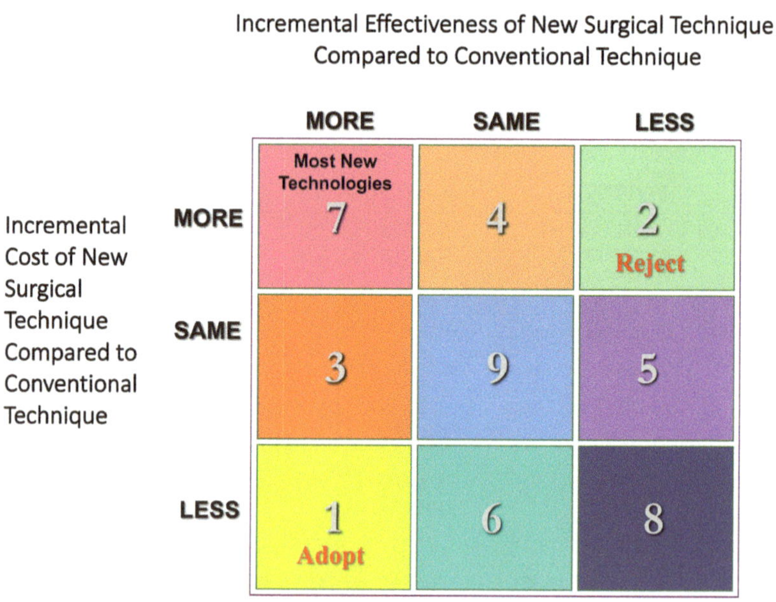

Fig. 23.2 Nine possible outcomes when comparing the new surgical technique and the conventional technique (the numbers within each cell are illustrative only). *Note* This figure was adapted, with permission, from Thoma et al. [17]

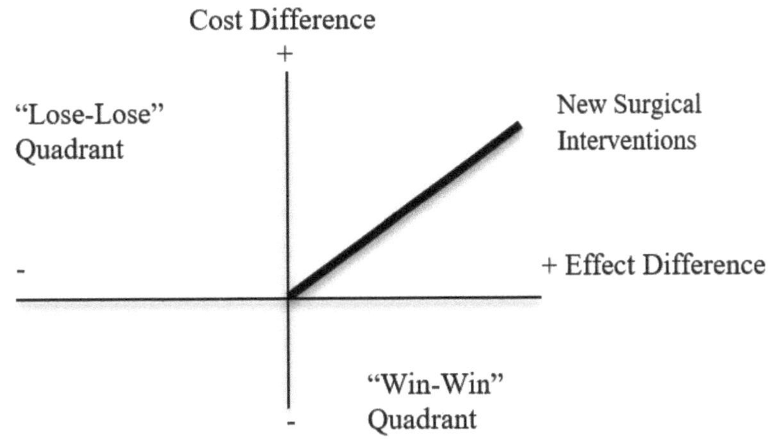

Fig. 23.3 Cost effectiveness plane. *Note* This figure was adapted, with permission, from Thoma et al. [18]

effective but also more costly. It is here that economic evaluations needs to be performed to find if indeed the novel interventions are cost-effective.

Another way of explaining these possibilities is the cost-effectiveness plane shown in Fig. 23.3, with the effectiveness on the x-axis and the cost on the y-axis. If the novel intervention falls in the right lower quadrant, we have a win–win situation meaning it is more effective and less costly. Alternatively, if it falls in the left upper quadrant, we have a lose–lose situation meaning it is less effective and costs more. The slope of this line will determine its acceptability or not. This slope is a ratio, which is precisely what the ICER/ICUR represents.

Will the Results Help Me in Caring for My Patients?

Are the Treatment Benefits Worth the Harms and Costs?

When we compare two surgical interventions (novel versus standard), surgeons need to understand that there are nine possibilities, as explained in Fig. 23.2. If the novel intervention falls in cell 1, we accept the novel intervention, as it is more effective and less costly. If it falls in cell 2, we reject it, as it is less effective and more costly. We use a similar reasoning for the other scenarios. In most cases of modern surgery however, most new innovations are more costly and at the same time more effective. This is similar to a new intervention falling in the right upper quadrant of the cost-effectiveness plane (Fig. 23.3). It is under these circumstances that we need to perform a CEA or CUA. In the past, if a new innovation had an ICUR of $20,000/QALY the recommendation was given to accept it [19]. In recent years, this figure has increased to $50,000/QALY [8]. The above were proposed thresholds in the literature. A more official threshold is the one proposed by The National Institute for Health and Clinical Excellence (NICE), which suggests anywhere from $27,000 to $41,000 to accept a new innovation [20].

Marsh et al. [11] found that arthroscopy was, in fact, less effective and more costly than nonoperative approaches. Surgery in itself also carries risks not encountered in nonoperative approaches, such as anesthetic complications, deep venous thrombosis, and pulmonary embolism [11]. Although these are uncommon, they can have lethal outcomes. In deciding on which approach to take, one may consider these risks.

Could a Clinician's Patients Expect Similar Health Outcomes?

In looking at Table 1 of the Marsh et al. article, and in particular, the demographic characteristics of their patients pertaining to age, BMI, and Kellgren–Lawrence osteoarthritis severity grade, we believe that their patients are similar to ours and therefore have no reason to dispute their findings. If on the other hand our patients were much older and the majority of our patients had a different ratio of severity, we may be more skeptical of the findings shown here.

Can I Expect Similar Costs?

The costs of arthroscopy and physical therapy may differ in different jurisdictions (provinces, states, and countries) and these should be considered seriously. If you believe that in your specific jurisdiction the costs are similar, then you should consider adopting the findings from this study. If on the other hand, the medical costs related to surgery or physical therapy are different in your geographic area, then you should recalculate the costs based on the health-related resource units provided by the authors of this paper. For example, you can calculate the cost of physical therapy for the average patient by multiplying the number of physical therapy visits by the cost in dollars per visit. It is therefore imperative for investigators not to just present the costs in an article but also state the resource units consumed for the two comparative interventions. From these data, we can recalculate the ICUR in our setting and decide for ourselves if the surgical option is cost-effective or not.

Resolution of the Scenario

Based on the baseline ICER and ICUR, we see that the surgical approach fell into the lose–lose quadrant of the cost-effectiveness plane and therefore we are not prepared to accept surgery over physical therapy for mild arthritis of the knee. We also believe that the young orthopedic surgeons' recommendation to spend more resources for this procedure is not supported by the evidence.

Final Thoughts and the CHEERS Statement

The EQUATOR network was established to enhance the quality and transparency of health research [21)]. They provide guidelines or checklists for various types of research including randomized trials, systematic reviews, and economic evaluations.

Clinical investigators who perform economic evaluations are encouraged to report their studies by following the CHEERS statement [21]. The CHEERS statement is a guideline specifically a checklist that covers all methodological aspects of an economic evaluation (title, introduction, methods, results, discussion, etc.). Although this guideline is not an appraisal instrument in itself, it does ensure that investigators cover all the elements of an economic evaluation. Familiarization with this guideline will ensure better quality study and eventual report.

References

1. Chatterjee A, Payette MJ, Demas CP, Finlayson SRG. Opportunity cost: a systematic application to surgery. Surgery. 2009 July;146(1):18–22.
2. Ziolkowski NI, Voineskos SH, Ignacy TA, Thoma A. Systematic review of economic evaluations in plastic surgery. Plast Reconstr Surg. 2013;132(1):191–203.
3. Gold MR, Siegel JE, Russell LB, Weinstein MC, editors. Cost-effectiveness in health and medicine. New York: Oxford University Press; c1996.
4. Drummond MF, Sculpher MJ, Torrance GW, O'Brien BJ, Stoddart GL. Methods for economic evaluation of health care programmes. 3rd ed. United Kingdom: Oxford University Press; 2005.
5. OECD. Tackling wasteful spending on health. [Internet]. Paris: OECH Publishing; 2018 [cited 2018 April]. Available from: http://dx.doi.org/10.1787/9789264266414-en.
6. Thoma A, Veltri K, Khuthaila D, Rockwell G, Duku E. Comparison of the deep inferior epigastric perforator (DIEP) and free transverse rectus abdominis myocutaneous (TRAM) flap in post-mastectomy

reconstruction: a cost-effectiveness analysis. Plast Reconstr Surg. 2004;113:1650–61.
7. Thoma A, McKnight L. Quality adjusted life year (QALY) as a surgical outcome measure. A primer for plastic surgeons. Plast Reconstr Surg. 2010;125 (4):1279–87.
8. Neumann PJ, Cohen JT, Weinstein MC. Updating COST-Effectiveness—the curious resilience of the $50,000-per-QALY threshold. N Engl J Med. 2014;371(9):796–7.
9. Thoma A, Kaur MN, Tsoi B, Ziolkowski N, Duku E, Goldsmith CH. Cost-effectiveness analysis parallel to a randomized controlled trial comparing vertical scar reduction and inverted T-shaped reduction mammaplasty. Plast Reconstr Surg. 2014;134(6):1093–107.
10. Waltho DA, Kaur MN, Haynes RB, Farrokhyar F, Thoma A. Users' guide to the surgical literature: how to perform a high-quality literature search. Can J Surg. 2015;58:349–58.
11. Marsh JD, Birmingham TB, Giffin JR, Isaranuwatchai W, Hoch JS, Feagan BG, et al. Cost-effectiveness analysis of arthroscopic surgery compared with non-operative management for osteoarthritis of the knee. BMJ Open. 2016;5:1–10.
12. Bellamy N, Buchanan WW, Goldsmith CH, Campbell J, Stitt LW. Validation study of WOMAC: a health status instrument for measuring clinically important patient relevant outcomes to antirheumatic drug therapy in patients with osteoarthritis of the hip or knee. J Rheumatol. 1988;15:1833–40.
13. Ehrich EW, Davies GM, Watson DJ, Bolognese Ja, Seidenberg BC, Bellamy N. Minimal perceptible clinical improvement with the Western Ontario and McMaster Universities osteoarthritis index questionnaire and global assessments in patients with osteoarthritis. J Rheumatol. 2000;27:2635–41.
14. Davies GM, Watson DJ, Bellamy N. Comparison of the responsiveness and relative effect size of the Western Ontario and McMaster Universities Osteoarthritis Index and the short-form Medical Outcomes Study Survey in a randomized, clinical trial of osteoarthritis patients. Arthritis Care Res. 1999;12:172–9.
15. Whitehead SJ, Ali S. Health outcomes in economic evaluation: the QALY and utilities. Br Med Bull. 2010;96(1):5–21.
16. Hoch JS, Briggs AH, Willan AR. Something old, something new, something borrowed, something blue: a framework for the marriage of health econometrics and cost-effectiveness analysis. Health Econ. 2002;11:415–30.
17. Thoma A, Sprague S, Tandan V. Users guide to the surgical literature: how to use an article on economic analysis. Can J Surg. 2001;44:347–54.
18. Thoma A, McKnight L, Knight C. The use of economic evaluation in hand surgery. Hand Clin. 2009;25:113–23.
19. Laupacis A, Feeny D, Detsky AS, Tugwell PX. How attractive does a new technology have to be to warrant adoption and utilization? Tentative guidelines for using clinical and economic evaluations. CMAJ. 1992;146(4):473–81.
20. McCabe C, Claxton K, Culyer AJ. The NICE cost-effectiveness threshold: what it is and what that means. Pharmacoeconomics. 2008;26(9):733–44.
21. Husereau D, Drummond M, Petrou S, Carswell C, Moher D, Greenberg D, et al. Consolidated Health Economic Evaluation Reporting Standards (CHEERS) statement. Eur J Health Econ. 2013;14 (3):367–72.

24 Studies Reporting Harm in Surgery

Robin McLeod

Clinical Scenario

You are the Surgical Quality Leader at your hospital, you and your colleagues are interested in implementing an Enhanced Recovery after Surgery (ERAS) program. From your reading, ERAS protocols lead to improved outcomes, fewer complications and decreased length of stay. You have organized several committees composed of individuals from all of the peri-operative groups that provide care to surgical patients. One of these groups is the Pain Management team which is recommending multimodality pain medication to decrease the need for opioids. The multimodal analgesia package includes the prescription of non-steroidal anti-inflammatory drugs (NSAIDs). While you are supportive of a multimodality analgesia package, you recently heard a discussion at a conference on the use of NSAIDs in patients undergoing a colorectal resection. While one of the colorectal surgeons supported the use of NSAIDs in this group of patients, another recommended being very cautious with the use of NSAIDs because of a possible increase in anastomotic leaks. You discuss this with your anaesthesiologist colleague who feels quite strongly that NSAIDs should be part of the regimen. He points out that NSAIDs decrease the need for opioids, which, in turn decrease the likelihood of post-operative ileus. Furthermore, with recent concerns of opioid addiction, there is merit in decreasing their use. While you agree with your colleague, you point out that an anastomotic leak can be life threatening. After this discussion, you both agree that you need to review the evidence before making a recommendation.

Introduction

While surgery is performed to improve the health and quality of life of patients, there always is a risk that patients having surgery may develop adverse side effects. In some cases, the likelihood of a negative consequence is small compared to the benefits of surgery. In others, however, the risk of harm may be more significant because of the severity or frequency of adverse events. Surgeons must always be aware of both the benefits and harm of surgery and strive to ensure that the benefits of surgery outweigh any potential harm. In addition, they need to ensure that patients themselves understand the risks so they can make decisions about their care. Just as surgeons must strive to use best evidence to assess the benefits of a surgical intervention, they should also use the best evidence to assess the risk of harm.

R. McLeod (✉)
Department of Surgery and the Institute of Health Policy, Management and Evaluation, University of Toronto, Toronto, ON, Canada
e-mail: robin.mcleod@cancercare.on.ca

A. Thoma et al. (eds.), *Evidence-Based Surgery*,
https://doi.org/10.1007/978-3-030-05120-4_24

In this clinical scenario, both the benefits and risks of NSAIDs require assessment. While this might not be considered a risk of surgery per se, the perioperative care of patients, which includes such interventions as pre-operative antibiotics, DVT prevention and pain management, is an essential part of the care of surgical patients. In this example, the use of post-operative NSAIDs, surgeons should be concerned because of the risk of an anastomotic leak which is definitely a surgical complication.

In line with the tenets of Evidence Based Surgery, the best evidence for determining harm is required as much as it is needed for assessing benefit. Ideally, evidence from a randomized controlled trial (RCT) is the best evidence for making decisions about harm. However, RCTs are generally designed to evaluate the effectiveness of a treatment to improve patient outcomes and only secondarily are they intended to measure complications or adverse events. It is certainly not ethical to randomize patients to determine which intervention is more harmful. In addition, some harmful effects may occur infrequently, and thus, the sample size would have to be very large to be able to make conclusions about the frequency of the harmful effects. Some side effects are not immediately apparent after treatment and therefore follow-up of patients participating in RCTs would have to be extended. For more information on RCTs see Chaps. 11–14.

Instead of using RCTs to ascertain the risk of harm, cohort and case-control studies are most often used. Case-control studies are observational studies which are often used in epidemiology. In these studies, individuals who have the medical condition (harmful side effect in this example) are identified (cases) and then a second cohort of patients who do not have the condition are matched to the cases. The advantage of these studies is that they require fewer resources and follow-up is not required but the evidence is weaker than that of a RCT (level 3 evidence) (see Chap. 5. As well, the characteristics of the case and control groups should be similar with the exception of the risk factor which is being studied.

Case-control studies are often used to study rare diseases or as a preliminary study where little is known about the association between the risk factor and the disease of interest. One of the most notable use of a case control study was the demonstration that smoking is associated with lung cancer [1]. For more information on case-control studies see Chap. 17.

The other method for determining whether a suspected risk factor leads to an adverse effect is to perform a cohort study (level 2 evidence). Cohort studies are longitudinal studies in which all patients are followed from a defined time but unlike RCTs, the patients are not randomized to the two groups but instead patients "choose" the group they are in. Cohort studies can be retrospective or prospective and are also used to assess the effect of exposure or protective factors on outcome. The limitation of cohort studies is that patients are not randomized and even if they are well matched there may be some differences which are not apparent or cannot be measured. The key strengths and limitations of the above study designs are summarized in Table 24.1. For more information on cohort studies see Chap. 16.

In this particular question, it may have been possible to do a RCT to assess the risk of anastomotic leak while assessing the efficacy of NSAIDs in controlling post-operative pain when NSAIDs were first introduced. However, when these studies were performed, there was no suggestion that NSAIDs might be associated with a risk of anastomotic leak. Now, it would be somewhat unethical to do a study looking at harm as the primary outcome.

Finding the Evidence

To identify the best evidence, we performed a literature search. We first formulated our research question using the PICOT (population,

Table 24.1 Description of the primary study designs

Characteristic	Study design		
	Randomized controlled trial	Prospective cohort study	Case-control study
Starting point	Intervention status	Intervention/exposure status	Event/outcome status
Group allocation	Randomization; groups are balanced for known and unknown confounding factors	Groups are selected to intervention or exposure; groups may not be balanced	Groups are selected to intervention or exposure; groups may not be balanced
Outcome measures	Incidence of disease	Incidence of disease	Prevalence of disease
Measure of risk	Relative risk; odds ratio, risk difference	Relative risk; odds ratio; risk difference	Odds ratio
Temporal relationship between exposure and disease	Easier to establish	Easier to establish	Harder to establish
Strength	Bias controlled	Bias uncontrolled	Bias uncontrolled
Validity (if well designed)	Level I evidence	Level II evidence	Level III evidence

Adapted from Levine et al. [2]

intervention, comparison, outcome, time horizon) format as seen below.

- Population: males and females undergoing an elective colorectal resection with anastomosis
- Intervention: NSAIDs
- Comparison: no NSAIDs prescribed
- Outcome: anastomotic leak
- Time horizon: seven days following surgery

Using the PICOT format your research question would be: "*Does the use of NSAIDs, as compared to no NSAIDS, lead to anastomotic leaks in elective colorectal resection with anastomosis seven days following surgery?*"

You perform a PubMed search based on the above-mentioned PICOT terms, you enter: "colorectal surgery" AND "non-steroidal anti-inflammatory drugs" AND "anastomotic leak" AND "postoperative". The original search yields 8 article (Appendix 1). You do a title and abstract review of each of the 8 articles; articles 2, 5 and 8 are not specific to your topic and article 7 is an abstract. Articles 1 and 3 are systematic reviews, and while they would be appropriate for your research question you are drawn to articles 4 and 6, which are cohort studies. Both cohort studies utilize prospectively collected data, however, a full text review reveals that the study by Klein et al. [3] use a Danish Colorectal Cancer Group database that has been validated and has a completeness rate of over 96%. You decide to go with the Klein et al. [3] study entitled, postoperative use of non-steroidal anti-inflammatory drugs in patients with anastomotic leakage requiring reoperation after colorectal resection: cohort study based on prospective data.

Study Appraisal

To properly understand, and present the information to your colleague, you have elected to use an article by Thoma et al. [4] to appraise your selected article. The questions used to appraise an article about harm in surgery are shown in Box 1.

Box 1. Questions Used to Appraise an Article Based on Harm

1. **Are the Results Valid?**

   a. Were patients similar in terms of prognostic factors that are known to be associated with the outcome (or was statistical adjustment necessary)?
   b. Were the circumstances and methods for detecting the outcome similar for patients and controls?
   c. Was the follow-up sufficiently complete?

2. **What are the Results?**

   a. How strong is the association between exposure and outcome?
   b. How precise was the estimate of the risk?

3. **How can I Apply the Results to my Patients or Clinical Practice?**

   a. Were the patients in the appraised study similar to the patients in my practice?
   b. Was follow-up sufficiently long?
   c. Is the exposure similar to what might occur in my patients?
   d. What is the magnitude of the risk?
   e. Are there any benefits that are known to be associated with exposure?

Critical Appraisal of the Article

A. Are the Results of the Study Valid?

Validity is a measure of the credibility of the research. Studies are valid if they actually measure what they set out to measure. There are two types of validity: (1) internal validity, whether the study itself is valid; and (2) external validity, whether the results of the study are generalizable. For example, if the goal of a study was to compare the effectiveness of two antibiotics in preventing wound infections it would be important that the patients in the two groups were similar. If there were a larger proportion of patients in one group who had perforated diverticulitis, compared to the other group, it would be difficult to conclude that the antibiotics were less effective or whether the difference was due to the group having a higher risk of infection. We would conclude that this study lacked internal validity. On the other hand, if both groups were similar but included only patients who had elective operations for diverticular disease, we would not be able to generalize the results to patients having emergency surgery for perforated diverticulitis. This refers to external validity.

Were patients similar in terms of prognostic factors that are known to be associated with the outcome?

The Klein et al. [3] study reported data from The Danish Colorectal Cancer Group, a national prospective database which holds data for over 96% of patients who have undergone surgery for colorectal cancer. Information from this database and electronically registered medical records were used; all orders in Denmark must be entered into the latter. For this study, only patients who had undergone an elective operation for colorectal cancer between January 1, 2006 and December 31, 2009 from the six major centers responsible for colorectal cancer surgery in eastern Denmark were included.

Demographic information, comorbidities, alcohol and tobacco use, tumour stage, intra-operative blood loss and transfusion and type of procedure (laparoscopic or open) and anastomotic leakage were collected in the Colorectal Cancer database using standardized definitions. The three groups appear to be similar with most variables (age, sex, ASA status, comorbidities including heart disease, hypertension, lung disease diabetes mellitus) as well as tumor status, resection type (rectal vs colonic) (Table 24.2).

Table 24.2 select patient characteristics

Demographic variables		Number of patients
Age	Median (interquartile range)	70 (62–77)
Sex	Male	1441
	Female	1315
ASA status	I	637
	II	1639
	III	428
	IV	20
Comorbidities	–	–
Ischaemic heart disease	Yes	341
	No	974
Hypertension	Yes	834
	No	478
Lung disease	Yes	196
	No	1984
Diabetes	Yes	259
	No	1060
Tumour T stage	1	161
	2	330
	3	1720
	4	516
Resection	Colonic	1988
	Rectal	768
Procedure	Open	1760
	Laparoscopic	996

However, there were differences in alcohol consumption and smoking, intraoperative blood loss and transfusion and whether the procedure was performed open or laparoscopically. Known risk factors for anastomotic leakage include gender (higher in males), smoking, obesity, alcohol abuse and preoperative steroid use [5].

Were the circumstances and methods for determining exposure similar for patients and controls?
Both circumstances and methods appear to be similar for both groups. In this prospective cohort study, the likelihood of bias is much lower than if this were a retrospective cohort study or a case-control study. We can assume that the exposure (i.e.: whether patients received NSAIDs) was well documented in the electronic medical records registry since all orders must be put into this register. In addition, if NSAIDs were ordered into the electronic medical record, three reviewers who were blinded as to whether the patient had/did not have an anastomotic leak reviewed the charts to determine if the patients actually received NSAIDs and if so, how many doses.

Was the follow-up sufficiently complete?
The standard follow-up to assess adverse events post-operatively in patients having colorectal surgery is 30 days. According to the literature, anastomotic leakage is most commonly detected 5–7 days following surgery [5]. In this study, there was complete follow-up in all but four patients at 30 days. You are therefore confident that the follow-up was an appropriate length, and sufficiently complete.

Was the correct temporal relationship demonstrated?
The authors do not report whether patients had used NSAIDs prior to surgery. While in some studies it would be important to document when the exposure occurred, it is unlikely that NSAIDs prior to surgery would have an effect because NSAIDs have a short half-life.

Was there a dose-response gradient?
Regular post-operative consumption of NSAIDs was defined as ingestion of at least 50 mg of diclofenac per day or ibuprofen 800 mg per day for at least two of the first seven post-operative days [3]. In reality, 95% of patients in the ibuprofen group ingested at least 1200 mg per day and 99% in the diclofenac group ingested at least 100 mg per day [3]. The authors did not do a dose-response analysis. However, in addition to the comparisons based on the definitions above, they reported that within the control group there were 231 patients (12.3%) who ingested less than two days of NSAIDs. The anastomotic leak rate

in this latter group was compared to those who received no NSAIDs and the anastomotic leak rates were similar (5.2% vs. 5.1%).

What are the Results?

How strong is the association between exposure and outcome?

The authors report that the anastomotic leak rate in the diclofenac group was 12.8%; in the ibuprofen group 8.2%; and 5.1% in the control group. Thus, the increased risk of an anastomotic leak in the diclofenac group was 7.8% (95% CI 3.9–12.8%) and in the ibuprofen group was 3.2% (95% CI 1.0–5.7%).

Odds Ratios (OR) measure how strong an association there is between the exposure (NSAIDs) and outcomc (anastomotic lcak). An Odds Ratio of greater than 1 indicates that the risk of the outcome (anastomotic leak) is higher when exposed to the risk factor (NSAID) whereas an OR equal to one indicates that there is no association.

In this study, multivariate logistic regression analyses were performed including the following risk factors: NSAID treatment, drug type, sex, intraoperative transfusion, hospital and type of resection (colonic or rectal operation. The authors report that the OR of an increased risk of an anastomotic leak for patients taking diclofenac was 7.2 (95% CI 3.8–13.4) and for those taking ibuprofen the increased risk was 1.5 (95% CI 0.8–2.9). In other words, the risk of an anastomotic leak was increased 7.2-fold in patients taking diclofenac and 1.5 times in those taking ibuprofen (although this was not statistically significant because the CI crossed 1.0).

Of note, the overall post-operative mortality was 3.3% but in patients who had a leak, the postoperative mortality was 9.5%. However, post-operative mortality was not increased in either the diclofenac (4.1%) or ibuprofen groups (1.8%) compared to the control group (3.2%).

How precise is the estimate of the risk?

The precision of the risk is mainly affected by the sample size. The 95% CI will be wider with a small sample size and narrower in studies with a large sample size. In this analysis, the risk of anastomotic leak for patients taking diclofenac was 7.2 and based on the 95% CI, we can be 95% certain that the risk lies somewhere between 3.8 and 13.4. In other words, we can be quite certain that taking diclenofac is associated with an increased risk of anastomotic leak. On the other hand, the 95% confidence intervals for ibuprofen ranged from 0.8 to 2.9 so while the OR for ibuprofen is above 1.0, in fact, the range could be from 0.8 to 2.9 and ibuprofen usage might or might not be associated with an anastomotic leak.

How can I Apply the Result to my Patients or Clinical Practice

Were the patients in the appraised study similar to the patients in my practice?

The characteristics of the patients in this study are representative of most patients you see for colorectal cancer surgery. However, there are some potential differences, although they likely do not affect the results. First, 36% of the patients had laparoscopic surgery; this analysis included patients who had surgery between 2006 and 2009; the proportion of patients having a laparoscopic approach would, most likely, be higher now in most jurisdictions [6]. Second, the outcome measure was patients who had an anastomotic leak and required reoperation; the proportion of patients who had an anastomotic leak and did not have a reoperation was not reported. Assuming that there were patients who had an anastomotic leak but did not require surgery, the rate of anastomotic leaks would likely be higher than expected. However, if there is a difference in the management of anastomotic leaks in Denmark so most or all patients are reoperated, there may not be a difference in the rate of anastomotic leaks. Instead there may be a difference in management since most patients who develop an anastomotic leak are treated non-operatively in North America.

Is the exposure similar to what might occur in my patient?

A variety of NSAIDs are available and may be prescribed to patients having elective colorectal surgery. This study suggests that further investigation is required to determine whether the risk of anastomotic leaks is lower in some NSAIDs and therefore may be safe for patients undergoing a colorectal resection. The exposure would therefore be similar for any patient that was prescribed NSAIDs; therefore your patient would have the same risk of exposure as those patients in the Klein et al. [3] article.

What is the magnitude of the risk?

The Number Needed to Harm (NNH) is similar to the Number Needed to Treat (NNT) . However, while the NNT is a measure of how many patients need to be treated in order for one patient to benefit from the treatment, the NNH is a measure of how many people need to be treated (or exposed to a risk factor) for one person to have a particular adverse effect [7]. To determine the clinical importance of the results, it is worthwhile to calculate the NNH If both are calculated, a low number for the NNT and a high number for the NNH would be the optimal finding [7]. For more information on magnitude and precision of treatment effects, please see Chap. 6.

The NNH is conceptually and mathematically simple for studies where there are distinct exposed and unexposed groups. In this study, it can be calculated by using the raw data for anastomotic leaks in the three groups or use the percentages. Using the latter, the anastomotic leak rates were 12.8% in the diclofenac group and 9.2% in the ibuprofen group compared to 5.1% in the control group. Thus, to calculate the NNH, the anastomotic leak rate in the control group (5.1%) can be subtracted from the diclofenac group leak rate: 12.8% minus 5.1% equals 7.1%. Then 100 divided by 7.1(%) is 14.1. So, that means that the NNH is 14.1 or in other words, for every 14 patients treated with diclofenac one patient would develop an anastomotic leak requiring reoperation and for every 50 patients treated with ibuprofen one patient would develop an anastomotic leak requiring reoperation.

Are there any benefits known to be associated with exposure?

After reviewing the evidence regarding harm, we must weigh the potential benefits against the potential adverse events with the use of post-operative NSAID use. There are certainly benefits to using NSAIDs for pain in patients having colorectal surgery. While this study did not present data on pain control and length of post-operative ileus, others have shown that NSAIDs are effective in decreasing pain post-operatively and the need for opioids [8]. However, this study does show that the risk of an anastomotic leak requiring surgery is also increased and it is well accepted that an anastomotic leak (especially those requiring re-operation) is one of the most common causes of post-operative mortality following a colorectal resection. Thus, this study provides evidence that there needs to be caution in prescribing NSAIDs post-operatively in patients who have had a colonic or rectal resection and anastomosis.

On the other hand, we also need more evidence to understand the benefits and risks of NSAIDs before our surgeon and anaesthesiologist who are making the ERAS guidelines can make strong recommendations. For instance, this study showed that the risk was much lower in patients receiving ibuprofen (NNH 50) than diclofenac (NNH 14 patients) so perhaps depending on its efficacy, ibuprofen may be recommended but diclofenac should be avoided. To be included in this evaluation, patients had to have taken NSAIDs for at least two days in the first seven days post-operatively. The authors did not do a temporal or dose related evaluation which might assist in making recommendations. Finally, we also know that the risk of anastomotic leaks is higher following rectal surgery than colonic resections so further evidence might change our recommendation in these cohorts of patients.

So what should the surgeon and anaesthesiologist recommend? As in many decisions in surgery, there is a balance between the benefit and the risk. However, given the seriousness of an anastomotic leak, a cautious approach should be taken in the recommendation of NSAIDS.

Conclusion

Surgeons are frequently relied upon to provide information about surgical procedures to patients or, as in this scenario, hospital policies. In both instances, decisions should be made based on the best evidence, taking into consideration the benefits and risks of surgery as well as the patient's wishes or demands. Virtually every surgical procedure is associated with some amount of harm. If there is strong evidence regarding both the benefits and harm of the intervention, it is important that these outcomes are discussed with patients. While the discussion should take into account the patients' desires, it is important that the information is provided in a way that can be understood by patients so they can make a decision.

Resolution of the Scenario

Although a RCT would provide stronger evidence, the methodology of this prospective cohort study is strong and there was no apparent bias between the two groups which could render the results invalid. There was a significantly positive association between one of the NSAIDs (diclofenac) and anastomotic leaks following colorectal surgery. Indeed, the OR was 7.2 (95% CI 3.8–12.4). On the other hand, there was not a significant association with ibuprofen (OR 1.5, 95% 0.8–2.9). Having this information, the surgeon and anaesthesiologist decided to recommend that diclofenac should not be used for pain control in patients having a colorectal resection and anastomosis. However, they also noted that further studies are needed to understand which NSAIDs are not associated with anastomotic leaks and can be used with greater confidence in this cohort of patients.

Appendix 1

1. Modasi A, Pace D, Godwin M, Smith C, Curtis B. NSAID administration post colorectal surgery increases anastomotic leak rate: systematic review/meta-analysis. Surg Endosc. 2018; EPub ahead of print. https://doi.org/10.1007/s00464-018-6355-1.
2. Gupta A, Bah M. NSAIDS in the treatment of postoperative pain. Curr Pain Headache Rep. 2016;20(11):62.
3. Slim K, Joris J, Beloeil H, Groupe Francophone de Réhabilitation Améliorée après Chirurgie (GRACE). Colonic anastomoses and non-steroidal anti-inflammatory drugs. J Visc Surg. 2016;153(4):269–75.
4. Paulasir S, Kaoutzanis C, Welch KB, Vandewarker JF, Krapohl G, Lampman RM, et al. Nonsteroidal anti-inflammatory drugs: do they increase the risk of anastomotic leaks following colorectal operations? Dis Colon Rectum. 2015;58(9):870-7.
5. Nepogodiev D, Chapman SJ, Glasbey JC, Kelly M, Khatri C, Fitzgerald E, et al. Multicentre observational cohort study of NSAIDs as risk factors for postoperative adverse events in gastrointestinal surgery.
6. Klein M, Gögenur I, Rosenberg J. Postoperative use of non-steroidal anti-inflammatory drugs in patients with anastomotic leakage requiring reoperation after colorectal resection: cohort study based on prospective data.
7. Kelin M. Postoperative non-steroidal anti-inflammatory drugs and colorectal anastomotic leakage. NSAIDs and anastomotic leakage. Dan Med J. 2012;59(3):B4420
8. Klein M, Krarup PM, Kongsbak MB, Agren MS, Gögenru I, Jorgensen LN, et al.

Effect of postoperative diclofenac on anastomotic healing, skin wounds and subcutaneous collagen accumulation: a randomized, blinded, placebo-controlled, experimental study. Eur Surg Res. 2012;48(2):73–8.

References

1. Doll R, Hill AB. Mortality in relation to smoking ten years' observations of British doctors. BMJ. 1964;1:1460–7.
2. Levine MAH, Ioannidis J, Haines AT, Guyatt G. Harm (observational studies). In: Guyatt G, Rennie D, Meade MO, Cook DJ, editors. Users' guide to the medical literature: a manual for evidence-based clinical practice. 2nd ed. New York: McGraw-Hill; 2008. p. 363–81.
3. Klein M, Gogenur I, Rosenberg J. Postoperative use of non-steroidal anti-inflammatory drugs in patients with anastomotic leakage requiring reoperation after colorectal resection: cohort study based on prospective data. BMJ. 2012;345:e6166.
4. Thoma A, Kaur MN, Farrokhyar F, Waltho D, Levis C, Lovrics P, Goldsmith CH. Users' guide to the surgical literature: how to assess an article about harm in surgery. Can J Surg. 2016;559(5):351–7.
5. Daams F, Luyer M, Lange JF. Colorectal anastomotic leakage: aspects of prevention, detection and treatment. World J Gastroenterol. 2013;19(15):2293–7.
6. Pascual M, Salvans S, Pera M. Laparocopic colorectal surgery: current status and implementation of the latest technological innovations. World J Gastroenterol. 2016;22(2):704–17.
7. Andrade C. The numbers needed to treat and the numbers needed to harm (NNT, NNH) statistics: what they tell us and what they do not. J Clin Psychiatry. 2015;76(3):e330–3.
8. Rutegård J, Rutegård M. Non-steroidal anti-inflammatory drugs in colorectal surgery: a risk factor for anastomotic complications? World J Gastroenterol. 2012;4(12):278–80.

25 Evaluating Surveys and Questionnaires in Surgical Research

Brian Hyosuk Chin and Christopher J. Coroneos

Introduction

Survey research is commonly used to gather information from a population of interest. When performed appropriately, surveys obtain important quantitative and qualitative data from a representative sample. In the surgical field, surveys are often used to assess the knowledge, perceptions, and attitudes of surgeons or patients [1–3]. These questionnaires can elucidate surgical practice patterns and potentially identify issues therein. Results are used to plan studies, for example: (1) a survey establishes a standard of care for the control group in a randomized controlled trial, and (2) a survey characterizes regional practice patterns to tailor an intervention in knowledge translation research. Although their use has been widely adopted, designing a survey involves rigorous planning to yield meaningful, unbiased results. The purpose of this chapter is to help surgeons understand the design and critical appraisal of surveys in the surgical literature.

Clinical Scenario

You are a Canadian general surgeon with a practice focusing on breast cancer. While attending a surgical conference in the United States, you listen to a presentation on variations in surgical breast-conserving therapy (BCT) for patients with early-stage breast cancer among American surgeons. This reminds you of a recent study demonstrating differences in breast cancer mortality for low socioeconomic populations between Canada and the United States. You begin to wonder what differences exist in the practice patterns between Canadian and American general surgeons for BCT.

Literature Search

You visit PubMed.gov to perform a literature search with the terms: "breast conservation therapy" AND "Canada" AND "United States" between 2008 and 2018. This yields 26 results in which two studies compare practice patterns

B. H. Chin · C. J. Coroneos (✉)
Department of Surgery, Division of Plastic Surgery, Faculty of Health Sciences, McMaster University, 1280 Main Street West, Hamilton, ON, Canada
e-mail: coronec@mcmaster.ca

B. H. Chin
e-mail: Hyosuk.chin@medportal.ca

A. Thoma et al. (eds.), *Evidence-Based Surgery*,
https://doi.org/10.1007/978-3-030-05120-4_25

Table 25.1 Key characteristics of the survey by Parvez et al. [5]

Characteristic	Survey
Survey development	Collaborative survey development by: • McMaster University • University of Toronto • Dalhousie University
Pilot testing	Conducted with ten respondents
Clinical sensibility testing	Not reported
Reliability and validity testing	Not reported
Sample	Canada: All general surgeons from *MedSelect* USA: Random sample of general surgeons from the *American Medical Association*
Method of administration	Physical mail survey
No. of contacts	Replacement surveys sent to all nonresponders at 4 weeks Canada: Two reminder letters USA: No reminder letters
Response rate	Canada: 730/1443 (51%) USA: 372/1447 (26%)
Breast cancer surgeons	Canada: 302/730 (41% of respondents) USA: 198/372 (53% of respondents)
Gender	Canada: Male (219/302, 72.5%); female (83/302, 27.5%) USA: Male (155/198, 79.9%); female (39/198, 20.1%)
Community practice	Canada: 242/302 (80%) USA: 178/198 (90.4%)
Surgical oncology fellowship	Canada: 40/302 (13.2%) USA: 18/198 (9.1%)
Years in practice	
≤ 10 years	Canada: 112/302 (37.1%) USA: 32/198 (16.2%)
11–20 years	Canada: 99/302 (32.8%) USA: 76/198 (38.6%)
>20 years	Canada: 91/302 (30.1%) USA: 89/198 (45.2%)

between Canada and the United States. The first study [4] examines environmental differences between Canada and the United States and how they influence rates of mastectomy. The second paper by Parvez et al. [5] is a survey comparing the perceptions and practice of Canadian and American general surgeons on breast-conserving surgery. Given its relevance, you decide to review the paper by Parvez et al. [5] and evaluate its methodology (Table 25.1).

Appraisal of a Surgical Survey

The appraisal of surgical surveys centers on evaluating the validity of the study, interpreting the results, and applying study findings clinically (Box 1) [6–8]. This framework will help readers determine whether the methodological development and execution of the survey are reliable to obtain accurate information, and whether the results are relevant to change practice.

Box 1. Framework for How to Evaluate a Surgical Survey [6–8]

I. **Are the results valid?**
Primary Guides

i. Is there a clear research question and objective?
ii. Was there an appropriate selection of the sampling frame?
iii. Was there appropriate development of the questionnaire (item generation, item reduction, formatting, and pretesting)?
iv. Was the administration of the questionnaire appropriate?

Secondary Guides

i. Was pilot testing performed?
ii. Was clinical sensitivity testing performed?
iii. Was reliability and validity testing performed?

II. **What are the results?**

i. Was there a sufficient response rate?
ii. Are appropriate statistical methods used?
iii. Is the reporting of the results transparent?
iv. Are the conclusions appropriate?

III. **Will the results change practice?**

i. Are the results generalizable to my practice?
ii. Will the conclusions from this survey change my practice/behavior?

I. Are the Results Valid?

Primary Guides

I. Are the Results Valid?

Primary Guides

i. *Is there a clear research question and objective?*

A clear research objective is essential to survey design. Each questionnaire should be guided by a primary research question that highlights the topic of interest and the target respondents [8]. Posing a clinically relevant and interesting question is more likely to attract attention and elicit responses. The survey by Parvez et al. [5] has a clear objective with appropriate context based on previous studies. Given differences between the Canadian and American healthcare systems, the investigators compare the reported BCT practice patterns by surveying Canadian and American general surgeons.

ii. *Was there appropriate selection of the sampling frame?*

The survey should have a clearly defined target population. In an ideal scenario, the survey is administered to the entire target population to obtain the most complete and accurate data. This is often impractical due to the large size of the population or study constraints; a sample of the target population is often surveyed (Fig. 25.1) [9]. The *sampling frame* can be defined as the empirically measurable members of the target population from which the sample is drawn [7–10]. The *sampling element* refers to the respondents of the sampling frame whose responses are collected and analyzed [10]. There may be individuals of the target population that cannot be surveyed and thus fall outside the sampling frame. Thus, it is important to select a

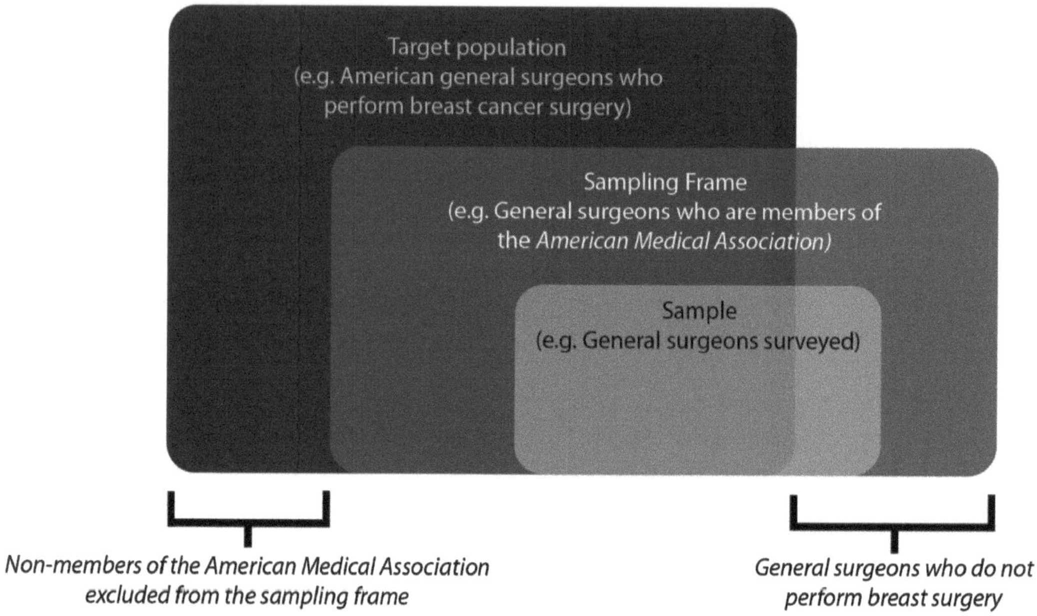

Fig. 25.1 Illustrative diagram of sampling strategy used by Parvez et al. [5] for American general surgeons. When selecting the sampling frame, consider individuals of the target population that may be potentially excluded and how it will affect the generalizability of the survey. Also consider potential inclusion of individuals that are not part of the target population within the sampling frame

specific sampling frame that best captures the target population of interest.

The reader should consider if the sampling frame appropriately represents the target population, and how the individuals within the population are identified to be respondents. If a membership registry is used, readers must consider if individuals outside of the target population (e.g., fellowship trainees, surgeons not in practice) may be included. Random sample selection is based on probability designs which include: simple random sampling, systematic random sampling, stratified random sampling, and cluster sampling [10, 11]. Deliberate nonprobability-based sampling is utilized to study populations that may be difficult to identify. Such designs include purposive sampling, quota sampling, chunk sampling, and snowball sampling [10]. Ultimately, the degree to which survey results can be generalized will depend on how similar the sample is to the target population of interest.

Parvez et al. [5] contacted all currently practicing general surgeons in Canada from a list obtained from *MedSelect* and a random sample of American general surgeons from the *American Medical Association* (Fig. 25.1). Given the research question, the target population would be general surgeons who perform breast cancer surgery. It is difficult to evaluate if *MedSelect* is an appropriate representative sampling frame for Canadian general surgeons; the resource itself is not described, nor how it compares to the membership from a professional group (e.g., the *Canadian Association of General Surgeons*), and it was not found with an Internet search. The sampling frame for American general surgeons is likely appropriate, but a justification of selecting the *American Medical Association* over surgical bodies such as the *American College of Surgeons* or *The American Society of General Surgeons* would strengthen the authors' methodology. Furthermore, given that a random sample of American general surgeons was surveyed, it would be important to report the proportion of surgeons sampled relative to the total obtained from the *American Medical Association*. This information is not provided by the authors. Another issue the investigators encountered in selecting the sampling frame is that not all general surgeons perform breast surgery. Therefore, the chosen sampling frame of all general surgeons likely overestimates the target population and underestimates the true response rate. Nevertheless, selecting a registry of general surgeons likely represents the best possible sampling frame from a pragmatic perspective.

iii. *Was there appropriate development of the questionnaire?*

The framework for survey questionnaire development includes four major phases: (1) item generation, (2) item reduction, (3) formatting, and (4) pretesting [8].

Item generation involves conceptualizing the research question and identifying all potential ideas and concepts that could be included. During the process, individual items are organized into broader themes or domains relevant to the research question to ensure all key aspects of the clinical problem are addressed. Items can be generated through a systematic review, discussion with potential responders, expert panels, and focus groups. The Delphi technique is a well-recognized process of item generation and ranking to develop a consensus that can be utilized in questionnaire development [12]. Once item generation is exhausted ("sampling to redundancy"), individual items are grouped into larger domains wherein questions are developed.

A large number of potential questions within domains is pruned for redundancy and consolidated during item reduction, without eliminating entire domains or important constructs. It is critical to limit the number of questions in a survey, as long questionnaires reduce response rates [13]. Item reduction is an iterative process achieved through ranking or rating of items with potential responders and content experts, or through external appraisal and statistical methods.

Survey questions should be formatted to be concise, easy to understand, and organized with a logical flow. The goal is to limit ambiguity in the question stem and response options. Question stems should be fewer than 20 words, with language appropriate for the lowest educational level in the cohort [12, 14]. Close-ended questions restricted to binary (e.g., yes or no) or limited responses (e.g., Likert scale: Never, Rarely, Sometimes, Frequently, Always) are ideal for analyses. In contrast, open-ended questions are challenging to aggregate and analyze [15]. Each question should focus on a single construct to avoid "double-barrel" or compound questions which involve more than one issue but only allow for one answer (e.g., How satisfied are you with your physician *and* medical care?) [7, 16]. When appropriate, indeterminate responses and "other" options should be included to allow for uncertainty [8, 14]. Terminology considered judgmental, biased or absolute (e.g., "always", "never") should be avoided as they may bias responses [17].

Lastly, pretesting should be conducted to ensure questions are interpreted appropriately and consistently by respondents. Pretesting is used to identify items that may be poorly worded, prone to misinterpretation, or difficult to answer [18, 19]. It is also an opportunity to check for unclear directions and assess the time to complete the questionnaire. Obtaining feedback from pretesters who are similar to prospective respondents allows for questions to be further refined. Specific methods of formal questionnaire testing are detailed in *Secondary Guides*.

The process of questionnaire development falls under the larger topic of measurement instruments which is beyond the scope of this chapter. Factors to consider in questionnaire design are an appropriate selection of the variable to measure, and the most suitable instrument to measure it. The COMET (Core Outcome Measures in Effectiveness Trials) initiative has made a significant effort to develop core outcome sets (COS) which should be measured for research on a specific condition [20]. In kind, the COSMIN (COnsensus-based Standards for the selection of health Measurement INstruments) initiative provides the best-validated instrument to measure a specific outcome [21]. Consider utilizing these or similar resources to guide development of surveys and strengthen its methodology.

Review of the methods reported by Parvez et al. [5] provides minimal detail on the process of questionnaire development. The authors state, "The survey was developed collaboratively by a group of researchers at McMaster University, Sunnybrook Health Sciences Centre and Dalhousie University" [5]. There is no information regarding item generation or reduction. Pretesting was completed with field experts whose feedback was used to revise the survey. Individual questionnaire items could not be assessed since the survey was not available for review, but the general format could be inferred based on study results. Questions utilized an ordinal response design for the definition of margin status and goals for gross resection margins. A five-point Likert scale for frequency was used for intraoperative techniques, skin and chest wall resection, recommendation for re-excision, and referral to radiation oncology.

iv. *Was the administration of the questionnaire appropriate?*

A variety of methods including postal, electronic, telephone and in-person interviews can be used to administer surveys. Selecting the method depends on factors such as the type of research question, design, amount and type of information needed, sample size and available resources. The method of administration must be carefully selected while considering how it will affect the representativeness of survey respondents [8]. There may be an element of selection bias in choosing telephone surveys (e.g., respondents must be home or in an office) or electronic surveys (e.g., respondents need a computer or Internet access, though this may now be historic). In-person interviews may contribute to response bias depending on the target population and research topic (e.g., interviewer bias, sensitive subject matter).

Postal and electronic delivery methods are the most common. While electronic methods are less labor-intensive, there is a recognized trade-off that response rates remain lower [22–24]. There are strategies to improve the response rate of postal and electronic survey questionnaires. Pre-notification, an interesting survey topic, monetary incentives, personalized questionnaires, and prepaid return envelopes all enhance response rates of mailed questionnaires [13]. Each mailed reminder can yield an additional 30–50% of the initial response for both postal [25] and electronic formats [26–28]. These strategies are critical when attempting to survey physicians, a population known to have a poor response rate [29, 30]. For additional in-depth discussion on this topic, see articles by Edwards et al. [13] and Sprague et al. [31].

Parvez et al. [5] distributed physical mail surveys to Canadian and American general surgeons between February and July of 2009. The survey was six pages long; the authors did not state how many questions were included in the questionnaire. Response enhancing techniques such as personalized cover letters and prepaid return envelopes were included. Although replacement surveys were sent to all nonresponders after 4 weeks, only Canadian general surgeons were sent two reminder letters. Reminders were not sent to American general surgeons due to a reported "mailing limitation" which may contribute to the American response rate of 26% compared to the 51% of Canadian surgeons.

Secondary Guides

v. *Was pilot testing performed?*

Following pretesting revisions, pilot testing is a small-scale rehearsal of the complete survey study. The purpose is to assess the dynamics of the questionnaire and test the research process (e.g., sampling, recruitment, administration, data collection, and analysis) in field conditions [7, 19, 32]. There may be unforeseen barriers or issues to troubleshoot during the pilot study that are important to resolve prior to the proper study. Respondents are also asked to evaluate the questionnaire for its overall relevance, flow and administrative ease [7]. Parvez et al. [5] report pilot testing with ten respondents and adjusted the wording of one question based on the responses.

vi. *Was clinical sensibility testing performed?*

While the focus of pretesting is primarily on the structure and understanding of individual questions, the goal of clinical sensibility testing is to evaluate the comprehensiveness, clarity, and face validity of the questionnaire [7]. The process evaluates how well the survey assesses the pertinent clinical domains identified during development. Clinical sensibility testing should be a structured assessment (e.g., use of a standardized assessment form) by independent evaluators. Parvez et al. [5] do not explicitly report clinical sensibility testing in their survey development.

vii. *Was reliability and validity testing performed?*

Reliability and validity testing essentially answer the following questions:

- Does my survey answer the question consistently? (reliability)
- Does my survey answer the correct question? (validity)

Reliability determines whether questions yield consistent answers over time and repeated administration [11, 33, 34]. A reliable test can also accurately differentiate respondents [12, 33]. The response to a given question should be alike among respondents who feel similarly, and divergent among respondents who differ [12]. For interrater reliability, two independent respondents will have similar responses where expected. Furthermore, internal consistency is determined when several questions that address the same domain produce similar answers [33]. In test–retest reliability, one individual will have consistent results when answering the same question at different times [11]. In other words, the results of a reliable questionnaire are consistent and reproducible.

Validity is defined as the extent to which an instrument (e.g., questionnaire) measures what it intends to measure. Face validity is a subjective assessment of survey validity by experts and participants, often conducted during clinical sensibility testing [7, 11]. Content validity is formal expert evaluation of whether the questionnaire items accurately evaluate all aspects of the topic (i.e., all pertinent clinical domains) [7, 11]. Construct validity is determined based on a conceptual inference and relationship between the instrument and object being measured (e.g., IQ test for intelligence) [7, 11]. Lastly, criterion validity compares the results of survey items to a "gold standard" or accepted existing measures [7, 11]. Validity assessments are important for future use of a given survey in a specific group and context. However, for most surveys, only face validity is warranted and it is completed during clinical sensibility testing.

Overall, reliability and validity testing are important to ensure that the questionnaire can attain the true answer to a research question. This is particularly vital when questions are used to infer conclusions for a different construct based on a theoretical association or relationship. For example, a survey developed to evaluate nutritional health can ask questions on diet habits (e.g., how often do you eat vegetables?). Although there is a scientific basis for the relationship between diet and nutrition, it would be important to empirically demonstrate that vegetable consumption is a valid measure of nutritional health through the methods described above. In contrast, face validity may be adequate when a survey is used for a descriptive purpose as in a cross-sectional design.

The survey by Parvez et al. [5] does not report assessment of reliability or validity. Although pretesting was completed, the absence of reliability and validity testing may affect the credibility of their results. However, this should also be considered in the context of its descriptive objective and cross-sectional design.

II. What are the Results?

i. *Was there a sufficient response rate?*

High response rates provide confidence that the survey results are representative of the target population. This reduces potential bias between responders and nonresponders, as well as improves the validity and generalizability of the study [7]. Response rates of 60–70% are considered acceptable and demonstrate face validity in the medical community [12, 35]. Given its importance, a proper sampling frame, selected sample, and techniques to enhance the response rate are critical to achieving a high response rate.

Parvez et al. [5] report response rates of 51% (730/1443) from Canadian general surgeons and 26% (372/1447) American general surgeons. This represents the *actual response rate*. However, only a proportion of responders performed breast surgery. Thus, the *analyzed response rate* was 21% (302/1443) for Canada and 14% (198/1447) for the United States. An issue previously identified is that the sampling frame is not precise to the target population (i.e., general surgeons who perform breast surgery). The result is that the chosen sampling frame likely underestimates the response rate. A reader should consider the generalizability of the results based on these factors.

ii. *Were appropriate statistical methods used?*

Surveys can collect descriptive (raw data) or explanatory (inference between constructs) data [6, 7]. Descriptive surveys present factual data and estimate a parameter of interest. In contrast, explanatory surveys generate connections between concepts to test a hypothesis. Surveys measuring one metric are considered unidimensional scales while those evaluating more than one metric are multidimensional scales [12]. Sample size calculation is as important for surveys as it is with other study designs, and is influenced by the research question, hypotheses, and overall design. For readers who plan to conduct a survey, we recommend consulting a biostatistician when developing your protocol.

Nonresponders and missing data can bias the results of the survey and affect its generalizability. Although strategies should be implemented during the survey design to maximize the response rate, nonresponse can be partially addressed through statistical methods such as multiple imputation [36]. The process and assumptions underpinning multiple imputation are beyond the scope of this chapter, but readers should consider if there was any attempt made to statistically address missing data.

Parvez et al. [5] completed a descriptive cross-sectional survey comparing BCT patterns between Canadian and American general surgeons. Appropriate statistical analyses were performed for categorical variables using chi-squared, and nonparametric ordinal variables using Mann-Whitney U test across seven domains. Baseline comparison of characteristics of the Canadian and American general surgeons was performed. Stepwise linear regression analysis was used to adjust for demographic variables that could influence group differences. Additionally, despite the overall low response rate, there was no attempt to adjust for missing data.

iii. *Is the reporting of the results transparent?*

The reported results of the survey should directly address the primary question. Sufficient detail is required to ensure that the findings are clear and transparent. The authors must also report methods used to handle and analyze missing data. The conclusion and implications of the study should be discussed and align with the data presented. Finally, whether the sample surveyed is representative of the population should be considered. Parvez et al. [5] present results in relative frequencies (%), but there is insufficient raw data for reanalysis if warranted. It is explicitly stated that results were included and analyzed for individual questions even if the survey was partially completed. The domains are adequately presented in tables and graphical format, but could also display the raw data that generated the percentile values. Access to the survey questionnaire would be valuable in an appendix to appraise individual question stems and responses.

iv. *Are the conclusions appropriate?*

The discussion should summarize the results and implications in a concise manner that aligns with the study data. Limitations of the study, particularly with respect to methodology, should be explored. Notably, the impact of the nonresponse rate to the validity of study findings should be discussed; unlike other forms of research, responders and nonresponders often cannot be compared. Finally, surveys are self-reported, and may not accurately reflect "real-world" clinical practice; results may reflect respondents' intentions or ideal practice instead of the care practically delivered. Parvez et al. [5] highlight several findings that demonstrate statistically significant variations in surgical practice, including decisions that deviate from the current standard of care. Study limitations are appropriately discussed with respect to low response rate, risk of response bias and missing data. Unfortunately, they do not discuss power calculation, nor the reliability and validity of the questionnaire. The authors indicate that the results may not be generalizable, but indicate a wide variety of practice patterns; this is an impetus for research and standardization in BCT.

III. **Will the Results Change Practice?**

i. *Are the results generalizable to my practice?*

The generalizability of the study describes how applicable the results are to the target population [6]. This is also known as the external validity. Even if a study is conducted with rigorous attention to its methodology, the results are not always generalizable. The sample being not representative of the target population is one contributing factor that is most often caused by a low response rate [7]. The survey by Parvez et al. [5] demonstrates a moderate response rate of 51% from Canadian surgeons, but a low 26% for American surgeons. This is likely explained by the fact that American surgeons were not mailed reminder letters. It should also be noted that the *analyzed* response rate was much lower as only a proportion of responders performed breast surgery: Canadian (21%, $n = 302$) versus American (14%, $n = 198$). Additionally, the 1466 American surgeons surveyed was a random sample of the *American Medical Association* (sampling frame). The proportion of American general surgeons surveyed from the sampling frame is not specified. This raises the question if the American sample is sufficiently representative and generalizable to the American surgeon population. This impacts the validity of the differences highlighted between Canadian and American surgeons.

ii. *Will the conclusions from this survey change my practice/behaviour?*

The survey by Parvez et al. [5] demonstrates statistically significant differences in surgical practice between Canadian and American surgeons. There is also statistically significant variation within the Canadian and American cohorts. The variations in the definition of a negative margin for ductal carcinoma in situ (DCIS) and recommending re-excision for <2 mm margin demonstrates a lack of consensus. Although there is no clear practice changing recommendations, findings highlight the need for a systematic standardization and guidelines for BCT.

Resolution of Clinical Scenario

You are surprised by the variations in BCT practice patterns between Canadian and American surgeons, but even more, struck by the variations within Canada. However, you recognize some methodological weaknesses with the survey that makes you cautious of its findings. The low response rate impacts the generalizability of the results. You remain unsure regarding the degree of variation between the two countries. You decide to present these findings at the next general surgery rounds and begin a new research project to identify the best-evidence underlying the practice patterns in breast-conserving therapy.

Conclusion

Survey research can uniquely gather information on the knowledge, beliefs, attitudes, and behaviors of a large cohort if they are properly conducted. The results of methodologically rigorous surveys can inform new trials, health policy, and effect change through knowledge translation interventions. Performing surveys can be challenging, and they must be carefully planned to obtain meaningful and unbiased results. We recommend consulting a biostatistician when developing the study design and methodology. This chapter demonstrates the importance of survey design, appropriate testing of questionnaires, methods of enhancing response rates, appropriate analysis of study results, and their interpretation.

References

1. Alderman AK, Hawley ST, Waljee J, Morrow M, Katz SJ. Correlates of referral practices of general surgeons to plastic surgeons for mastectomy reconstruction. Cancer [Internet]. 2007;109(9):1715–20. Available from: http://www.ncbi.nlm.nih.gov/pubmed/17387715.
2. Mathes DW, Schlenker R, Ploplys E, Vedder N. A survey of north american hand surgeons on their current attitudes toward hand transplantation. J Hand Surg Am [Internet]. 2009;34(5):808–14. Available from: http://www.ncbi.nlm.nih.gov/pubmed/19410983.
3. Coroneos CJ, Roth-Albin K, Rai AS, Rai AS, Voineskos SH, Brouwers MC, et al. Barriers, beliefs and practice patterns for breast cancer reconstruction: a provincial survey. Breast [Internet]. 2017;32:60–5. Available from: http://www.ncbi.nlm.nih.gov/pubmed/28038321.
4. Covelli AM, Baxter NN, Fitch MI, Wright FC. Increasing mastectomy rates-the effect of environmental factors on the choice for mastectomy: a comparative analysis between Canada and the United States. Ann Surg Oncol [Internet]. 2014;21(10):3173–84. Available from: http://www.ncbi.nlm.nih.gov/pubmed/25081340.
5. Parvez E, Hodgson N, Cornacchi SD, Ramsaroop A, Gordon M, Farrokhyar F, et al. Survey of American and Canadian general surgeons' perceptions of margin status and practice patterns for breast conserving surgery. Breast J [Internet]. 2014;20(5):481–88. Available from: http://www.ncbi.nlm.nih.gov/pubmed/24966093.
6. Thoma A, Cornacchi SD, Farrokhyar F, Bhandari M, Goldsmith CH. Evidence-based surgery working group. How to assess a survey in surgery. Can J Surg [Internet]. 2011;54(6):394–402. Available from: http://www.ncbi.nlm.nih.gov/pubmed/21939608.
7. Burns KEA, Duffett M, Kho ME, Meade MO, Adhikari NKJ, Sinuff T, et al. A guide for the design and conduct of self-administered surveys of clinicians. CMAJ [Internet]. 2008;179(3):245–52. Available from: http://www.ncbi.nlm.nih.gov/pubmed/18663204.
8. Burns KEA, Kho ME. How to assess a survey report: a guide for readers and peer reviewers. CMAJ [Internet]. 2015;187(6):E198–205. Available from: http://www.ncbi.nlm.nih.gov/pubmed/25691790.
9. Rubenfeld GD. Surveys: an introduction. Respir Care [Internet]. 2004;49(10):1181–85. Available from: http://www.ncbi.nlm.nih.gov/pubmed/15447800.
10. Aday LA, Cornelius LJ. Designing and conducting health surveys: a comprehensive guide. 3rd ed. San Francisco: Jossey-Bass; 2006.
11. Hulley SB, Cummings SR, Browner WS, Grady DG, Newman TB. Designing clinical research. 4th ed. Philadelphia: Lippincott Williams & Wilkins; 2013.
12. Passmore C, Dobbie AE, Parchman M, Tysinger J. Guidelines for constructing a survey. Fam Med [Internet]. 2002;34(4):281–86. Available from: http://www.ncbi.nlm.nih.gov/pubmed/12017142.
13. Edwards PJ, Roberts I, Clarke MJ, Diguiseppi C, Wentz R, Kwan I, et al. Methods to increase response to postal and electronic questionnaires. Cochrane Database Syst Rev [Internet]. 2009;(3):MR000008. Available from: http://www.ncbi.nlm.nih.gov/pubmed/19588449.
14. Stone DH. Design a questionnaire. BMJ [Internet]. 1993;307(6914):1264–66. Available from: http://www.ncbi.nlm.nih.gov/pubmed/8281062.
15. Jones TL, Baxter MAJ, Khanduja V. A quick guide to survey research. Ann R Coll Surg Engl [Internet]. 2013;95(1):5–7. Available from: http://www.ncbi.nlm.nih.gov/pubmed/23317709.
16. Babbie E. Survey research methods. 2nd ed. Belmont: Wadsworth; 1973.
17. Fox J. Designing research: basics of survey construction. Minim Invasive Surg Nurs [Internet]. 1994;8(2):77–9. Available from: http://www.ncbi.nlm.nih.gov/pubmed/7812386.
18. Collins D. Pretesting survey instruments: an overview of cognitive methods. Qual Life Res [Internet]. 2003;12(3):229–38. Available from: http://www.ncbi.nlm.nih.gov/pubmed/12769135.
19. Ruel E, Wagner WEJR, Gillespie BJ. The practice of survey research: theory and applications. Thousand Oaks: SAGE Publishing; 2015.
20. Williamson PR, Altman DG, Bagley H, Barnes KL, Blazeby JM, Brookes ST, et al. The COMET handbook: version 1.0. Trials [Internet]. 2017;18(Suppl 3):280. Available from: http://www.ncbi.nlm.nih.gov/pubmed/28681707.

21. Mokkink LB, Terwee CB, Patrick DL, Alonso J, Stratford PW, Knol DL, et al. The COSMIN checklist for assessing the methodological quality of studies on measurement properties of health status measurement instruments: an international Delphi study. Qual Life Res [Internet]. 2010;19(4):539–49. Available from: http://www.ncbi.nlm.nih.gov/pubmed/20169472.
22. Kim HL, Hollowell CM, Patel RV, Bales GT, Clayman RV, Gerber GS. Use of new technology in endourology and laparoscopy by American urologists: internet and postal survey. Urology [Internet]. 2000;56(5):760–65. Available from: http://www.ncbi.nlm.nih.gov/pubmed/11068295.
23. Raziano DB, Jayadevappa R, Valenzula D, Weiner M, Lavizzo-Mourey R. E-mail versus conventional postal mail survey of geriatric chiefs. Gerontologist [Internet]. 2001;41(6):799–804. Available from: http://www.ncbi.nlm.nih.gov/pubmed/11723348.
24. Braithwaite D, Emery J, De Lusignan S, Sutton S. Using the Internet to conduct surveys of health professionals: a valid alternative? Fam Pract [Internet]. 2003;20(5):545–51. Available from: http://www.ncbi.nlm.nih.gov/pubmed/14507796.
25. Sierles FS. How to do research with self-administered surveys. Acad Psychiatry [Internet]. 2003;27(2):104–13. Available from: http://www.ncbi.nlm.nih.gov/pubmed/12824111.
26. Fischbacher C, Chappel D, Edwards R, Summerton N. Health surveys via the Internet: quick and dirty or rapid and robust? J R Soc Med [Internet]. 2000;93(7):356–59. Available from: http://www.ncbi.nlm.nih.gov/pubmed/10928022.
27. McLean SA, Feldman JA. The impact of changes in HCFA documentation requirements on academic emergency medicine: results of a physician survey. Acad Emerg Med [Internet]. 2001;8(9):880–85. Available from: http://www.ncbi.nlm.nih.gov/pubmed/11535480.
28. Schleyer TK, Forrest JL. Methods for the design and administration of web-based surveys. J Am Med Inform Assoc [Internet]. 2000;7(4):416–25. Available from: http://www.ncbi.nlm.nih.gov/pubmed/10887169.
29. Asch DA, Jedrziewski MK, Christakis NA. Response rates to mail surveys published in medical journals. J Clin Epidemiol [Internet]. 1997;50(10):1129–36. Available from: http://www.ncbi.nlm.nih.gov/pubmed/9368521.
30. Cummings SM, Savitz LA, Konrad TR. Reported response rates to mailed physician questionnaires. Health Serv Res [Internet]. 2001;35(6):1347–55. Available from: http://www.ncbi.nlm.nih.gov/pubmed/11221823.
31. Sprague S, Quigley L, Bhandari M. Survey design in orthopaedic surgery: getting surgeons to respond. J Bone Joint Surg Am [Internet]. 2009;91(Suppl 3):27–34. Available from: http://www.ncbi.nlm.nih.gov/pubmed/19411497.
32. Bowden A, Fox-Rushby JA, Nyandieka L, Wanjau J. Methods for pre-testing and piloting survey questions: illustrations from the KENQOL survey of health-related quality of life. Health Policy Plan [Internet]. 2002;17(3):322–30. Available from: http://www.ncbi.nlm.nih.gov/pubmed/12135999.
33. Streiner DL, Norman GR. Health measurement scales: a practical guide to their development and use. 4th ed. Oxford: Oxford University Press; 2008.
34. Kirshner B, Guyatt G. A methodological framework for assessing health indices. J Chronic Dis [Internet]. 1985;38(1):27–36. Available from: http://www.ncbi.nlm.nih.gov/pubmed/3972947.
35. Elder JP, Artz LM, Beaudin P, Carleton RA, Lasater TM, Peterson G, et al. Multivariate evaluation of health attitudes and behaviors: development and validation of a method for health promotion research. Prev Med (Baltim) [Internet]. 1985;14(1):34–54. Available from: http://www.ncbi.nlm.nih.gov/pubmed/4034513.
36. Rubin DB. Multiple imputation of nonresponse in surveys. Toronto: Wiley; 1987.

Opinion Pieces in Surgery

26

M. Torchia, D. Austin and I. L. Gitajn

Clinical Scenario

You are a young orthopedic surgeon in a community practice. One night while on call, you are consulted about a 56-year-old female who presents with a complex four-part proximal humerus fracture after a low-speed bike accident. Further imaging shows the fracture to have a mild degree of posteromedial comminution but no "head-splitting" components. The fracture is closed, there is no associated neurovascular compromise, and the patient has no other injuries. The patient is in good health and is very active, playing tennis at least three times per week with her husband and participating in aerobic exercise like biking and hiking at least once per week. While you believe that reconstructing the bone by open reduction and internal fixation (ORIF) may help the patient you want to ensure there is not a nonoperative option. You turn to the literature to examine the underlying evidence behind this treatment modality in hopes of counseling your patient regarding the best treatment plan.

M. Torchia · D. Austin · I. L. Gitajn (✉)
Division of Orthopaedics, Dartmouth-Hitchcock, Lebanon, NH, USA
e-mail: Ida.Leah.Gitajn@hitchcock.org

A. Thoma et al. (eds.), *Evidence-Based Surgery*,
https://doi.org/10.1007/978-3-030-05120-4_26

Literature Search

Based on the above clinical scenario, you form a research question using the PICOT format:

Population: patients with displaced proximal humerus fractures
Intervention: open reduction and internal fixation (ORIF)
Comparative Intervention: nonoperative management
Outcome: clinical outcome scores
Time Horizon: any time after intervention.

Using the PICOT format your research question becomes: *In patients with displaced proximal humerus fractures, does open reduction and internal fixation result in better outcome scores as compared to non-operative management after surgery?* Using the following search terms: "displaced proximal humerus fracture" AND "ORIF" AND "nonoperative" AND "outcome" you perform a literature search in MEDLINE. Your search yields three articles (Appendix 1); the first article compares three different surgical techniques; the second article is a survey between surgeons and orthopedic traumatologists, however, does not include outcomes of patients; and the third is in elderly patients. You are not confident that the three articles identified are appropriate for your patient. Feeling discouraged, you decide to bring up this clinical dilemma with colleagues, one of who directs you to an expert opinion article by Sperling et al. [1], entitled; the difficult proximal humerus fracture: tips and techniques to avoid complications and improve results. The article provides opinions on techniques to fix displaced proximal humerus fractures, especially those with displaced tuberosities and comminution, which your patient has.

Expert Opinion in the Context of Evidence-Based Medicine and Surgery

Scrutiny of the evidence behind clinical decisions is becoming increasingly pervasive. While the term "evidence-based medicine" (EBM) was first attributed to Gordon H. Guyatt at McMaster University in 1991 [2], the origins of the term can be traced back much further to the eighteenth-century European enlightenment period [3]. Perhaps no example better illustrates the thought of this era than the Scottish naval surgeon James Lind's controlled trial of oranges and lemons for the prevention of scurvy, published in 1753 [4].

A popular definition of EBM was proposed by what many consider the father of the field, Sackett [5], "the conscientious, explicit, and judicious use of current best evidence in making decisions about the care of individual patients". As EBM grew in prominence and popularity [6], most of the focus and subsequent criticism was aimed at the creation, content and application of what was deemed to be "evidence" [7]. Specifically, while double-blind, randomized placebo-controlled trials were deemed to be the highest standard in clinical research [8, 9], many researchers expressed concerns regarding the external validity of these trials [10–13] and quality of the studies [14–16]. Moreover, the limit s of evidence in clinical practice was recognized by Naylor [17], who articulated "grey zones of clinical practice where the evidence about risk-benefit ratios of competing clinical options are incomplete or contradictory."

Such criticisms of evidence in particular, and EBM more broadly, may induce a false dichotomy between those who would practice EBM to exclusion of clinical reality and those who would rely on accumulated clinical experience to the exclusion of published evidence. Yet returning ad fontes, or "to the original sources", to use a term popularized by the Renaissance humanists, the early descriptions of EBM viewed the clinical experience as a necessary aspect of incorporating external evidence into clinical practice. As Sackett [5] states, "Good doctors use both individual clinical expertise and the best available external evidence, and neither alone is enough. Without clinical expertise, practice risks becoming tyrannized by evidence, for even excellent external evidence may be inapplicable to or inappropriate for an individual patient. Without current best evidence, practice risks becoming rapidly out of date, to the detriment of patients" [5]. Thus, even though "expert opinion" is relegated to the bottom of most evidence hierarchies [18–20], it remains an integral aspect to the practice of EBM, and even more so when there is a gap in evidence regarding a particular clinical situation.

What Is the Value of Expert Opinion?

Perspective in the presence of evidence gaps
One of the certainties of clinical medicine is uncertainty [21, 22]. Given that medical knowledge involves multiple "ways of knowing" [23], many in medicine decry the elevation of EBM as a "new paradigm" which replaces "intuition, unsystematic clinical experience, and physiologic rationale" [24]. Indeed, there is a large body of literature which documents the role of personal experience and judgment, rather than clinical practice guidelines or algorithms, when physicians make complex medical decisions [25–29]. The aggregate of this literature points to the accumulation of clinical expertise as an iterative process of hypothesis generation, discovery and refinement; not dissimilar to the scientific method that undergirds published evidence. Seen from this perspective, expert "opinion" is an unfortunate misnomer.

Beyond the epistemological questions of what exactly physicians know and how they know it, there is the additional consideration that there are evidence gaps in nearly all aspects of medicine [30]. Understanding that published evidence will not and cannot answer all the nuances that accompany each clinical situation; expert opinion can offer valuable perspective. This is particularly relevant in the surgical fields, where evidence often focuses on the outcomes of the surgical treatment rather than the intraoperative details on which many of the outcomes depend. Hard-won clinical expertise, refined over many years, and thousands of patient encounters, can bring perspective and practicality to clinical decisions that exist at the fringes of published evidence.

Expertise when available published research is flawed

In 2005, Dr. John Ioannidis published a provocative article titled Why Most Published Research Findings Are False [31]. In it, the author laid out a mathematical explanation for why published research is more often false than true. In the same year, he published another article showing that of 49 highly cited research articles (cited more than 1000 times) in three major medical journals, over a third were subsequently contradicted by future studies or found effects stronger than those of future studies. Moreover, less than half (44%) of the studies had been replicated [32]. In this way, the paper refuted with real-world examples the mathematical model that was originally proposed [31, 32]. While Dr. Ioannidis's results may be the most rigorous to examine the dynamic of contradicted medical research, his work echoes the concerns that many investigators have previously raised; namely, that incorrect inferences are being drawn based on a flawed understanding of statistics [33–35], that selective reporting of results biases the published literature [36], and that pervasive and underreported conflicts of interest in the medical research can further increase bias [37, 38]. Ironically, these are many of the criticisms that have been levied at expert opinion.

When faced with evidence that is flawed or with conclusions that are grossly inconsistent with observations from years of clinical practice, expert opinion can provide a check to the potential "tyranny of evidence" [5], which, can result when research is not subject to the realities of day-to-day clinical care. Seen from the original perspective of EBM as a harmony of individual clinical expertise and the best available external evidence [5], turning to expert opinion in the context of flawed studies is consistent with practicing EBM.

What Are the Limitations of Expert Opinion?

Expert opinion has been shown to be unreliable when compared to accepted gold standards of evidence [39]. One potential reason for this unreliability is the sheer volume of medical evidence available. A MEDLINE search revealed that 869,666 citations were added to the index in 2016, while another study estimated that the global scientific output doubles every 9 years [40]. While these figures are only rough point estimations, the orders of magnitude involve attesting to the difficulty of staying current in the age of scientific "information overload" [41].

Another reason why expert opinion can be unreliable is due to introduced bias from conflicts of interest. Although many physicians feel as if they can resist financial conflicts of interest [42], empirical evidence would imply otherwise [43–46]. That financial conflicts of interest can introduce bias into the research process is self-evident, and matters of opinion are particularly ripe for such manifestation. Yet conflicts of interest are not always so obvious. Clinicians may be biased due to an ardent belief in a particular medical theory or be particularly attached to their own findings [31]. Moreover, many experts who write expert opinion pieces in the literature also serve as editors and reviewers of journals; such experts could have a perverse incentive to downplay or reject research that is deemed contrary to their viewpoints, thus introducing bias into the peer-reviewed process and potentially propagating a false body of evidence.

Expert Opinion in the Context of the Surgical Literature

Surgical practice relies heavily on the motor skills (technical ability) and intraoperative decision-making (non-technical skills) of the surgeon in the operating room for the outcomes that are commonly reported in the surgical literature. Neither has been studied extensively in the peer-reviewed literature, despite the intraoperative environment being the location where often the most consequential acts and decisions are made that affect the outcomes which are reported. For many surgical procedures, there are several, perhaps even dozens, of different ways to achieve the same outcome, and the nuances of each method are rarely discussed in the formal literature. Moreover, there are thousands of different decisions that must be made during the course of even the simplest operation. Expert opinion in the surgical literature, perhaps to a greater degree than the medical literature, provides a means to discuss and disseminate the nuances of technique and decision-making that are both unique to the surgical field and rarely able to be discussed within other venues.

Seen in this way, expert opinion provides a way for surgeons who have years of clinical experience, often with the most complex cases, to prioritize and clarify the goals of surgery and the intraoperative decision-making processes. Given the extraordinary number of intraoperative decisions that need to be made and the multiple means to achieve the same goal, surgeons with less experience can often feel overwhelmed by these demands. When covering the content of surgical technique and decision-making, therefore, expert opinion can provide clinically relevant information.

Beyond the topics of surgical technique or decision-making, expert opinion can also help to guide other clinicians through the hazards of interpreting research on their own. Beyond simply keeping up with the latest research findings, physicians must also understand how to critically appraise and correctly interpret the published evidence. This task is complicated by the emergence of advanced statistical methods employed on massive data sets, new statistical techniques of combining results in meta-analyses, and the opaque reporting of methodology in manuscripts. Thus, clinicians may be simultaneously aware of new research while lacking the skills to interpret and apply the evidence. This may partially explain why the large regional variations in medical practice first documented decades ago [47–50] are still observed [51–53] despite significant changes in the evidence base in most medical fields. Expert opinion can clarify the main findings of a study and how it applies to a population of interest. Of course, this presumes that the expert has no ulterior motive or biases in interpreting the literature and also assumes that the expert has the skills necessary to correctly interpret and apply the evidence. Nonetheless, with the emergence of ever-increasing statistical and methodological complexity in published studies, expert opinion can be used to guide readers through potential pitfalls.

Does Expert Opinion Apply to Me?

Surgical outcomes are intimately related to the technical ability of the surgeon. Indeed, one study demonstrated that greater surgical skill as measured by blinded, independent surgeons judging a videotape of surgeons conducting bariatric surgery was associated with fewer postoperative complications, readmission, and visits to the emergency department [54]. Additionally, there are documented associations between increased hospital and surgeon volume and better outcomes across several surgical specialties [55–58]. Therefore, in the surgical literature, not all evidence is equally applicable to surgeons and practice environments. In a similar fashion to evaluating the external validity of a study, one must also ask whether expert opinion is relevant to one's particular surgical training and practice environment.

Should I Trust an Expert Opinion

The questions in Box 1 can help a reader determine if the opinions of author or authors can be trusted. Box 1 has a number of different items that a reader can consider when appraising the validity of an opinion piece. It is important to note that not all the questions will be relevant to all opinion pieces. The authors of this chapter and editors of this book developed the below questions using material from Sackett et al. [5], McCracken and Marsh [59] as well as their years of experience contributing to, and utilizing medical literature. The questions are broken down into four categories to measure the knowledge, experience, reputation, and background of the author(s) of an opinion piece. Answering these six questions will help give the reader more information about the author(s) and, therefore, help them determine if they feel like they can trust, and apply their opinion to a specific clinical scenario.

Box 1. Questions to Appraise an Article Based on Expert Opinion

Clinical Knowledge

1. What relevant training does the author (s) have?
2. What relevant clinical experience does the author(s) have?

Technical Knowledge

3. Has the author(s) published material on the subject matter in your clinical scenario before?
4. Has the author(s) previous publications shown successful outcomes in similar cases as that in your clinical scenario?
5. Has the author(s) reported the results with a credible time horizon (i.e.: were the results measured early, late or at the appropriate time)?

Perception as an Expert

6. What is the perception of the author(s) by others? (i.e.: are they considered an expert by their colleagues? Do people turn to them for an opinion? Have they been invited as key speakers at specialty conferences?)

Conflict of Interest

7. Is there any conflict of interest between the author(s) and any type of industry (i.e., Pharmaceuticals)?
8. Have they declared this or any other type of conflict of interest in previous publications?

Answers to the questions in Box 1, specific to our selected article are listed below. You are confident, given these answers, that the authors are experts in their field and that their opinions are trustworthy.

Clinical Knowledge

What relevant training does the author(s) have? The primary author is a fellowship-trained shoulder and elbow surgeon. Therefore, the primary author has formal subspecialty training on the topic of the article. Additionally, all authors of the article were invited by their primary professional organization (the American Academy of Orthopaedic Surgeons) to contribute to the article based on their reputation as experts in the topic.

What relevant clinical experience does the author(s) have?

The primary author is an established academic shoulder and elbow surgeon with over 240 publications on shoulder and elbow conditions. Further, all authors, including the primary author, were recognized by their professional organization for their expertise in the subject matter under consideration and thus invited to contribute to the article.

Technical Knowledge

Has the author(s) published material on the subject matter in your clinical scenario before?
Yes

Has the author(s) previous publications shown successful outcomes in similar cases as that in your clinical scenario?
Yes

Has the author(s) previous publications shown successful outcomes in similar cases as that in your clinical scenario?
Yes. The article in question extensively discusses the relevant literature and cites multiple articles with variable follow-up time periods.

Perception as an Expert

What is the perception of the author(s) by others? (i.e.: are they considered an expert by their colleagues? Do people turn to them for an opinion? Have they been invited as key speakers at specialty conferences?)
All the authors of the article were asked by their specialty society to contribute their expertise to the subject matter based on their reputation as experts in the field. The authors were therefore selected from their peers as those with exceptional experience and knowledge that would be valuable to share with the greater orthopaedic surgery community.

Conflict of Interest

Is there any conflict of interest between the author(s) and any type of industry (i.e., Pharmaceuticals)?
The article states that one or more of the authors or the departments with which they are affiliated have received something of value from a commercial or other party-related directly or indirectly to the subject of the article. Although this disclosure does not specify which author or authors received something of value, the disclosure is clearly visible on the first page of the article.

Have they declared this or any other type of conflict of interest in previous publications?
A quick review of the literature does not reveal other conflict of interest disclosures in previous publications.

Resolution of Case

After an extensive discussion with the patient regarding her options, she elects to proceed with ORIF of her proximal humerus fracture. Utilizing techniques emphasized in the opinion paper you found prior to the case, you are able to focus on providing stability to the posteromedial region of metaphyseal bone and obtaining an anatomic reduction of the greater and lesser tuberosity. The patient tolerates the surgery without any complications, and after a course of physical therapy can participate in all of her previous activities without issue. At her latest follow-up one year from surgery she is satisfied with her results and you discharge her from your care.

Appendix 1: Articles Identified in Literature Search

1. LaMartina J 2nd, Christmas KN, Simon P, Streit JJ, Allert JW, Clark J, et al. Difficulty in decision making in the treatment of displaced proximal humerus fractures: the effect of uncertainty on surgical outcomes. J Shoulder Elbow Surg. 2018;27(3):470–77.
2. Bhat SB, Secrist ES, Austin LS, Getz CL, Krieg JC, Mehta S, et al. Displaced proximal humerus fractures in older patients: shoulder surgeons versus traumatologists. Orthopedics. 2016;39(3):e509–13.
3. Li Y, Zhao L, Zhu L, Li J, Chen A. Internal fixation versus nonoperative treatment for displaced 3-part or 4-part proximal humeral

fractures in elderly patients: a meta-analysis of randomized controlled trails. PLoS One. 2013;8(9):e75464.

References

1. Sperling JW, Cuomo F, Hill JD, Hertel R, Chuinard C, Boileau P. The difficult proximal humerus fracture: tips and techniques to avoid complications and improve results. Instr Course Lect. 2007;56:45–57.
2. Guyatt GH. Evidence-based medicine. ACP J Club. 1991;114(2):A16–A16.
3. Howard MR. Review: to improve the evidence of medicine: the 18th century British origins of a critical approach. J R Soc Med. 2001;94(4):204–5.
4. Lind J. A treatise of the scurvy. In: Stewart CP, Guthrie D, editors. Edinburgh: Edinburgh University Press; 1953.
5. Sackett DL, Rosenberg WM, Gray JM, Haynes RB, Richardson WS. Evidence based medicine: what it is and what it isn't. BMJ. 1996;312(7023):71–2.
6. Godlee F. Milestones on the long road to knowledge. BMJ. 2007;334(suppl 1):s2–3.
7. Feinstein AR, Horwitz RI. Problems in the "evidence" of "evidence-based medicine". Am J Med. 1997;103(6):529–35.
8. Sackett DL, Haynes RB, Guyatt GH, Tugwell P. Clinical epidemiology: a basic science for clinical medicine. 2nd ed. Boston: Little, Brown; 1991.
9. Starfield B. Quality-of-care research: internal elegance and external relevance. JAMA. 1998;280(11):1006–8.
10. Zarin DA, Young JL, West JC. Challenges to evidence-based medicine: a comparison of patients and treatments in randomized controlled trials with patients and treatments in a practice research network. Soc Psychiatry Psychiatr Epidemiol. 2005;40(1):27–35.
11. Begg CB. Cancer clinical trials in the USA: patient eligibility, generalizability of results and technology transfer. Bull Cancer. 1987;74(2):197–203.
12. Tannock IF. Assessment of study design in clinical trials for bladder cancer. Urol Clin North Am. 1992;19(4):655–62.
13. Mulrow CD, Cornell JA, Herrera CR, Kadri A, Farnett L, Aguilar C. Hypertension in the elderly. Implications and generalizability of randomized trials. JAMA. 1994;272(24):1932–8.
14. Egglin TK, Horwitz RI. The case for better research standards in peripheral thrombolysis: poor quality of randomized trials during the past decade. Acad Radiol. 1996;3(1):1–9.
15. Detsky AS, Naylor CD, O'Rourke K, McGeer AJ, L'Abbé KA. Incorporating variations in the quality of individual randomized trials into meta-analysis. J Clin Epidemiol. 1992;45(3):255–65.
16. Moher D, Jadad AR, Nichol G, Penman M, Tugwell P, Walsh S. Assessing the quality of randomized controlled trials: an annotated bibliography of scales and checklists. Control Clin Trials. 1995;16(1):62–73.
17. Naylor CD. Grey zones of clinical practice: some limits to evidence-based medicine. Lancet. 1995;345(8953):840–2.
18. Wright JG, Swiontkowski MF, Heckman JD. Introducing levels of evidence to the journal. J Bone Joint Surg Am. 2003;85-A(1):1–3.
19. Howick J, Chalmers I, Glazious P, Greenhalgh T, Heneghan C, Liberati A, et al. The 2011 Oxford CEBM evidence levels of evidence (introductory document). Oxford Centre for evidence-based medicine [Internet]. [cited 2018 Sept 6]. Available from https://www.cebm.net/index/aspx?o=5653.
20. Chung KC, Swanson JA, Schmitz D, Sullivan D, Rohrich RJ. Introducing evidence-based medicine to plastic and reconstructive surgery. Plast Reconstr Surg. 2009;123(4):1385–9.
21. Beresford EB. Uncertainty and the shaping of medical decisions. Hastings Cent Rep. 1991;21(4):6–11.
22. Gorovitz S, MacIntyre A. Toward a theory of medical fallibility. Hastings Cent Rep. 1975;5(6):13–23.
23. Tanenbaum SJ. What physicians know. N Engl J Med. 1993;329(17):1268–71.
24. Guyatt G, Cairns J, Churchill D, Cook D, Haynes B, Hirsh J, et al. Evidence-based medicine: a new approach to teaching the practice of medicine. JAMA. 1992;268(17):2420–5.
25. Polanyi M, Prosch H. Meaning. Chicago: University of Chicago Press; 1977.
26. Tanenbaum SJ. Knowing and acting in medical practice: the epistemological politics of outcomes research. J Health Polit Policy Law. 1994;19(1):27–44.
27. Gordon DR. Clinical science and clinical expertise: changing boundaries between art and science in medicine. In: Lock M, Gordon D, editors. Biomedicine examined. Culture, illness and healing, vol. 13. Dordrecht: Springer; 1988.
28. Dreyfus H, Dreyfus SE, Athanasiou T. Mind over machine: the power of human intuition and expertise in the era of the computer. New York: The Free Press a Division of Macmillian, Inc.; 2000.
29. Wartofsky MW. Clinical judgment, expert programs, and cognitive style: a counter-essay in the logic of diagnosis. J Med Philos. 1986;11(1):81–92.
30. Buchan H. Gaps between best evidence and practice: causes for concer. Med J Aust. 2004;180(6 Suppl):S48.
31. Ioannidis JP. Why most published research findings are false. PLoS Med. 2005;2(8):e124.

32. Ioannidis JP. Contradicted and initially stronger effects in highly cited clinical research. JAMA. 2005;294(2):218–28.
33. Sterne JA, Smith GD. Sifting the evidence—what's wrong with significance tests? Phys Ther. 2001;81 (8):1464–9.
34. Wacholder S, Chanock S, Garcia-Closas M, El Ghormli L, Rothman N. Assessing the probability that a positive report is false: an approach for molecular epidemiology studies. J Natl Cancer Inst. 2004;96(6):434–42.
35. Risch NJ. Searching for genetic determinants in the new millennium. Nature. 2000;405(6788):847–56.
36. Chan AW, Hrobjartsson A, Haahr MT, Gotzsche PC, Altman DG. Empirical evidence for selective reporting of outcomes in randomized trials: comparison of protocols to published articles. JAMA. 2004;291 (20):2457–65.
37. Krimsky S, Rothenberg L, Stott P, Kyle G. Scientific journals and their authors' financial interests: a pilot study. Psychother Psychosom. 1998;67(4–5): 194–201.
38. Papanikolaou GN, Baltogianni MS, Contopoulos-Ioannidis DG, Haidich AB, Giannakakis IA, Ioannidis JP. Reporting of conflicts of interest in guidelines of preventive and therapeutic interventions. BMC Med Res Methodol. 2001;1(1):3.
39. Antman EM, Lau J, Kupelnick B, Mosteller F, Chalmers TC. A comparison of results of meta-analyses of randomized control trials and recommendations of clinical experts. Treatments for myocardial infarction. JAMA. 1992;268(2):240–8.
40. Bornmann L, Mutz R. Growth rates of modern science: a bibliometric analysis based on the number of publications and cited references. ASIS&T. 2015;66(11):2215–22.
41. Landhuis E. Scientific literature: information overload. Nature. 2016;535(7612):457–8.
42. Boyd EA, Cho MK, Bero LA. Financial conflict-of-interest policies in clinical research: issues for clinical investigators. Acad Med. 2003;78 (8):769–74.
43. Wazana A. Physicians and the pharmaceutical industry: is a gift ever just a gift? JAMA. 2000;283 (3):373–80.
44. Bekelman JE, Li Y, Gross CP. Scope and impact of financial conflicts of interest in biomedical research: a systematic review. JAMA. 2003;289(4):454–65.
45. Dana J, Loewenstein G. A social science perspective on gifts to physicians from industry. JAMA. 2003;290(2):252–5.
46. Ezzet KA. The prevalence of corporate funding in adult lower extremity research and its correlation with reported results. J Arthroplasty. 2003;18(7 Suppl 1):138–45.
47. Wennberg J, Gittelsohn A. Small area variations in health care delivery: a population-based health information system can guide planning and regulatory decision-making. Science. 1973;182 (4117):1102–8.
48. Wennberg JE, Freeman JL, Culp WJ. Are hospital services rationed in New Haven or over-utilised in Boston? Lancet. 1987;1(8543):1185–9.
49. Wennberg JE, Gittelsohn A. Health care delivery in Maine I: patterns of use of common surgical procedures. J Maine Med Assoc. 1975;66(5):123–49.
50. Wennberg JE, Gittelsohn A, Soule D. Health care delivery in Maine II: conditions explaining hospital admission. J Maine Med Assoc. 1975;66(10):255–61, 269.
51. Birkmeyer JD, Reames BN, McCulloch P, Carr AJ, Campbell WB, Wennberg JE. Understanding of regional variation in the use of surgery. Lancet. 2013;382(9898):1121–9.
52. Deyo RA, Mirza SK. Trends and variations in the use of spine surgery. Clin Orthop Relat Res. 2006;443:139–46.
53. Song Y, Skinner J, Bynum J, Sutherland J, Wennberg JE, Fisher ES. Regional variations in diagnostic practices. N Engl J Med. 2010;363(1): 45–53.
54. Birkmeyer JD, Finks JF, O'Reilly A, Oerline M, Carlin AM, Nunn AR, et al. Surgical skill and complication rates after bariatric surgery. N Engl J Med. 2013;369(15):1434–42.
55. Katz JN, Losina E, Barrett J, Phillips CB, Mahomed NN, Lew RA, et al. Association between hospital and surgeon procedure volume and outcomes of total hip replacement in the United States Medicare population. JBJS. 2001;83(11):1622–9.
56. Sosa JA, Bowman HM, Tielsch JM, Powe NR, Gordon TA, Udelsman R. The importance of surgeon experience for clinical and economic outcomes from thyroidectomy. Ann Surg. 1998;228(3):320.
57. Kalkanis SN, Eskandar EN, Carter BS, Barker FG. Microvascular decompression surgery in the United States, 1996 to 2000: mortality rates, morbidity rates, and the effects of hospital and surgeon volumes. Neurosurgery. 2003;52(6):1251–62.
58. Birkmeyer JD, Sun Y, Wong SL, Stukel TA. Hospital volume and late survival after cancer surgery. Ann Surg. 2007;245(5):777.
59. McCracken SG, Marsh JC. Practitioner expertise in evidence-based practice decision making. Res Soc Work Pract. 2008;18(4):301–10.

Simple Statistical Tests and *P* Values

27

Charles H. Goldsmith, Eric K. Duku, Achilles Thoma and Jessica Murphy

Clinical Scenario

A 75-year-old retired surgeon is seen in your office after a recent colonoscopy identified a malignant polyp in his colon. As a colorectal surgeon, you recommend a segmental colon resection. You are concerned, however, by his overall poor physical condition. He is overweight, has hypertension, and more importantly has dyspnea. His medical history notes that he was a former smoker for 30 years. You guess that he has a score III/IV on the American Society of Anesthesiologists (ASA) scale. You inform him that you will be asking for an anesthesia consult before surgery. He asks you if you would consider a prehabilitation program for him before surgery. You inform him that you are not certain if this helps but you are willing to consider it. You promise to check if there is any evidence to support this approach. You are very skeptical of published studies that proclaim the superiority of some novel intervention and show a *P* value to justify their claim.

Literature Search

As stated in previous chapters, the first step to finding the best available evidence is to formulate a research question based on the PICOT format as given below:

- Population: High-risk patients for abdominal surgery
- Intervention: Prehabilitation intervention.
- Comparative intervention: Standard care.
- Outcome: Complications.
- Time: Any time after surgery.

Using the PICOT format terms, your clinical research question is: in high-risk patients who undergo abdominal surgery, does a prehabilitation intervention, compared to standard care,

C. H. Goldsmith (✉)
Faculty of Health Sciences, Simon Fraser University, Burnaby, BC, Canada
e-mail: cgoldsmi@sfu.ca

C. H. Goldsmith
Department of Occupational Science and Occupational Therapy, Faculty of Medicine, The University of British Columbia, Vancouver, BC, Canada

C. H. Goldsmith · A. Thoma
Department of Health Research Methods, Evidence and Impact, McMaster University, Hamilton, ON, Canada
e-mail: athoma@mcmaster.ca

E. K. Duku
Department of Psychiatry and Behavioral Neurosciences, McMaster University, Hamilton, ON, Canada
e-mail: duku@mcmaster.ca

A. Thoma · J. Murphy
Department of Surgery, Division of Plastic Surgery, McMaster University, Hamilton, ON, Canada
e-mail: murphj11@mcmaster.ca

A. Thoma et al. (eds.), *Evidence-Based Surgery*,
https://doi.org/10.1007/978-3-030-05120-4_27

reduce the chance of postoperative complications any time after surgery?

To answer your research question, you conduct a literature search on June 10, 2018, using PubMed. From the PICOT format terms mentioned above, you choose the following for your search: High Risk AND Abdominal Surgery AND Prehabilitation AND Complications; you narrow your search to the last 10 years. Your search yields six articles (see Appendix 1). You screen the articles by title, and then by abstracts. Following this screening, you feel as though the article by Barberan-Garcia et al. [1] appears to be the best suited for the research question. This article focuses on a personalized prehabilitation program for high-risk patients. It is recent (2018) and it utilizes a randomized, blinded controlled study design. The other articles found in your search focus on general and digestive surgery populations, sarcopenia, are two or more years old, or are systematic reviews; because of this, you are confident in using the Barberan-Garcia et al. [1] article.

Chapter Goal

The authors of this chapter would recommend that readers consider reading Chap. 29 as some of the overlapping ideas are discussed there.

Reporting of studies in the surgical literature usually contains the use of statistical principles such as estimation and hypothesis testing. These ideas are often displayed using equations and mathematically oriented ways of doing calculations with a calculator; however, statistical software has been widely developed to do these calculations. The goal of this chapter is to describe the statistical principles in English; leaving the mathematical symbolism to a minimum. We have decided to keep our estimation and hypothesis testing to a few simple methods, which are often seen in the surgical literature. We leave the detailed statistical and mathematical descriptions to the statistics literature. Some of the references listed throughout the chapter have more detailed discussions of these statistical ideas to make them more explicit for the mathematically inclined reader.

The clinical article that the authors have selected to illustrate the statistical principles is a randomized controlled trial (RCT) with two arms (or groups): control and intervention. The primary outcome measure is complication rates in the two groups. Two secondary outcome measures are stated as the number of complications per patient and severity of these complications. The paper by Barberan-Garcia et al. [1] reports other findings using other statistical tests and *P* Values; however, these are not described in this chapter. Our discussion will focus on those used in comparing these two groups with descriptive statistics, test statistics with their names, and how they can be computed with reliable statistical software. We will then reproduce these statistical test results and compare our results with those reported in the Barberan-Garcia et al. article [1]. Along the way, we will comment on the assumptions that go with these tests. We do not produce tests of these assumptions, just whether the paper's authors [1] have provided enough detail to convince us that the tests used and conclusions drawn from them support the findings we need to resolve the clinical scenario. We include confidence intervals (CIs) and *P* values to help interpret the findings in the appraised paper [1]. [For more information, readers may consult Chap. 28 or work by Cadeddu et al. [2].] Numbers, tables, and text will be used to describe the statistical output from the cited software as well as how the software does the computations. Graphs, although they often can be helpful to our understanding of these ideas, will not be used.

Critical Evaluation of the Paper for Reporting RCTs

This chapter uses the validity checklist for scoring meta-analysis articles by Cochrane [3] as it seemed to be most relevant to this scenario (see Appendix 3). The interventions in our scenario are not surgical; they compare prehabilitation to no prehabilitation (standard care), which seem to be used with surgery, however, are mostly exercise related and not surgical.

The risk of bias tool was scored by CHG. Of the items in the list, one [randomization] was scored Yes, indicating it was done well. However, the rest were either scored No or Unsure, which usually gets interpreted as a No. So, in summary, Barberan-Garcia et al. [1] article was Considered Flawed, as it was not reported up to the standards usually seen in the RCT literature.

CI: Confidence Interval, SD: Standard Deviation

From the information in Table 27.1, there are some different statistical tests and CIs used that

Table 27.1 Summary of findings in the paper [1] that use text to display things relevant to the outcome

Study element	Information	Pg.
Study objectives		
Main outcome	Proportion of patients suffering postoperative complications (any deviation from the normal postoperative course)	50
Secondary outcomes	Mean number of complications per patient and severity of postoperative complications	52
Methods		
Sample size justification	– Complication rate of similar patients: 30% – α-risk of 0.05 – β-risk of 0.2 – two-sided test – anticipated 20% dropout rate – Minimal clinically important difference: decrease in percentage of patients with complication (intervention vs. control) of 20% or more *Total needed: 70 participants per group*	52
Excluded patients	19: due to the changes in surgical plan	50
Dropout rate	19/144 = 13.2% (less than the 20% used in the sample size justification)	52
Randomization	71 in control arm; 73 in intervention arm	50
Modified intention-to-treat analysis	63 from control; 62 from intervention group were included	50
Results		
Statistical tests	Categorical variables: Chi-square or Fisher exact tests. Numerical variables: Student's or Wilcoxon tests	52
Presentation of data	Mean and standard deviation, or count and percentage, as indicated	52
Baseline characteristics	Characteristics were balanced, including: – Complexity of the surgical approach, in the modified intention-to-treat patients – Intraoperative variables	52
By group	The intervention group had a lower rate of complication (31%) as compared to the control group (62%) ($P = 0.001$)	53
Relative risk (RR)	Estimated RR of 0.5 (CI 0.3–0.8) for complications suggested that prehabilitation has a protective role for postoperative complications	53
Mean (SD) by group	The intervention group had a lower complication mean (SD) 0.5 (1.0) as compared to the control group 1.4 (1.6) ($P = 0.001$)	55
Severity	No effects on severity of complications, as measured by the Clavien–Dindo classification (data not shown)	53

(continued)

Table 27.1 (continued)

Study element	Information	Pg.
Conclusion		
Prehabilitation	Prehabilitation-enhanced clinical outcomes following surgery	50
Complications	The incidence of complications in patients was 46%	53

These findings in Table 27.1 are taken from the Barberan-Garcia et al. [1] paper; the results have been organized by study element and page number (Pg.) where this information can be found

we will discuss. Then, we will use software to recompute the findings in the Barberan-Garcia et al. [1] article. These recomputed findings can be compared to what the Barberan-Garcia et al. [1] article stated. Last, we will look at the impact of the conclusion for our clinical scenario. Along the way, we will refer to available resources which can be found in the reference list that may provide readers with more details of the statistical issues and maybe helpful to readers who like additional information or want another viewpoint than we present.

Statistical Tests and *P* Values

In Table 27.2, we list the test statistics, the null hypothesis, and their reference distributions for computing the associated *P* values that will be encountered in the resolution of the clinical scenario. These tests can also be analyzed using confidence intervals to test the null hypotheses listed. Both chi-square and Student's t reference distribution need to know the degrees of freedom (DF) from a test statistic for a *P* value computation. The Fisher exact test provides a way to get the *P* value by direct computation from a table of counts like Table 27.3 without creating any intermediate numerical test statistic. While the statistical literature contains many thousands of different statistical tests, we will keep to those that are needed to be able to understand and interpret the test statistics and their *P* values to compare with the output from the Barberan-Garcia et al. paper [1].

In Table 27.1, it is clear that a chi-square test was done to compare the proportions (or percentages) between the trial arms as well as the relative risk comparing the two groups, although which test was used to report the findings was NOT reported in each of the result tables. This choice came from the statistical software (cited later when used) that was used to recompute the findings that are reported. Each test statistic has a corresponding confidence interval (CI), although just the 95% CI was reported in the paper. These CIs were recomputed with the statistical software, although the confidence coefficient (the 95) usually can be changed in many statistical software packages. The criterion used to judge statistical significance (the level of statistical

Table 27.3 Primary outcome counts with modified ITT analysis

Complications\Arm	*I*	*C*	Total
Yes	19	39	58
No	43	24	67
Total	62	63	125

Table 27.2 Test statistics, null hypotheses, and reference distributions

Test statistic	Null hypothesis	Reference distribution
Chi-square	Statistical independence	Chi-square
Two independent sample Student's t	0 (zero)	Student's t
Two independent sample proportions	0 (zero)	Normal (0, 1)
Relative risk	1 (one)	Normal (0, 1) on the $\log_e$ scale
Fisher exact	Statistical independence	Hypergeometric

significance) was set at $\alpha = 0.05$ in Table 27.1. The confidence coefficient is computed from the α value by determining its compliment and expressing it as a percentage, or $(1 - \alpha)$ 100%, in this case, 95%. From Table 27.1, we also saw that the authors reported two-sided tests; this also means that the confidence intervals are two tailed, showing a minimum and a maximum as two numbers, usually reported as (minimum to maximum) to avoid using a dash (–) to separate them if the data could be reported as negative numbers, such as with differences.

The chi-square test can be computed from a 2×2 contingency table illustrated in Table 27.3. The rows in the table designate complication counts (Yes) and non-complication counts (No) with the bottom margin of the table showing total counts for each column. The first two total counts in the last row come from the header in Table 4 of the Barberan-Garcia et al. [1] article. The columns in the table show *I* (intervention) counts, *C* (control) counts, as well as total counts for each row of the table.

The Yes row was derived from Table 4 of the appraised article [1], the total by adding 19 + 39 = 58. The total in the bottom right corner is obtained by adding the two sample sizes 62 + 63 = 125, the number of patients that Barberan-Garcia et al. [1] claims is the intention-to-treat (ITT) total. However, the paper's authors [1] have misused this term, it should be "Modified ITT" as it leaves out the 19 patients that were randomized, Table 27.1, but did not get surgery. We are NOT told details of these 19 patients as they were also left out of Table 27.1 in the original article [1], and no complications were recorded or presented for them; even though the intervention patients could have had complications resulting from the prehabilitation intervention, and the control patients may have had complications in any event.

Using the data in Table 27.3, the overall rate of complications is 58/125 = 0.464 or 46.4%, which the authors report as 46% but not as a proportion, Table 27.1. [While it is simple to convert proportions to percentages and vice versa, they can matter when you enter them into statistical software when one or the other is specifically required.] For the control group, the rate of complications is 39/63 = 0.619 or 61.9%; for the intervention group, the rate of complications is 19/62 = 0.306 or 30.6%. The paper authors reported these as integer percentages: 62 and 31%, Table 27.1. [Reporting to more decimal places is not reasonable for these sample sizes; however, the extra decimal places should be used to do further calculations such as with a relative risk. We use the statistical software to compute these here.]

Could All of This Be Due to the Play of Chance?

To consider the role of chance in our results, the sample size calculation, Table 27.1, used by Barberan-Garcia et al. [1] is based on percentages, not proportions, Table 27.1. A background complication rate of 30% using colorectal patients which could be considered as the control group rate was used. Also, the reduction in the rate was stated to be at least 20% and so this implied either a difference in percentages of that size to be considered as a clinically important minimum important difference (MID) [4], with similar interpretations for ratios such as the relative risk. From proportions (percentages), the variance and standard deviation can be computed, so they are not needed to be stated separately. Also, α and β are defined, so all four Greek letters: α, β, δ, and σ are specified along with the two-sided or two-tailed tests [Ts], Table 27.1, and the study design (D). While the software used to calculate the sample size needed for the trial is specified, the outcome measure [O] and test statistic [Tt] were not specified among the four tests that Barberan-Garcia et al. [1] planned to use, Table 27.1. Therefore, six of the eight criteria for a sample size calculation (Recall $n = f(\alpha, \beta, \delta, \sigma, \mathrm{D}, \mathrm{O}, \mathrm{Ts}, \mathrm{Tt})$ from Chap. 29) were specified by the paper's authors [1]. The paper's authors also inflated the computer output to accommodate 20% dropouts, to get the 70 needed per group. [Of the 140 required, the authors randomized 144.] For our discussion here, we assume that the outcome (primary) was the rate of complications and the test statistic was the chi-square test.

Computing the Test Statistic

The data in Table 27.3 were entered into Minitab 18 [5] using the "Chi-square Test for Association." The output is shown in Table 27.4. [We do not show here that the output included the data in Table 27.3 which is useful to check that the data entry step was correct.]

For this discussion, we will use the Pearson method for computing the value of the chi-square test statistic. [If there is a choice in statistical software output, surgical researchers should state which one was chosen and why.] In this case, the value of the test statistic is 12.277, it was computed with 1 DF and the *P* value was 0.000. [It is important that researchers be careful with statistical software output.] The number of decimal places printed can be modified in most software packages. Minitab 18 [5] produces three decimal places by default. This does not mean that you should blindly report this *P* Value in your paper, it should be reported as "< 0.001", Table 27.1. [If you are interested in the other method for computing the chi-square test statistic, Minitab 18 [5] has a help file to explain the differences between the two methods.]

What Does the Number Mean to a Reader?

For the data in Table 27.3, when we compute a chi-square test statistic, this is the value of the number used to judge whether the null hypothesis being tested is true. Association in the null hypothesis is statistical independence between the arms of the trial as columns in the table and the rows that have the numerators/denominators for the percentages (or proportions) of complications, such as in Table 27.3. For a test statistic with 1 DF, we expect numerical values in the region of the mean = 1, so the 12.277 seems bigger than the mean; it is in the right-hand tail of what we would expect.

We can also use the data in Table 27.3 to do a statistical test that compares two proportions (or percentages) where we compute a difference between the two proportions as the test statistic and its associated CI. Here, the null hypothesis is that the population difference between the two arms is 0 (zero) and the test statistic has a sampling distribution of the test statistic that is normal with a mean of 0 (zero) and variance (and standard deviation) of 1 (one). However, since differences can be negative or positive, the sampling distribution has two tails that we could decide to test a one-tail test to get a *P* value as 1P or as P1, depending on which tail is to be set by the alternative hypothesis. We will use both tails because we would like to detect either harm or benefit for the intervention of prehabilitation, i.e., compute P2. The sample size justification also appears to be claiming a MID of a least a 20% difference in complications rates to be credible as well as detectable in the trial justification, Table 27.1. Because Barberan-Garcia et al. [1] did not mention which test statistic or the outcome measure explicitly, one might surmise that the paper's authors meant the testing of equal proportions (percentages) of complications from the two arms of the trial.

Table 27.4 Numerical chi-square test results

Tests/values	Chi-square	DF	*P* value
Pearson	12.277	1	0.000
Likelihood ratio	12.495	1	0.000

Where Do *P* Values Come from?

For each test statistic, if we were to repeatedly sample, say, hundreds of times, the data from the study as we have here [nobody ever does this in reality; however, that is what the statistical theory postulates], a two-arm trial on the prehabilitation intervention, there would be hundreds of different numbers for that test statistic in these samples. For a large number of samples, statistical theory tells us the distribution of these chi-square test statistics that has a Chi-square distribution with 1 DF. This distribution is sometimes called a reference distribution as *P* values are computed from this reference distribution considering the numerical value that corresponds to the significance level specified for the study; here, $\alpha = 0.05$. With the chi-square test statistic, both positive and negative deviations are computed from what would be expected by the null hypothesis. The "square" part of the chi-square test statistic indeed squares computationally these numbers so both the large negative deviations and large positive deviations from the null hypothesis get relegated to the right-hand tail of the reference distribution. There are two tails to the set of test statistics, but they get forced into a single right-hand tail of this reference distribution. Even so, from the original data there are two tails involved so this becomes a two-tail test, as required by Barberan-Garcia et al. [1] and for our clinical scenario. One way to see this is to have stated this as P2 to indicate a two-tail test, P1 as a one-tail test in the right-hand part of the departure from the null hypothesis and 1P as a one-tail test in the left-hand part of the departure from the null hypothesis. So, in this case, we could just as easily reported that P2 < 0.001, rather than the notation that the paper's authors used.

The chi-square reference distribution with 1 DF has a mean of 1, variance of 2, and standard deviation as the square root of 2 or 1.414 to 3 dp (decimal place). So the computed test statistic of 12.277 seems to have many standard deviations [(12.277 − 1)/1.414 = 7.97, around 8] above the mean in the reference chi-square distribution. To make this more specific, given the size of level of significance of 0.05 and the area under the reference distribution of one, the chance or probability that the reference distribution exceeds 12.277 will be the area in the right-hand tail. Minitab 18 [5] has computed this as 0.000 in Table 27.4 and it should be reported as P2 < 0.001. Because this P2 value is less than the significance level, these complication rate data are declared to be statistically significant.

Many times, there are standard assumptions that need to be met, if the sampling distribution for the test statistic is well described by the reference distribution. These should be reported as being checked in any paper using these distributions. For example, the assumptions for the chi-square test statistic to have a chi-square reference distribution for *P* value calculation are: two independent arms, each patient in each arm should be independent of each other, and the allocation of patients to arms should be random and have complete reporting. The first three seem to be satisfied; however, not the last one, as the authors use a modified ITT, leaving out those 19 patients who were randomized but did not get surgery, Table 27.1. A sensitivity analysis could be used in this case to compare the results of those randomized to those used in the modified ITT analysis; which we report later. Multiple imputation [6] is not sensible here because the baseline variables for the 19 patients left out from the results were not available to be used for the imputations.

There is currently much controversy about using *P* values to judge the importance of research findings. Some of the debate is cited in the references: [7–13]. Some of the remedies to help include using CIs to express the study findings. Please see Chap. 28, for more information.

A second way of reporting the findings in Table 27.3 is to use a null hypothesis related to relative risk (RR) of complications in the intervention group compared to the control group. An RR compares the rate of complications in the intervention group to the rate in the control group using the ratio with intervention in the numerator and control in the denominator. The null hypothesis here is that the population RR is 1 (one). [Be careful with the data entry into the software used as the reverse for the numerator and denominator can give the inverse of RR as 1/RR instead.] To do the computation here, we are using statistical software called CIA for confidence interval analysis [14] to do the computations with confidence intervals rather than *P* values. Using the 2 × 2 entries in Table 27.3, we use "Relative Risk for parallel groups," with results are shown in Table 27.5.

To report these values like in the Barberan-Garcia et al. [1] paper, Table 27.1, the estimate and the boundaries of the 95% CI are rounded to 1 dp as 0.5; 0.3–0.8. Using the

Table 27.5 Proportions for relative risk calculations with Minitab [5]

Statistic	Estimate	95% CI	Minitab P+	Fisher exact P+
RR	0.495	0.325–0.755	0.000	0.001

Notes +Computed with proportions test in Minitab 18 [5], reported as P2 < 0.001 for the normal test of the difference in proportions as well as the Fisher exact test as P2 = 0.001. However, the latter is not usually used since all of the counts in Table 27.3 exceed 5

Table 27.6 Secondary outcome: results per patient by group using Minitab [5]

Group	*n*	Mean	SD	SE mean++
Control	63	1.40	1.60	0.20
Intervention	62	0.50	1.00	0.13
Total+	125			

Notes +Added to the table by CHG with calculator computation with these entries. ++ is added by Minitab 18 [5], not in Barberan-Garcia et al. [1]. The rest of the results may have been rounded to 1 dp by Barberan-Garcia et al. [1]; the raw data were not in the appraised article [1] to check their veracity. Having a distribution of the counts of complications for all patients by group would have permitted their recomputation

output, we could choose normal approximation of the logarithms of the RR null hypothesis test and this can be reported P2 < 0.001 for it or P2 = 0.001 for the Fisher exact test. This compares favorably with Table 27.1, except for which test was used. Our computations would agree with the Barberan-Garcia et al. [1] using the two proportions test statistic, but NOT with the normal approximation since the Fisher exact test was not needed. The event rates were not rare or highly skewed where the Fisher exact test gets used. The reference distribution for the Fisher exact test is the hypergeometric distribution. The assumptions for the relative risk tests are the same as for the chi-square test; however, the normal approximations for the test statistic depend on the proportions being between 0.2 and 0.8 as they were here. Otherwise, the values could be highly dependent on the distance away from 0.5 in the tails of the proportion distribution. Sensitivity analysis shown in Appendix 2 for the chi-square test should be similar for the comparison of the ratio of proportions called RR as well as the Fisher exact test. The one corner shown to be bigger than $\alpha = 0.05$ and so not statistically significant should be the same as the RR in Appendix 2, although we do not show these.

Now, what about the secondary outcomes computed from the complications; their mean and standard deviations with a *P* value shown in Table 27.1. These are called rates and are computed from the total count of complications divided by the sample size values per patient rather than whether or not a patient had at least one complication, the Yes row in Table 27.3. They could be then tested with a two independent sample Student's *t* test. Computations are done in Minitab 18 [5]. However, the SDs are both bigger than the means and suggests that the distribution of the number of complications is skewed right. It is also possible that the SD for the control group is larger than the intervention group so might violate the variance homogeneity assumption of the usual Student's *t* test. We may have to use the Welsh variation of the Student's *t* test which does not assume variance homogeneity. [CHG's rule without testing variance homogeneity is doubling of one SD over the other, which is not true here.] The assumptions of randomness are still a problem, but independence between and within the groups is still satisfied (Table 27.6).

The equal variance assumption for the Student's *t* test computed the mean difference as 0.900, pooled SD of 1.337 with a 95% CI: 0.427–1.373. Since the null hypothesis here would be 0 (zero), it is clear that the 95% CI does not contain the null value. The pooled Student's *t* test is 3.76 with 123 DF and a *P* value of 0.000. This could be reported as P2 < 0.001 and is lower than the significance level of $\alpha = 0.05$, so the results are statistically significant. We were not given what Barberan-Garcia et al. [1] consider to be the MID for this measure, so the clinical meaning may not be possible without other data.

The Welsh *t* test does not assume that the variances or SDs of the two groups are equal, and so Minitab 18 [5] does not report the pooled standard deviation in its output. The mean difference is still 0.900, with a 95% CI: 0.428–1.372. Since the null hypothesis here would also be 0 (zero), it is clear that the 95% CI does not contain the null value. The Welsh t test is 3.78 with 104 DF and a *P* value of 0.000. This could be reported as $P2 < 0.001$ and is lower than the significance level of $\alpha = 0.05$, so the results are statistically significant.

The impact of the variance homogeneity assumption is small. The 95% CIs are different in the third dp, and test statistics are different by 0.02, a small amount and the DF are quite different suggesting that the reference Student's *t* distribution for computing the *P* value is different; however, to 3 dp, the *P* values are both 0.000 and regardless of which one was chosen it still would be reported a $P2 < 0.001$. Hence, the variance homogeneity assumption would not make any difference to the interpretation of the tests.

Like the other tests, the two independent sample Student's *t* test would have been nice to be able to do a sensitivity analysis to counter the modified ITT that was reported in the appraised article [1]. The one thing that we could do is to assume that all data from the 19 patients left out of the analysis had some specific number of complications, which were not reported.

Last, the third way to consider the complications was to analyze the severity data on the complications. However, we were not given any data on the severity except how they were coded with no reference citation of how. Barberan-Garcia et al. [1] claimed that there was no difference in the severity, Table 27.1. However, leaving out these 19 patients, this claim does seem credible given the large differences shown in enhanced aerobic capacity with ΔET, $P < 0.001$ and the reduced length of stay in the ICU shown in Table 4 of the appraised article [1], even though $P = 0.078$. Data should have been provided to support this finding.

Confidence Intervals

Just like hypothesis tests and *P* values, confidence intervals can be one or two tailed. Our discussion here uses two-tailed confidence intervals, although Minitab 18 [5] and CIA [14] allow one-tailed confidence intervals if they make sense. Readers are advised to read Streiner's article [15] for a discussion of the reasoning for the choices between one- and two-tailed tests.

Software

Below are three commonly used, and easily accessible statistical software options that readers may consider utilizing.

R: This software is free and is supported by statisticians all over the world under the creative commons license. As this chapter is being written, it has survived for 25 years, currently contains 12,900 expansion packages and 220,000 additional functions. As an example, 251 new packages were added to the CRAN [16] network in July 2018. All of these are available for anyone to try for their personal and study usage. Package authors tend to be very responsive to sensible questions. Readers wanting more information are invited to consider the references [6, 21–23].

CIA: This software is specifically for computation of confidence intervals [14]. It comes as part of the book when purchased.

Minitab [5]: The current version of this software is 18.1. Academic and student versions available for those with appropriate academic affiliations.

Those who choose to use software such as Microsoft Excel, web, cell phone, and cloud apps for their statistical calculations should be wary of their poor computational validity as suggested by many different peer-reviewed publications [17–20]. Your collaborative biostatistician should help you find the reviews of software in these as different new devices and locations that you can cite when you use such questionable sources to support your surgical research.

Sensitivity Analysis

A credible RCT needs to report all the data for all patients randomized to conduct an ITT analysis, which is considered the Gold Standard way to report study findings. When that does not happen as in the Barberan-Garcia et al. [1] paper, variations from ITT such as a modified ITT reported in the appraised paper [1] need to be supplemented with a sensitivity analysis for any assumption that has not been met to make the statistical analysis valid. We conducted such a sensitivity analysis by comparing the modified ITT reported in the appraised paper [1] and making some assumptions about the 19 patients randomized but removed from the tables in the Barberan-Garcia et al. [1] paper. For these 19 patients, we are not given any baseline data on them in Table 27.1 of the original paper [1], so we do not know any of their baseline characteristics. This prevented us from doing multiple imputations of these data related to these 19 patients to see if it had any impact on the study conclusions. Such imputations can be conducted using R software [6, 21–23] and should be used to study the missing data impact on the conclusions as outlined in the New England Journal of Medicine [22] that summarizes a 2010 National Science Foundation report. A NEJM editorial published with the article suggests NEJM does not want to see manuscripts if this is not done; the surgical literature should take heed.

We have created a sensitivity analysis shown in Appendix 2 that measures the veracity of the group difference analysis done with the primary outcome of rates of complications as they are reported in Table 27.3. To do so, we create four different uses of whether the 19 patients would have an impact on the analysis and reporting by including these patients as have complication Yes or No between the two arms of the trial data making tables that contain all 144 patients randomized versus Table 27.3 which has 125 and excludes these 19 patients. Notice that all the created tables have a total of 144 patients, with 73 in the intervention group and 71 in the control group, exactly as randomized. The P values created by the chi-square tests as done for Table 27.3 show that three of these analyses have P values that are below the level of significance, so these sensitivity analyses also show statistically significant findings, and effect sizes denoted by Δ that are larger than the MID of 20%. However, one of the sensitivity analyses, *c*, showed P values that are larger than the significance level, and the Δ of 14% is smaller than the stated 20% so this case is NOT statistically significant, nor a clinically important finding.

In summary, three of the four sensitivity analyses support the modified ITT analysis and one of the four does not. The dashes in the *e* part of the tables were not computed, yet in the right-hand corner of the 3×3 tables, there maybe other cases apart from *c* where the sensitivity data do not support the modified ITT analysis. This suggests that the fact of the discrepancy among these sensitivity analyses created by the missing 19 patients casts serious doubt about the clinical importance as well as the statistical significance of the prehabilitation reported in the Barberan-Garcia et al. paper [1]. Although we do not show it here, we anticipate that the relative risk analysis and the proportions analyses would also NOT pass the sensitivity analyses of these assumptions using tables similar to those in Appendix 2; however, using these other test statistics.

If we had access to Table 27.1 data at baseline for the 19 deleted patients, a strategy called multiple imputation analysis could be conducted with the package called *mice* (multiple imputation using chained equations) in R as outlined by van Buuren [6]. What imputation does is produce models that are fitted to the available data using variables in the study to make multiple predictions for all the missing data. Next, for each imputed data set, do a complete planned analysis as described in a statistical analysis plan for the study, to measure the impact of missingness on the conclusions and this impact should be reported as part of the Barberan-Garcia et al. paper [1], as now some journals require [24].

Multiplicity

When there is more than one source of data that reflect on a single outcome variable such as the Barberan-Garcia et al. paper [1] with complications measured in three ways: counts, mean per patient, and severity. It means a reader trying to decide about a clinical scenario needs to consider which of the three to use in the resolution of the scenario. We already know that the paper's authors claimed that the counts was considered to be the primary outcome measure and presumably that is what was used in the sample size justification, although not stated by the appraised paper authors [1]. What other choices could be made using this multiplicity of outcome measures. Multiplicity leads to consideration of how one might use the risk of a Type I error called α, which we now know drives the *P* values to determine whether the test statistics used are statistically significant. One common way is to consider the three ways judged separately with the Bonferroni adjustment of the level used by having each of the outcomes compared to $\alpha/3 = 0.05/3 = 0.0266$. With our scenario, this will not work since the adjusted level has an assumption of statistical independence, which is not true since there are three ways all of which are derived from the same outcome, and hence are highly correlated. Because of this, we chose NOT to make any level adjustment for the interpretation of the test statistics. If all three of these ways are to be judged simultaneously, then the proper way to do so with a multivariate test statistic, called Hotelling's *T*-squared test; however, we could NOT consider doing this due to lack of data reporting by the paper's authors.

However, there is statistical literature on the multiplicity issue that is not followed well in the health sciences journals, including those from surgery. Readers are directed references [8, 25–29] for more information. Again, we would like to emphasize that, if you are a surgical researcher, your collaborative biostatistical colleague can help with the selection of a suitable method, and provide references to support what was used.

Resolution of Clinical Scenario

Recall that in the PICOT we created, the outcome was complications. However, in the paper, there are three ways of considering complications: their rate, mean per patient, and their severity. The first of these was the primary outcome of the trial, so might be the most important for the patient and discussions with the patient. Barberan-Garcia et al. [1] report using a chi-square test and a *P* value of 0.001, which was statistically significant at the 0.05 level, although the authors did not report the value of the chi-square statistic. Using the same data as the authors, we showed how to compute the chi-square statistic and found the *P* value was indeed less than 0.001! A flaw in this thinking is that the authors thought they were doing an ITT analysis; however, they were incorrect because they excluded 19 patients who were randomized from their analysis. A subsequent sensitivity analysis was not totally convincing since one of the analysis suggested that the *P* value was around 0.1 and so it would not be statistically significant. Thus, the benefit of the prehabilitation intervention would be 14% which was less than what paper's authors had considered as the minimum important difference of 20% in the sample size justification. The appraised paper's authors [1] also show the results of a relative risk analysis that was reported with a 95% confidence interval as their test statistic method. However, the numerical value of this test statistic was not reported. The paper's authors [1] report stated that the RR was 0.5, 95% CI: 0.3–0.8, $P = 0.001$. We were able to use the same data as the paper's authors and our calculation gave 0.495, 95% CI: 0.325–0.755, which when rounded to one decimal place gave the same results as the authors [1]; however, with a *P* value of less than 0.001, just like we obtained with the chi-square test. Note, both of these CIs excluded 1 (one) which is the value assumed in the null hypothesis. We were able to redo the sensitivity analysis with the 19 patients who were left out and came to the same conclusion. However, one of the four extremes computed had a confidence interval that included 1 (one) from the null hypothesis. This provides doubt about the veracity of the data shown by the authors; suggesting that there maybe no benefit to the patients.

For the mean complication per patient analysis, we were unable to do a sensitivity analysis, because we were not given any data on the 19 patients excluded, nor did we have their baseline characteristics to do a multiple imputation analysis. We were able to redo the analyses of the means found in the paper. The analysis of the means reported in the Barberan-Garcia et al. [1] paper was very similar to our computations.

For the severity of the complications, the authors report no data, Table 27.1, to support the sentence that they claimed there was no difference in the severity of complications. This is not quite credible as the large increases are seen in physical performance in the intervention group as well as the much shorter ICU length of stay. We do not find this conclusion of the authors credible.

Finally, the fact that there are three different ways of expressing the complications; they would be derived from the same patients and so would be highly correlated measures of outcome, yet there was no mention of how these three analyses would reflect on the conclusions of this study. Certainly, individual *P* values would not lead to the same conclusion for all three variables, even though that is what was reported, apart from severity. Here is where the multiplicity of testing issue should be discussed by Barberan-Garcia et al. [1] and how they proposed to handle it statistically, and if that had an important impact on their conclusion for the outcome of complications.

Our overall conclusion is that the PICOT question could not be answered by the results of the appraised study [1]. Better evidence should be found that does not have the same methodological flaws as the paper we found seems to have. Maybe a trial older than 2018 would have used ITT properly and the complications would not have been coded in three different ways to confuse the reader.

Reporting Statistical Findings in the Surgical Literature

When summarizing the information that was reported in Table 27.1, many ideas were written about statistical issues that displayed a lack of reporting clarity, and we often disagreed with what Barberan-Garcia et al. [1] had said. The most serious issue from our viewpoint is the claim that an "Intention-To-Treat" analysis was done. This was NOT correct because the authors [1] chose to ignore the 19 patients that were randomized to the prehabilitation arm or not, and reported on a total sample of 125 patients instead of the 144 randomized. We also could not identify from the author list in the appraised paper [1], a biostatistical collaborator. To rectify these concerns in the future, we suggest that surgical researchers always have a highly trained statistical collaborator as part of their research team to help write about the statistical issues more cogently. Readers interested in statistical reporting guidelines maybe interested in references [25, 30–34].

Appendix 1: Articles Identified in the Literature Search

1. Barberan-Garcia A, Ubré M, Roca J, Lacy AM, Burgos F, Risco R, Momblan D, Balust J, Blanco I, Martinez-Palli G. Personalized prehabilitation in high-risk patients undergoing elective major abdominal surgery: a randomized blinded controlled trial. Ann Surg. 2018;267(1):50–6. https://doi.org/10.1097/00000000000002293.
2. Berkel AEM, Bongers BC, vanKamp M-JS, Kotte H, Weltevreden P, deJongh FHC, Eijvogel MMM, Wymenga ANM, Bigirwamungu-Bargeman M, vander Palen J, van Det MC, van Meeteren NLU, Klasse JM.

The effects of prehabilitation versus usual care to reduce postoperative complications in high-risk patients with colorectal cancer of dysplasia scheduled for elective colorectal resection: study protocol of a randomized controlled trial. BMC Gastroenterol. 2018;18:29. https://doi.org/10.1186/s12876-018-0754-6.

3. Mayo NE, Feldman L, Scott S, Zavorsky G, Kim DJ, Charlebois P, Stein B, Carli F. Impact of preoperative change in physical function on postoperative recovery: argument supporting prehabilitation for colorectal surgery. Surgery. 2011;150(3):505–14. https://doi.org/10.1016/j.surg.2011.07.045.
4. NCT02024776. Effectiveness of prehabilitation program for high-risk patients underwent abdominal surgery. [Registration]. Online Publication Date: 2018. Available from: http://clinicaltrials.gov/show/nct02024776. 2013. [This is the registration for A1-1.]
5. NCT02934230. The prehabilitation study: exercise before surgery to improve patient function in people. [Registration]. Online Publication Date: 2018. Available from: http://clinicaltrials.gov/show/nct02934230. 2016.

Appendix 2: Sensitivity Analysis for Table 27.3 Using Chi-Square Test and Minitab 18

(a) Assume outcomes for missing patients were all NO, for both arms

Comps\Arm	*I*, %	*C*, %	Total, %	Δ	Pearson X^2, LR X^2	DF	*P* values	Report P2
Yes	19, 26	39, 55	58.40	29	12.499, 12.793	1	0.000, 0.000	< 0.001, < 0.001
No	54	32	86					
Total	73	71	144					

Comps = complications, Δ = %*C* − %*I*, LR = Likelihood Ratio, X^2 = computed chi-square statistic, DF = degrees of freedom, P2 = two-tailed *P* value; also for b, c, and d.

(b) Assume outcomes for missing patients were all NO for *I* and Yes for *C*

Comps\Arm	*I*, %	*C*, %	Total, %	Δ	Pearson X^2, LR X^2	DF	*P* values	Report P2
Yes	19, 26	47, 66	66.46	40	23.394, 24.077	1	0.000, 0.000	< 0.001, < 0.001
No	54	24	78					
Total	73	71	144					

(c) Assume outcomes for missing patients were all NO for *C* and Yes for *I*

Comps \Arm	*I*, %	*C*, %	Total, %	Δ	Pearson X^2, LR X^2	DF	*P* values	Report P2
Yes	30, 41	39, 55	69.48	14	2.760, 2.769	1	0.097, 0.096	No change
No	54	32	86					
Total	73	71	144					

(d) Assume outcomes for missing patients were all Yes, for both arms

Comps\Arm	*I*, %	*C*, %	Total, %	Δ	Pearson X^2, LR X^2	DF	*P* values	Report P2
Yes	30, 41	47, 66	77.53	25	9.115, 9.219	1	0.003, 0.002	No change
No	43	24	67					
Total	73	71	144					

(e) Sensitivity analysis summary of all four tables above: think checkerboard! Using a 3 × 3 board

	I No		*I* Yes
C No	**< 0.001, < 0.001**, a	–	0.097, 0.096, c
	–	–	–
C Yes	**< 0.001, < 0.001**, b	–	**0.003, 0.002**, d

Entries are P2 values, letters indicate the tables above, and dashes (–) indicate parts of the sensitivity that we did not compute. Notice that the bolded cells, a, b, and d are all less than $\alpha = 0.05$, so are statistically significant, while c cell that is not bolded so is not statistically significant.

Appendix 3: Risk of Bias Scoring of the Barberan-Garcia et al. [1] Paper

Risk of Bias

A	**Was the method of randomization adequate?**	Yes
B	**Was the treatment allocation concealed?**	No
Was knowledge of the allocated interventions adequately prevented during the study?		
C	*1. Was the patient blinded to the intervention?*	No
D	*2. Was the care provider blinded to the intervention?*	No
E	*3. Was the outcome assessor blinded to the intervention?*	Unsure
Were incomplete outcome data adequately addressed?		
F	*1. Was the dropout rate described and acceptable?*	No, No
G	*2. Were all randomized participants analyzed in the group to which they were allocated?*	No
H	**Are reports of the study free of suggestion of selective outcome reporting?**	Unsure
Other sources of potential bias:		
I	*1. Were the groups similar at baseline regarding the most important prognostic indicators?*	Unsure
J	*2. Were co-interventions avoided or similar?*	Unsure
K	*3. Was the compliance acceptable in all groups?*	Unsure
L	*4. Was the timing of the outcome assessment similar in all groups?*	Unsure
M	**Is there a serious and fatal flaw with this study?** (focus on the impact of selection bias, information bias, reporting errors, and confounding)	Flawed
	Are other sources of potential bias unlikely? - funding bias, conflict of interest statement - outcome measure not valid	Unsure

The Cochrane risk of bias tool is available from Higgins et al. [3].

References

1. Barberan-Garcia A, Ubré M, Roca J, Lacy AM, Burgos F, Risco R, et al. Personalised prehabilitation in high-risk patients undergoing elective major abdominal surgery: a randomized blinded controlled trial. Ann Surg. 2018;267(1):50–6.
2. Cadeddu M, Farrokhyar F, Levis C, Haines AT, Thoma A for the Evidence-Based Surgery Working Group. Users' guide to the surgical literature; understanding confidence intervals. Can J Surg. 2012;55(3):207–11.
3. Higgins JPT, Altman DG, Gøtzsche PC, Jüni P, Moher D, Oxman AD, et al. The Cochrane

Collaboration's tool for assessing risk of bias in randomised trials. BMJ. 2011;343:d5928.
4. Schunemann HJ, Guyatt GH. Commentary—goodbye M(C)ID! Hello MID, where do you come from? Health Serv Res. 2005;40:593–7.
5. Minitab Inc. Minitab [Internet]. [cited 2018 Sep 6]. Available from: http://www.minitab.com/en-us/.
6. van Buuren S. Flexible imputation of missing data, 2nd ed. Boca Raton, FL: Chapman & Hall/CRC; 2018.
7. Goodman SN. p values, hypothesis tests, and likelihood: implications for epidemiology of a neglected historical debate. Am J Epidemiol. 1993;137(5):485–96.
8. Fraser DAS, Reid N. Crisis in science? Or crisis in statistics! Mixed messages in statistics with impact on science. J Statist Res. 2016;48–50(1):1–9.
9. Wasserstein RL, Lazar NA. The ASA's statement on p-values: content, process, and purpose. Am Stat. 2016;70(2):129–33.
10. Mark DB, Lee KL, Harrell FE Jr. Understanding the role of P values and hypothesis tests in clinical research. JAMA Cardiol. 2016;1(9):1048–54.
11. Ioannidis JPA. The proposal to lower P values thresholds to .005. JAMA. 2018;319(14):1429–30.
12. Wild CJ, Pfannkuch M, Regan M. Towards more accessible conceptions of statistical inference. J Roy Statist Soc A. 2011;174(Part 2):1–23.
13. Hurlbert SH, Lombardi CM. Lopsided reasoning on lopsided tests and multiple comparisons. Aust NZ J Stat. 2012;54(1):23–42.
14. Altman DG, Machin D, Bryant TN, Gardner MJ, editors. Statistics with confidence, 2nd ed. BMJ Books; 2011.
15. Streiner DL. One-tailed and two-tailed tests. Statistics commentary series; commentary #12. J Clin Psychopharmacol. 2015;35(6):628–9.
16. CRAN (Comprehensive R Archive Network). The Comprehensive R Archive Network [Internet]. [cited 2018 Sep 6]. Available from: http://CRAN.R-project.org.
17. Wheatley M. 5 key considerations when choosing open source statistical software. Data informed. Big data and analytics in the enterprise. http://data-informed.com/author/nadaeum/ [It worked for CHG.].
18. Edwards H. A review of probability and statistics apps for mobile devices. In: Maker K, de Sousa B, Gould R, editors. Sustainability in statistics education. Proceedings of the ninth international conference on teaching statistics (ICOTS July). Flagstaff AZ: Voorburg; 2014. p. 1–4.
19. McCullough BD, Yalata AT. Spreadsheets in the cloud—not ready yet. J Stat Softw. 2013;52(7). Available from: https://www.jstatsoft.org/article/view/v052i07/v52i07.pdf.
20. Melard G. On the accuracy of statistical procedures in Microsoft Excel 2010. Comput Stat. 2014;29(5):1095–128.
21. The R Foundation. The R project for statistical computing [Internet]. Available from: https://www.r-project.org. Accessed 24 Jul 2018.
22. Pearson RK. Exploratory data analysis using R. Boca Raton FL: Chapman & Hall/CRC; 2018.
23. Thieme N. R generation. The story of a statistical programming language that became a subcultural phenomenon. Significance. 2018;15(4):14–9.
24. Little RJ, D'Agostino R, Cohen ML, Dickersin K, Emerson SS, Farrar JT, et al. The prevention and treatment of missing data in clinical trials. NEJM. 2012;367:1355–60.
25. Mayo-Wilson E, Fusco N, Li T, Hong H, Canner JK, Dickersin K for the MUDS Investigators. Multiple outcomes and analyses in clinical trials create challenges for interpretation and research synthesis. J Clin Epidemiol. 2017;86:39–50.
26. Perneger TV. What's wrong with Bonferroni adjustments? BMJ. 1998;316(7137):1236–8.
27. Cook RJ, Farewell VT. Multiplicity considerations in the design and analysis of clinical trials. J Roy Statist Soc A. 1996;159(1):93–110.
28. US Department of Health and Human Services, Food and Drug Administration, Center for Drug Evaluation and Research (CDER), Center for Biologics Evaluation and Research (CBER). Multiple endpoints in clinical trials [Internet]. [cited 2018 Sep 6]. Available from: https://www.fda.gov/downloads/drugs/guidancecomplianceregulatoryinformation/guidances/ucm536750.pdf.
29. Bland JM, Altman DG. Multiple significance tests; the Bonferroni method. Statistics notes. BMJ. 1995;310:170.
30. Livingston EH. Introducing the JAMA guide to statistics and methods. NEJM. 2014;312(1):35.
31. Aslan D, Sandberg S. Simple statistics in diagnostic tests. J Med Biochem. 2007;26:309–13.
32. Lydersen S. Statistical review: frequently given comments. Ann Rheum Dis. 2015;74:323–5.
33. Lang TA, Altman DG. Basic statistical reporting for articles published in biomedical journals: the "Statistical Analyses and Methods in the Published Literature" or "the SAMPL guidelines". In: Smart P, Maisonneuve H, Polderman A, editors. Science editors' handbook. European Association of Science Editors; 2013. p. 1–8.
34. Wan X, Wang W, Liu J, Tong T. Estimating the sample mean and standard deviations from the sample size, median, range and/or interquartile range. BMC Med Res Methodol. 2014;14:13.

28 Confidence Intervals

Jessica Bogach, Lawrence Mbuagbaw
and Margherita O. Cadeddu

Confidence Intervals (CI) have become essential in most journals for researchers to communicate their study results. Understanding CIs gives clinicians the ability to assess both the results of a study as well as the uncertainty surrounding these results [1]. It is therefore crucial for surgeons to understand what CIs are, how they can inform our assessment of study results and whether the study results are useful for our patients.

Surgeons are familiar with statistical significance and the use of *p*-values but less so with CIs. Having a deeper understanding of what CIs can tell us about study results will allow a surgeon to better assess the certainty of the study results and whether they are likely to be clinically relevant. To understand this in a clinical context, we present a scenario to demonstrate key points relating to CIs.

Clinical Scenario

You are a General Surgeon scheduling an operation for an elective laparoscopic sigmoid resection for a patient with recurrent diverticulitis and a known colo-vesicular fistula. As per your routine practice, you have asked a Urologist to place lighted ureteric catheters (UC). When booking the case, a nurse asks if the catheters are necessary, as they add about 30 min to the procedure time. Your understanding is that ureteric catheters may not prevent injury but can help identify a ureteric injury at the time of surgery. You decide to perform a literature review to satisfy yourself that what you are planning has merit.

You develop a clinical question in the PICOT format (See Chap. 3)

P Patients undergoing elective sigmoid resection for diverticulitis
I Use of ureteric catheters (UC)
C Surgery without UC
O Ureteric injury
T Within 30 days from surgery.

Research question: In patients undergoing elective sigmoid resection for diverticulitis, does

J. Bogach · M. O. Cadeddu (✉)
Department of Surgery, Faculty of Health Sciences, McMaster University, 1280 Main Street West, Hamilton, ON L8S 4K1, Canada
e-mail: mcadeddu@stjosham.on.ca

J. Bogach
e-mail: Jessica.bogach@medportal.ca; bogachj@mcmaster.ca

L. Mbuagbaw
Department of Health Research Methods, Evidence and Impact, McMaster University, Biostatistics Unit/FSORC, 50 Charlton Avenue East, St Joseph's Healthcare—Hamilton, 3rd Floor Martha Wing, Room H321, Hamilton, ON L8N 4A6, Canada
e-mail: mbuagblc@mcmaster.ca

A. Thoma et al. (eds.), *Evidence-Based Surgery*,
https://doi.org/10.1007/978-3-030-05120-4_28

the use of ureteric catheters compared to no catheters decrease the risk of ureteric injury within 30 days from surgery?

The Literature Search

Using the key words 'diverticulitis', 'ureteric catheters' and 'ureter injury' combined with the Boolean operator AND, you perform a literature search in EMBASE (see Appendix 1). Four articles [2–5] (Appendix 2) were reviewed, and after abstract review, you found that one was a review article, one was a single centre's experience and one did not look at ureteric injury as an outcome. The article you selected: Prophylactic Ureteral Catheters for Colectomy: A National Surgical Quality Improvement Program-Based Analysis by Coakley et al. [2] addressed your question and was from an administrative database which can increase generalizability [6].

As an overview, this was an administrative database study looking at prophylactic ureteric catheter placement (PUCP) and ureteric injury (UI). While it is not recommended to make clinical decisions based on the results on one study, but rather on systematic reviews, this is the only and best available evidence you find. The study by Coakley et al. [2] looked at patients undergoing elective colon resection and a large proportion of the patients were having surgery for diverticulitis. The primary outcome was the rate of ureteric injury and whether UC placement impacted this rate. Given this, you feel your PICOT question will be addressed with these results (Table 28.1).

In multivariable analysis, when controlling for all other factors (the effects of other factors held constant), the study found PUCP was associated with a lower rate of UI with an Odds Ratio (OR) of 0.45 [2]. The study also reported a 95% Confidence Interval (CI) of 0.25–0.81. You interpret this to mean that PUCP is associated with less ureteric injury but would like to understand better what this confidence interval means.

Understanding Confidence Intervals

Within any research question, we are attempting to fill a void of knowledge [7]. One approach to surgical research is to take a sample of patients within the population and analyse it with the aim of generalizing the results to a broader patient population. The Coakley et al. [2] study is trying to determine if prophylactic ureteric catheters prevent ureteric injury. Although this study has a very large sample size, and we believe it to represent the population we are interested in, the true population value (by how much is UI prevented in the presence of PUCP) is unknown. The only way to know the true population value would be to study the entire patient population; this is almost always impossible, so the next best approach is having a population sample that is representative of the true population without systematic biases (Table 28.2).

For our scenario, we want to determine the true odds of a ureteric injury with PUCP compared to the odds of injury without PUCP in *all* patients undergoing resection for diverticular disease. Because we cannot know this true odds ratio, we use our study patients as a sample to help estimate the truth. Recognizing that our estimate is based on a sample and not the entire population, we expect that the value we obtain is not identical to the true, unknown, population value, and the confidence interval is a measure of imprecision and reflects how confident we are that the true population value lies within a spectrum of estimates. CIs are essentially the expression of the variability and uncertainty of the study results. The imprecision of our estimate can come from multiple sources, including sampling error, sample size, inaccurate measurement, and the prespecified chance that we have selected (i.e. 99 vs. 95%) [9].

To understand how we get to CIs from raw study data, an understanding of the standard deviation (SD) is necessary. For a certain characteristic that is being studied in a random sample of a population, there will be variation in the

Table 28.1 Demographics of patients included in Coakley et al. study [2]

	No PUCP ($N = 46{,}639$)	PUCP ($N = 2486$)	P-value
Age (mean)	61	58	<0.001
Diverticulitis	5.8	10.9	<0.001
Ureteral injury %	0.65	0.6	NS
Ileus %	13.9	16	0.002
Wound infection %	1.7	2.3	0.03
Urinary tract infection %	2.5	3.5	0.002
30-day readmission %	9.9	12.4	<0.001

PUCP prophylactic ureteric catheter placement, *NS* not significant, $p < 0.05$ defined as statistically significant by Coakley et al. [2]

Table 28.2 Sources of selection bias (addresses internal validity of a study)[a]

Possible systematic errors and bias	Example
Systematic differences between the intervention group and the control group	Those that received PUCP were more often in academic centres
Differences in prognostic characteristics between intervention group and control group	More complicated diverticulitis in the intervention group
Different administration of the intervention	Method of ureteric catheters placement different in a certain group of patients
Target outcome definition biases the results	Definition of a complication is too broad
Placebo effect (for subjective outcomes)	Patients who knew they received PUCP were more likely to report urinary symptoms
Co-intervention if not blinded	When no UC placed, surgeon takes extra precaution dissecting around the ureter
Loss to follow up	Delayed ureteric injury may not be identified

[a]Created using information from Guyatt et al. [8]

results. For example, if wound infection rates are being measured in 10% of the hospital's surgical population, and each month a random sample of patients is measured, this estimate will vary each month around a central value. This creates a distribution of values. From each month, a mean wound infection rate can be calculated along with a standard deviation (SD) which shows how much the estimates varied from the mean infection rate [10]. The SD is the square root of the variance of the estimate. The calculation used for variance depends on the function you are using (mean, odds ratio, etc.) to measure effect. Gardner and Altman present the different variance and Confidence Interval calculations in their paper 'Confidence intervals rather than *P*-values: estimation rather than hypothesis testing' [11]. The larger the sample size, the more the estimate approximates the population and the smaller our SD will be. For hypothesis testing and estimation, the SD is a key component in CI calculation.

Why Are CI's Different from *p*-Values?

Biomedical literature has a generally accepted level of significance, with an alpha of 0.05. Although this is convention, it is somewhat arbitrary [11]. Using a *p*-value alone, we tend to dichotomize outcomes as significant or non-significant, even if *p*-values are very similar. For example, with a *p*-value of 0.049, we would reject a null hypothesis, but with a *p*-value of 0.051, we would not reject it [12]. Walsh et al. [13] showed that in major randomized control trials published in high impact journals, it is often a single event that can push the *p*-value into statistical significance. Additionally, even with a statistically significant result, there is no information about the magnitude of difference and clinical relevance [11].

Confidence intervals do suffer from the same fragility, in that if the confidence interval covers our 'null value', we reject a statistically significant difference. This interval can also be influenced by single data points. However, by using confidence intervals, we are informed about the direction and magnitude of the effect, and the interval may contain clinically relevant effects.

Getting to Estimation

Our background in the scientific method has allowed us to be very familiar with the concept of hypothesis testing and the null hypothesis [14]. In developing a study, the null hypothesis is essential for determining power and sample size. However, for interpreting and using the results of a study the estimation approach can give more clinically useful information. For more information on hypotheses and power, please see Chap. 29.

Estimation can be presented in two ways: as point estimates or interval estimates. The point estimate is our single 'best guess' estimate of a population parameter but gives no information about how confident we are in this estimate or how much it may vary. In other words, we have no idea how precise it is.

In contrast, the second estimation approach is the 'Interval Estimation' approach [9]. Once the study value is calculated, an interval of values that takes into account uncertainty from sampling and variation is calculated. This interval of values is intended to contain the population value with a certain degree of confidence and is called the Confidence Interval. In effect, point estimates in a study are calculated and then CIs are generated around that estimate to demonstrate the confidence that this interval contains the true value. CIs have traditionally been calculated for 95% confidence, but they do not have to be. Some studies use 90% CIs or 99% CIs, but most studies typically use 95% CIs for results and calculations.

We must remember that the true population value will never change. If the same study was repeated, the predicted value and CI would change depending on the results, sample size etc. If you did the experiment or study multiple times in the same population, you would expect that the CI would cover the true value 95% of the time. Figure 28.1 demonstrates this concept.

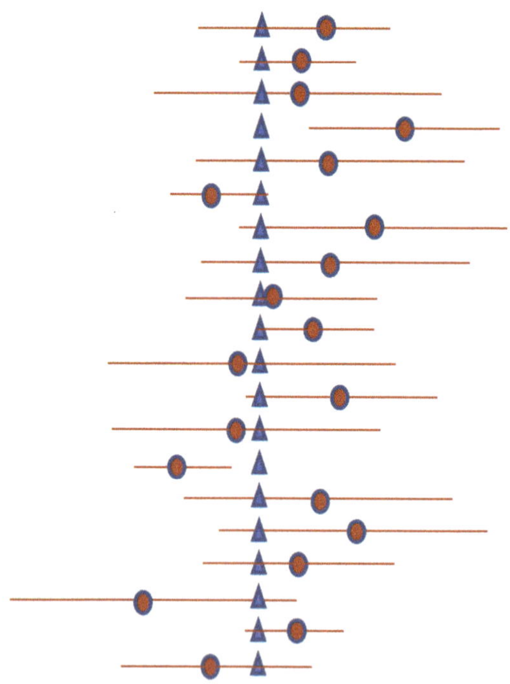

Fig. 28.1 95% confidence intervals covering a mean value. Triangles represent the true, unknown population mean value. Here, there are 20 different measurements attempting to estimate a mean. The circle represents the estimate, and the line is the 95% confidence interval. We see that in 19/20 (95%) estimates, the confidence interval covers the true population value

Hypothesis Testing

The null hypothesis does enter into our discussion of CIs since the value used for generating the null hypothesis value may or may not be included in the interval calculated for the results of the study. Similar to *p*-values, we can use the 95% CI to test a null hypothesis [1]. It is important to recognize what the null hypothesis of a study is to interpret the results. In the study used for our scenario, the null hypothesis would be that the odds of UI are the same with and without the placement of PUCs. The Odds Ratio for this would be 1. So, if our 95% CI crosses our null value of one, we cannot reject our null hypothesis and there is no difference in UI with or without PUCP. However, in our example, PUCP reduces the odds of UI by 54% and the 95% CI of 0.25–0.81 suggests that this reduction can be as large as 75% or as small as 19%. This shows that the point estimate and the CIs include only benefits. In another example, if we were not using an odds ratio, but a difference in values, we would be looking to see if the confidence interval crosses 0 (zero). For example, Gianotti et al. [15] looked at oral carbohydrate loading prior to major abdominal surgery in reducing postoperative infection. The experimental group received a preoperative carbohydrate load and had a postoperative infection rate of 16.3% while the placebo arm had an infection rate of 16.0%. Here, they calculated a risk difference of 0.003 (95% CI −0.053 to 0.059) [15]. The null hypothesis would be that the difference between the groups is 0 (zero), and because that is included in the confidence interval, we do not reject the null hypothesis. We then interpret that there is no difference in postoperative infection rates using a preoperative carbohydrate load.

We must also consider to what we are comparing our estimate. For example, if we are taking a single sample and comparing it against a known value (i.e. is the mean of our sample greater than the expected population mean?), our only source of variability is our estimation from the sample. If the population mean value is included within the CI we can say that there is no statistically significant difference between our sample and the population [16].

However, when comparing two groups, we are introducing more sources of variability. Often when reading literature, when faced with overlapping CIs, clinicians instinctively think that the two populations are not significantly different. However, when the two values are formally tested (i.e. a *t*-test), it is possible with overlapping CIs that they will show a statistically significant difference. In fact, the 95% CIs can overlap up to 29% and still have significant *p*-values at the 5% level [16]. Therefore, we must be careful in our interpretation of CIs that are overlapping when comparing two estimated values (Table 28.3). When comparing groups, it is more useful to create an estimate and CI for the relationship between the two results (i.e. mean difference, relative risk) rather than comparing the CIs for each result, as this will be less susceptible to misinterpretation [9].

Lastly, we should consider the Minimum Clinically Important Difference (MCID). MCID is a useful concept in determining whether a result has clinical relevance. MCID is the smallest effect of a treatment that patients would perceive as valuable without any side effects having been incurred [21]. This can be specified overtly or clinicians can determine this independently. Figure 28.2 shows four hypothetical study results for comparing PUCP and effect on UI. A difference of 20% in 30-day incidence of ureteric injury is assumed to be the minimum clinically important difference (MCID). The null hypothesis is that the difference in UI between PUCP and no placement is zero (vertical line drawn through zero). For each study, the dot represents the mean difference (point estimate) and the line represents the corresponding 95% CI.

From Fig. 28.2, when the results of a study are positive (statistically significant), the CIs would exclude the value indicated for null hypothesis (zero) which we see with Study 1 and Study 2. We still need to check the boundaries of the confidence interval. If the MCID of 20% falls outside of the lower (the smallest plausible treatment effect compatible with results)

Table 28.3 Examples of 95% confidence intervals and their appropriate interpretation

Study	Type of result	Null value	Result	Reported confidence interval (CI)	Interpretation
Coakley et al. [2]	Odds Ratio	1	0.45	95% CI 0.25–0.81	The use of PUCP decreases the risk of UI
Columbo et al. [17] A Meta-analysis of the Impact of aspirin, clopidogrel, and dual antiplatelet therapy on bleeding complications in noncardiac surgery [18]	Relative risk	1	0.96	95% CI 0.76–1.22	There is no difference in bleeding rates requiring re-intervention with the use of aspirin
Gianotti et al. [15] Preoperative carbohydrate load versus placebo in major elective abdominal surgery (PROCY)	Relative difference	0	0.003	95% CI −0.053 to 0.059	The use of oral carbohydrate load does not decrease the risk of wound infection
Koullouros et al. [19] The role of oral antibiotic prophylaxis in prevention of surgical site infection in colorectal surgery (Two studies from the meta-analysis)	Odds Ratio	1	1.27	Espin-Basany et al. [18]: CI = 0.48–3.38	In the first study, there is no difference in surgical infection rate with the use of oral antibiotic prophylaxis. In the second study, there is a reduction in surgical infection rate. However, we cannot infer any difference between the two studies because of the overlapping confidence intervals without a formal statistical test
			0.30	Sadahiro et al. [20]: CI = 0.11–0.79	

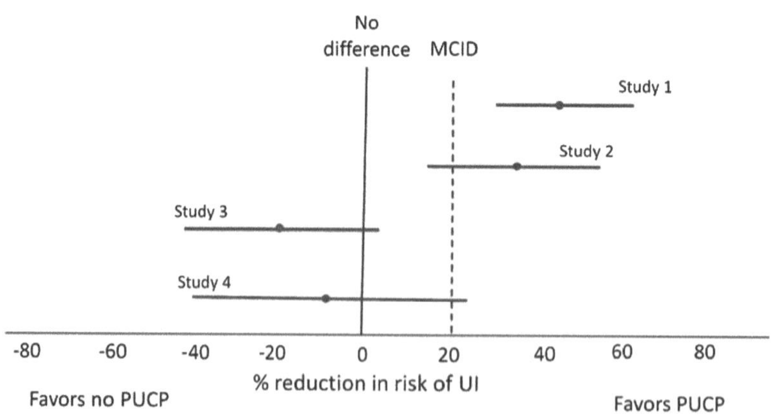

Fig. 28.2 Results of 4 hypothetical studies comparing PUCP versus control and outcome on UI, where a 20% reduction in UI is the minimal clinical important difference (MCID). The vertical straight line above the *x*-axis at zero represents the null hypothesis of no difference, MCID is represented by the dashed line. For each study, the dot represents the mean difference (point estimate) and the line represent the boundaries of the 95% confidence intervals around the point estimate

boundary of confidence interval, we could confidently conclude in this study PUCP reduces UI, and we would institute use of PUCP (Study 1). If a study's mean difference is greater than the MCID of 20%, but the MCID falls inside of the lower boundary of CI (Study 2), there is still uncertainty as to whether PUCP has a clinically relevant benefit that would change practice. Studies 3 and 4 show results of a point estimate favouring no PUCP use, but both CIs contain 0 in the interval so that the null hypothesis cannot be rejected. The difference between study 3 and 4 is that the MCID is outside of the CI in study 3, so the study was adequately powered and thus a truly negative study. In study 4, the CI includes the MCID, indicating that the study was underpowered and so the results are inconclusive, and more research would be required to answer the question of PUCP and UI.

How Do We Calculate Confidence Intervals?

The way to calculate the CI depends on what type of estimate you are creating the interval for: is it a point estimate or a ratio? If the interval is for a mean, compared to an odds ratio, the calculation is done differently. However, each calculation takes into account two important factors: the variance and the degree of confidence (i.e. 95%) [11] (See Table 28.4).

- Variance: This helps determine the precision of the sample estimate compared to the population parameter. The calculations vary depending on what type of estimate we are using (i.e. 'a mean or an odds ratio') [11].
- Degree of confidence—we choose a pre-specified degree of confidence
  - 90% smaller interval
  - 99% larger interval

  The higher our confidence, the larger our interval.

The larger interval will be more likely to contain the true population value but will also be more likely to cross into 'no difference in effect' territory.

Why Use Confidence Intervals?

Cumming and Finch [22] propose 4 reasons why CIs should be reported:

1. By giving point and interval information, it facilitates understanding and interpretation and allows us to look at the original data units
2. CIs allow us to perform null hypothesis testing, but by looking at the interval of values we can look at other hypotheses as well, not just the null hypothesis
3. CIs are very useful in meta-analysis and evidence synthesis where we are comparing and combining different data
4. They provide information about precision

Back to Our Scenario

Based on your understanding of confidence intervals, you review the article by Coakley et al. [2]. This was a retrospective administrative database study looking at the rate of ureteric

Table 28.4 Factors that impact the width of your confidence interval

Narrows confidence interval	Widens confidence interval
Large sample size	Small sample size
Smaller standard error	Larger standard error
Low degree of confidence (i.e. 90%)	High degree of confidence (i.e. 99%)
Homogeneous data	Large amount of variability

Table 28.5 Questions about article validity and applicability [23]

Question	Answer
Is this study valid?	
Were the groups similar?	—Study was retrospective and not randomized; however, baseline demographics were similar
Was the method for detecting the outcome the same in both groups?	—Administrative data limits knowledge on how outcomes were detected
What are the results?	
How strong is the association between exposure and outcome?	—The OR suggests that placement of ureteric catheter decreases the odds of ureteric injury by 55% (100–45%)
How precise is the estimate?	—The confidence interval (95% CI = 0.25–0.81), does not include our null value [1] therefore, we interpret this as a statistically significant result that includes our MCID (20% reduction)
Can I apply them to my practice?	
Were the patients in the study similar to the patients in my practice?	—Diverticulitis was the third most common indication for surgery in the study group, so the results are generalizable to your patient
Were all important outcomes considered?	—The study included relevant surgical complications (UI, infections, bleeding, reoperation, cardiorespiratory events)
Are the likely benefits worth the potential harms?	—There was a higher rate of UTIs (3.5% vs. 2.5%), ileus (16% vs. 13.9%), and readmission for UTIs (3.3% vs. 1.6%) in the group that underwent PUCP. These risks must be weighed against the decreased risk of ureteric injury

injury with and without prophylactic ureteric catheter placement (PUCP). It reports an odds ratio for ureteric injury with PUCP of 0.45, (95% CI 0.25–0.81) [2]. You ask yourself whether you can apply this article to your patient (Table 28.5).

Since the results apply to your patient and show a statistically significant and clinically relevant decrease in rate of UI, you decide to take the time to have ureteric catheters placed, understanding that you will need to be aware of certain postoperative harms such as UTIs and ileus.

Appendix 1

Database: Embase <1980 to 2018 Week 32>
Search Strategy:

1. diverticulitis.mp. or diverticulitis/(8893)
2. ureteric catheter.mp. or ureter catheter/(1308)
3. ureter injury/or ureteric injury.mp. (3087)
4. 1 and 2 and 3 [4]

Appendix 2

1. Coakley KM, Kasten KR, Sims SM, Prasad T, Heniford BT, Davis BR. Prophylactic ureteral catheters for colectomy: a national surgical quality improvement program-based analysis. Dis Colon Rectum. 2018;61(1):84–8.
2. Yang D, Miller A, Avant R, Tollefson M, Viers B, editors. Indocyanine green for ureteral identification during non-urologic robotic surgery: mayoclinic pilot experience. In: 2018 Annual Meeting, American Urological Association, AUA 2018; 2018 Apr 2018, United States.
3. Tsujinaka S, Wexner SD, DaSilva G, Sands DR, Weiss EG, Nogueras JJ et al. Prophylactic ureteric catheters in laparoscopic colorectal surgery. Tech Coloproctol. 2008; 12(1):45–50.
4. da Silva G, Boutros M, Wexner SD. Role of prophylactic ureteric stents in colorectal surgery. Asian J Endosc Surg. 2012;5(3):105–10.

References

1. Akobeng AK. Confidence intervals and p-values in clinical decision making. Acta Paediatr. 2008;97(8): 1004–7.
2. Coakley KM, Kasten KR, Sims SM, Prasad T, Heniford BT, Davis BR. Prophylactic ureteral catheters for colectomy: a national surgical quality improvement program-based analysis. Dis Colon Rectum. 2018;61(1):84–8.
3. Yang D, Miller A, Avant R, Tollefson M, Viers B, editors. Indocyanine green for ureteral identification during non-urologic robotic surgery: mayoclinic pilot experience. In: 2018 Annual Meeting, American Urological Association, AUA 2018; 2018 Apr 2018, United States.
4. Tsujinaka S, Wexner SD, DaSilva G, Sands DR, Weiss EG, Nogueras JJ, et al. Prophylactic ureteric catheters in laparoscopic colorectal surgery. Tech Coloproctol. 2008;12(1):45–50.
5. da Silva G, Boutros M, Wexner SD. Role of prophylactic ureteric stents in colorectal surgery. Asian J Endosc Surg. 2012;5(3):105–10.
6. Anoushiravani AA, Patton J, Sayeed Z, El-Othmani MM, Saleh KJ. Big data, big research: implementing population health-based research models and integrating care to reduce cost and improve outcomes. Orthop Clin North Am. 2016;47(4):717–24.
7. Hazra A. Using the confidence interval confidently. J Thorac Dis. 2017;9(10):4125–30.
8. Guyatt G, Rennie D, Meade MO, Cook DJ. In: Evidence J, editor. Users' guides to the medical literature: a manual for evidence based clinical practice. 2nd ed. McGraw Hill; 2008.
9. Altman DG. Why we need confidence intervals. World J Surg. 2005;29(5):554–6.
10. Sedgwick P. Standard deviation or the standard error of the mean. BMJ. 2015;350:h831.
11. Gardner MJ, Altman DG. Confidence intervals rather than P values: estimation rather than hypothesis testing. Br Med J (Clin Res Ed). 1986;292(6522):746–50.
12. Piccirillo JF. Improving the quality of the reporting of research results. JAMA Otolaryngol Head Neck Surg. 2016;142(10):937–9.
13. Walsh M, Srinathan SK, McAuley DF, Mrkobrada M, Levine O, Ribic C, et al. The statistical significance of randomized controlled trial results is frequently fragile: a case for a fragility index. J Clin Epidemiol. 2014;67(6):622–8.
14. Cadeddu M, Farrokhyar F, Thoma A, Haines T, Garnett A, Goldsmith CH et al. Users' guide to the surgical literature: how to assess power and sample size. Laparoscopic vs open appendectomy. Can J Surg. 2008;51(6):476–82.
15. Gianotti L, Biffi R, Sandini M, Marrelli D, Vignali A, Caccialanza R, et al. Preoperative oral carbohydrate load versus placebo in major elective abdominal surgery (PROCY): a randomized, placebo-controlled, multicenter, Phase III Trial. Ann Surg. 2018;267(4): 623–30.
16. Austin PC, Hux JE. A brief note on overlapping confidence intervals. J Vasc Surg. 2002;36(1): 194–5.
17. Columbo JA, Lambour AJ, Sundling RA, Chauhan NB, Bessen SY, Linshaw DL, et al. A meta-analysis of the impact of aspirin, clopidogrel, and dual antiplatelet therapy on bleeding complications in noncardiac surgery. Ann Surg. 2018;267(1): 1–10.
18. Espin-Basany E, Sanchez-Garcia JL, Lopez-Cano M, Lozoya-Trujillo R, Medarde-Ferrer M, Armadans-Gil L et al. Prospective, randomised study on antibiotic prophylaxis in colorectal surgery. Is it really necessary to use oral antibiotics? Int J Colorectal Dis. 2005;20(6):542–6.
19. Koullouros M, Khan N, Aly EH. The role of oral antibiotics prophylaxis in prevention of surgical site infection in colorectal surgery. Int J Colorectal Dis. 2017;32(1):1–18.
20. Sadahiro S, Suzuki T, Tanaka A, Okada K, Kamata H, Ozaki T, et al. Comparison between oral antibiotics and probiotics as bowel preparation for elective colon cancer surgery to prevent infection: prospective randomized trial. Surgery. 2014;155(3): 493–503.
21. McGlothlin AE, Lewis RJ. Minimal clinically important difference: defining what really matters to patients. JAMA. 2014;312(13):1342–3.
22. Cumming G, Finch S. A primer on the understanding, use, and calculation of confidence intervals that are based on central and noncentral distributions. Educ Psychol Measur. 2001;61(4):532–74.
23. Thoma A, Kaur MN, Farrokhyar F, Waltho D, Levis C, Lovrics P, Goldsmith CH. Users' guide to the surgical literature: how to assess an article about harm in surgery. Can J Surg. 2016;59(5):351–7.

Power and Sample Size

29

Jessica Murphy, Eric K. Duku, Achilles Thoma and Charles H. Goldsmith

A frequent criticism of published surgical studies pertains to whether or not there is adequate sample size. In other words, readers are hesitant that the chosen sample size would enable the trial to detect a clinically meaningful difference between surgical interventions, if one exists. This criticism applies to all study designs, however, is particularly relevant to the randomized controlled trial (RCT), which, is touted to produce the highest level of evidence. While RCTs are the preferred study design, they can be incredibly difficult to implement in surgery. Many reasons have been given for the small number of RCTs performed in surgery, with recruitment difficulties being one of the most common obstacles [1, 2]. Regardless of these difficulties, when a RCT proclaims that a new surgical innovation is superior, or equal to, the standard approach (standard care), we need to be certain that this proclamation is valid.

This chapter will explain the methodological issues that pertain to sample size calculation and provide the reader with the necessary skills to appraise an RCT based on its sample size. Readers will find definitions to the bolded terms, and more information regarding the factors that influence power and sample size in Appendix 1.

Clinical Scenario

At the last minimal access surgery rounds, a junior surgical faculty member recommended that the service start using a preoperative ultrasound-guided transversus abdominis plane (TAP) block to control pain after laparoscopic surgery for colorectal cancer. She claimed that at the center where she did her fellowship, TAP blocks were used all the time.

A cynical senior surgeon commented that such an approach is useless; it will only lengthen the procedure, enrich the anesthetist, and do

J. Murphy · A. Thoma (✉)
Department of Surgery, Division of Plastic Surgery, McMaster University, Hamilton, ON, Canada
e-mail: athoma@mcmaster.ca

J. Murphy
e-mail: murphj11@mcmaster.ca

E. K. Duku
Department of Psychiatry and Behavioral Neurosciences, McMaster University, Hamilton, ON, Canada
e-mail: duku@mcmaster.ca

E. K. Duku · A. Thoma · C. H. Goldsmith
Department of Health Research Methods, Evidence and Impact, McMaster University, Hamilton, ON, Canada
e-mail: cgoldsmi@sfu.ca

C. H. Goldsmith
Faculty of Health Sciences, Simon Fraser University, Burnaby, BC, Canada

C. H. Goldsmith
Department of Occupational Science and Occupational Therapy, Faculty of Medicine, The University of British Columbia, Vancouver, BC, Canada

A. Thoma et al. (eds.), *Evidence-Based Surgery*,
https://doi.org/10.1007/978-3-030-05120-4_29

nothing to improve a patient's pain! Furthermore, he lamented that most of the conclusions presented in the surgical literature are suspect as they are based on studies with inadequate sample size.

The program director challenged the fellow to return to the rounds the following week and present evidence supporting her recommendation from a study with a large enough sample size.

A disclaimer to our readers:

The aim of this chapter was to attempt to describe the factors impacting, and the calculations associated with power and sample size. The authors suggest the use of software and the help of a trusted biostatistician when calculating sample size.

The Importance of Power and Sample Size

Sample size is incredibly important in clinical research; because of this, surgeons and surgeon-researchers should be familiar with its influencing factors. Box 1 summarizes the factors that inform sample size; whether one is calculating the required sample size by hand, or using statistical software, the factors in Box 1 will be needed.

For the community surgeons, having an understanding of sample size, is important before applying reported conclusions of studies to their practice. For the research-minded surgeons, this knowledge provides the foundation for a well-executed and credible clinical trial.

Box 1. Factors Informing Sample Size

Factor	Further information
Outcome of interest	Page 312
Minimal clinically important difference (MCID)	Page 313
Standard deviation	Page 313
Level of significance/chance of Type I error	Page 314 and Fig. 29.1
Chance of Type II error	Page 315 and Fig. 29.1
Number of tails	Page 315
Study design	Page 315
Test/test statistic	Page 316

How the factors informing sample size presented in Box 1 interact can be best understood using the formula below:

$$n = f(\alpha, \beta, \delta, \sigma, D, O, T_s, T_t)$$

n = sample size; f = function of; α = significance level or chance of Type I error; β = chance of type II error ($1 - \beta$ = power); δ = MCID; σ = standard deviation; D = study design, O = outcome measure; T_s = test statistic; T_t = test tails.

Therefore, we can think of sample size as a function of the factors presented on the right side of the equation. Because of this interrelationship between the factors and sample size, if we are interested in obtaining the MCID, δ, for example, we can do so by rearranging the function so that MCID or δ is on the left side of the equation and show that δ is a different function, g, of the other terms and sample size, n. Therefore, the relationship between MCID and the other terms can be represented in a formula as

$$\delta = g(\alpha, \beta, \sigma, D, O, T_s, T_t, n)$$

In surgical research, the clinical scenario or research question informs both the outcome(s) to be measured and the target population to be studied. In research studies, there is a primary and sometimes a secondary outcome. The primary outcome is the endpoint that is of greatest importance, while the secondary outcome is used to measure additional effects of the intervention [3]. In the above-mentioned scenario, the primary outcome would be pain following surgery with and without the use of TAP Blocks; the target population would be colorectal patients undergoing laparoscopic surgery.

Once the outcome and the target population are determined, the next step is to decide on the appropriate outcome measure (the scale or instrument) to be used. A literature review can be used to ensure that the outcome measure is: (1) relevant; (2) meaningful; (3) reliable; (4) valid and (5) responsive to change. Next, one would determine the type of data measurement the outcome measure would produce (nominal, ordinal, interval or ratio) as this has a bearing on the type of statistical analysis that will be performed. The outcome measure for the current scenario would be the Numerical Rating Scale (NRS) pain score, which is continuous (interval) in nature.

The next step is to review previous literature to determine the **MCID** (δ) for your specific outcome measure. The concept of MCID was introduced in 1989 by Jaeschke et al. MCID is defined as the smallest difference in the outcome of interest perceived generally by patients (or physicians) as beneficial. In other words, the MCID refers to the smallest amount of difference in an outcome measure considered meaningful [4–7]. For surgeons, it means the smallest difference between a novel and standard approach that will persuade them to adopt the novel intervention. If no information on the MCID for your outcome measure is available, the MCID could be computed using **effect size** (ES), defined as the number of **standard deviation units** of change to be expected (ES = δ/σ).

For an RCT, effect size can be calculated as the difference in the means between two chosen times, divided by the standard deviation of scores at the first time point [7]. We can also think of the effect size in terms of the degree to which a specified nonzero difference can be observed in the population under study. The larger the value of ES, the greater the degree to which manifestation of the difference is found in the population.

As noted by Cohen [8], the ES is a very important factor in determining power and required sample size. A small effect size can be expected in patients reporting minimal or no difference in the outcome of interest. Alternatively, a large effect size is expected in patients reporting large differences in the chosen outcome. Where there is nothing in the literature, we can use the suggestions by Cohen that categorizes effect sizes as proxies, i.e., small effect = 0.2; medium effect size = 0.5 or large effect size = 0.8 as proxies for our MCID [8]. The formula for calculating effect size is shown below [7]

$$\mathrm{ES} = \frac{[\mathrm{Mean}(X_{\mathrm{Initial}}) - \mathrm{Mean}(X_{\mathrm{Final}})]}{\sigma_{\mathrm{baseline}}}$$

X: Observed Value; X_{initial}: values at baseline; X_{Final}: values following treatment/procedure; $\sigma_{\mathrm{baseline}}$: standard deviation of the baseline values.

It is important to note that, in clinical research, it is possible to have a positive or a negative value for ES. Therefore, it is important to consider your research question when interpreting data. In other words, if we are comparing Health-Related Quality of Life (HRQOL) scores in a sample from baseline to 6 months following surgery, then we would expect to see an improvement in HRQOL, and therefore a negative ES. For example, a baseline score of 50 on the HRQOL scale SF-36 that increases to 80 at 6 months will give a negative ES based on the above formula. However, if we are measuring pain, we would expect a decrease from baseline to 6 months, and therefore a positive ES; for example, a preoperative pain score of 8 on a Visual Analog Scale (VAS) of 0–10 postoperatively improves to a score of 3.

With the MCID for your specific outcome in mind, the research question is reframed into a clinical hypothesis, a statement about the expected relationship between two variables [9]. In the above scenario, the clinical hypothesis would address the suspected relationship between pain and TAP blocks ("*There will be an important decrease in pain score for those patients who had TAP Blocks, as compared to those who did not*"). The clinical hypothesis can then be stated as a statistical hypothesis, also known as the null hypothesis, which states the lack of relationship between the two variables (*There will be no difference in pain scores between groups*) [9]. The null hypothesis is essentially the hypothesis we would like to reject or nullify.

Once you have formulated your hypotheses, you must determine the best way to answer your research question. As it is often difficult, or impossible, to study everyone in a population, a subgroup (sample) of individuals from the population can be drawn [10]. The *population* is a group of individuals within a geographic region or institution (e.g., city, country, hospital, or school) [10]. The *sample*, which is also known as the study group, comprises those individuals that will actually be a part of the study [10]. The aim of sampling is to gather a diverse group of individuals from the population so that as many individuals are represented as possible. A representative sample allows more confidence when generalizing results found within the sample back to the population of interest.

Generalizing the results from a sample back to the population is referred to as statistical inference. Generalization is subject to some errors, one of which is making a false positive statement; this is known as Type I error [5, 10] (see Fig. 29.1). Type I error occurs when the null hypothesis is rejected, when in fact, it is true. In other words, if the results of a study indicate that there is a difference between two treatment groups when in reality there is not; a Type I error was committed. The chance of a Type I error is referred to as the level of statistical significance and is denoted by the first Greek letter α [5, 10]. For example, a level of significance of 0.05 indicates that we have a 5% risk of making a conclusion that there is a difference even if there is no difference. If we feel it is very important that a Type I error is not made, then we can choose a level of significance lower than 0.05, say 0.01. To reduce the chance of adopting interventions or procedures that are not effective, it is necessary for us to control our Type I error rate.

The other type of error associated with making inferences from a sample to the population is known as a Type II error, represented by the second Greek letter β. It is referred to as the chance of not rejecting the null hypothesis when it is not true, or the chance of not detecting a difference when it exists [5, 10]. Type II error is related to the concept of power, the chance of rejecting the null hypothesis when it is not true (Fig. 29.1) [5, 10]. This works out computationally to $1 - \beta$ and is the same as the chance of detecting a difference when there is a difference to detect. For example, power of 0.80 or 80% indicates that if a difference exists between two groups in a study, there is a 20% chance the study will not detect it.

Power should be measured or calculated before (a priori) a trial begins and not after. As Farrokhyar et al. [5] explain, a priori power and sample size calculations can reduce the risk of Type II error (false-negative result). Through conducting a power calculation a priori, researchers are aware of the sample size required to reach power and can then ensure that the

Fig. 29.1 Explanation of Type I and Type II error

		Reality in Target Population	
		Alternative Hypothesis is True	**Null Hypothesis is True**
Results of Research	**Reject the Null (there is a difference)**	**CORRECT**	**Type I Error** *(You determined there was a difference when in fact there is not)*
	Did Not Reject the Null (there is no difference)	**Type II Error** *(You determined there was no difference when in fact there is)*	**CORRECT**

necessary number of participants are recruited. When power is calculated a priori, researchers can be confident in the results of their study knowing that they had the power to detect a difference if one existed. Conversely, if power is calculated post hoc (after the completion of a study) and power was not adequate the researchers may have less confidence in their results. For example, after having completed a trial, researchers conclude no statistical difference in their outcome of interest between two groups; however, if the study was found to have inadequate power, these results may be false (Type II Error).

The next steps are to determine the directionality of our hypothesis and the variability in the outcome measure of interest. Standard deviation, the dispersion of data, helps us to understand how different an individual's score is from the others [11]. Standard deviation is represented by the Greek letter σ (in the population and s in the sample). Information on variability of specific outcome measures, within the target population, may be found in the literature. However, usually, it is the variability found within a sample that is reported, not the variability of the entire population. If this information is not available, a pilot study may need to be carried out to obtain this information. In addition to reviewing the literature for variability, the literature can also be used to determine if your hypothesis needs to be tested using one-tailed or two-tailed testing. A one-tail test involves unidirectional testing of the hypothesis; meaning, it tests for the possibility of a relationship in one direction and ignores the possibility of a relationship in the other direction [12]. For example, if we are interested in the improvement of Health-Related Quality of Life (HRQOL) with a new surgical intervention, we may expect that there will only be a change in one direction (improvement). However, by doing this, we may be ignoring the fact that this new intervention may be worsening HRQOL or even causing death in some situations. A two-tail test, on the other hand, involves a bidirectional testing of the hypothesis and tests for the possibility of a relationship in both directions [12]. Two-tailed tests are most often used in research, as we are usually not sure of the directionality of the relationship when designing the study.

Once your null hypothesis is formulated and directionality decided on, you must decide on the type of study design to use to test your hypothesis. The most appropriate type of study design depends on: (1) The research question or goal of the study; (2) Whether or not an intervention or random allocation is needed; and (3) When the outcomes are to be measured and what outcome measure to use. Surgeon-researchers should be familiar with the different study designs and the hierarchy of evidence (see Chap. 5) comprehensive web-sites on study designs are available and beyond the scope of this chapter [13–15].

Study design can impact sample size [5], for example, if the participants are being assigned into different study groups using a random allocation mechanism, such as using a random number generator, this will impact the overall number of participants needed. In the case of random allocation, one needs to properly determine the overall required sample size, as well as how many participants are needed in each group so that the study has adequate power. The final required sample size is also contingent on the allocation ratio, sample loss, or attrition during the study. Thus, the computed sample size of the study (n) needs to be increased by a factor of $1/(1 - p)$ to give us a sample of size n' [16]. That is, $n' = n/(1 - p)$; where p is proportion lost, and n' is rounded up to the integer multiple of the number of arms or groups in the trial [16]. More complicated study designs, such as those utilizing stratification through predetermined subgroups (e.g., grouping by recruitment site or gender) require larger sample sizes to maintain power [5]. Calculation of power and sample size for these types of study designs are beyond the scope of this chapter. If readers would like more information on subgroups, please see Chap. 30 more detailed information on the adjustments needed to calculate sample size in more advanced study designs can be found elsewhere (see Appendix 3).

Generally, the analysis of the study data is dependent on the study design, the study hypothesis, the type of data collected, and the outcome measures. After we translate the study hypothesis into a statistical hypothesis, we then test for the chance that the study would have obtained a value/result that we are interested in or something more extreme using a test statistic. The choice of a statistical test, and hence the test statistic used, depends on the study hypothesis and data collected. The test statistic can be defined as a statistic computed from the data in the study and used in a statistical test to support or reject the null hypothesis. From our scenario, the hypothesis involves a comparison of the means of the NRS between two groups, the test is the independent samples t-test of the means, and the test statistic is the t-statistic. Other tests and test statistics are available to use depending on the hypothesis tested using more complicated models that consider stratification and covariate adjustment.

While there are ways of calculating power and sample size by hand, there are many software options such as commercially available PASS software from NCSS Statistical Software [17] or freely available software such as G*Power version 3.1 [18, 19] or R [20]. In Appendix 2, we have included an assortment of screenshots using G*Power to illustrate the effects that the factors summarized in Box 1 have on power and sample size.

In summary, the required sample size will increase if a smaller effect size is chosen, if power or standard deviation is increased, or as significance level (α), or β are decreased. However, even when calculations are done a priori, and the most valiant of efforts are made, in reality, the proper sample size cannot always be attained. In such cases, it is best for the investigators to disclose this in the limitation section of their manuscript. In most situations, if the study was performed with the appropriate methodology, it can still contribute to the literature by being combined with similar work in systematic reviews or meta-analyses (see Chap. 15).

Article Selection

To address the clinical dilemma described in the clinical scenario, you will need to consult the available evidence within the surgical literature. To do so, you form a clinical research question using the PICOT format (see Chap. 3) and use these terms to perform a literature search (see Chap. 4). Since you have already identified your outcome, target audience, and outcome measure, completing a research question using the PICOT format is quite simple. The PICOT format terms for this scenario would be as follows:

- **P**opulation: Colorectal Cancer Patients undergoing laparoscopic surgery
- **I**ntervention: TAP Blocks
- **C**omparative Intervention: No use of TAP Blocks
- **O**utcome: Pain
- **T**ime Horizon: 24 h following surgery

Therefore, your research question is, "*In colorectal patients undergoing laparoscopic surgery, does the use of TAP Blocks affect pain, as measured by the Numerical Rating Scale (NRS) compared to no TAP blocks at 24 h following surgery?*"

You enter "Colorectal Cancer AND Laparoscopic surgery AND TAP Blocks AND Pain" into Cochrane Library; your search yields three published articles (article 1, 3, 4) and one conference abstract (article 2) (see Appendix 4). A title and abstract screening reveals the most appropriate article for your research question, "*Effects of preoperative ultrasound-guided transverse abdominus plane block on pain after laparoscopic surgery for colorectal cancer: a double-blind randomized controlled trial*", by Oh et al. [21]. Of the three available studies, this study is chosen as it is the most recent study that focuses specifically on colorectal cancer patients, and the comparison of two groups (patients with and without TAP Blocks). The chosen article is summarized below:

Summary of the Appraised Article by Oh et al. [21]

A sample size of 25 patients per group was obtained by the authors with the assumption that there would be 30% difference in pain between patients measured using a Numeric Rating Scale (NRS). Allowing for potential sample loss of 10%, the authors calculated they would need 28 patients per group.

The authors report no statistically significant differences between the two groups in age, Body Mass Index (BMI), ASA classifications, surgical duration, anesthesia duration or comorbidities. However, there were statistically significant differences reported in sex distribution between groups (82:17.9% M:F in the TAP group and 51.9:48.2% M:F in the control; $p = 0.017$), and operation type (39.3:60.7% colon:rectum in the TAP group and 66.7:33.3% colon:rectum in the control group; $p = 0.042$). While Oh et al. [21] stated whether statistically significant differences existed, the authors did not report if differences between groups were clinically important. The inclusion of this information is common in RCTs, however, as recommended by Altman [22], it is more impactful to state if there are clinically important differences between groups. Altman [22] states that it is not good practice to infer from the lack of statistical significance that the variable under question had no effect on the outcome of interest. In other words, even though subjective assessment requires prior knowledge of the prognostic impact of the variables of interest, this should be used in place of statistical analysis to determine the similarity between two randomized groups [22]. With this in mind, it would have been more effective for Oh et al. [21] to comment on the known prognostic importance of those variables compared between groups (age, BMI, ASA, surgical and anesthesia duration, and comorbidities).

There are no statistically significant differences in NRS scores both at rest and on coughing at 1 h postanesthetic recovery (PAR) although the mean score for patients in the TAP group was slightly lower than that for the control group (see Table 29.1). Postoperative results showed no statistically significant differences in NRS scores at 24, 48, and 72 h after surgery. Full results are available in the original publication [21]; Table 29.1 summarizes the data for pain at rest and when coughing for postanesthetic recovery and 24 h postoperatively. If readers wish to see full results by Oh et al. [21], including pain scores for 48 and 72 h, please see the original publication.

Questions Used to Appraise

You believe that this is an appropriate article to answer the clinical dilemma posed in the scenario; however, before presenting the evidence to your supervisor and colleagues, you want to ensure its credibility. You uncover an article by Caddedu et al. [23] that provides a set of questions to appraise a randomized controlled trial (RCT) based on power and sample size. The Caddedu et al. [23] article has general questions on how to appraise an RCT, however, this chapter is going to focus on those questions specific to assessing power (Box 2).

Box 2: Key Questions to Assess Power Within a Study [23]

1. Was a power analysis performed?
2. Was the sample size calculation detailed for the primary outcome?
3. Is the effect size clinically relevant?
4. Would the stated difference in treatment effect result in a change in practice?
5. Is the effect size precise and consistent with your clinical experience and previously published trials?
6. If no power analysis was completed, are the results reported appropriately to estimate power?
7. Are confidence intervals included so that the estimation of the treatment effect can be determined?

Question 1: Was a power analysis performed?

As power and sample size are directly related to each other, it is important to perform a power analysis a priori. After reviewing the Oh et al. [21] article,

Table 29.1 Pain outcomes between patient groups at four follow-up periods [21]

		Postanesthetic recovery (PAR) mean, SD	24 h post-operative (POD1) mean, SD
Pain at rest	TAP block (n = 28)	5.3, 1.9	4.0, 1.6
	Control (n = 27)	5.9, 2.0	3.9, 1.7
	p value[a]	0.24	0.87
Pain when coughing	TAP block (n = 28)	6.8, 1.9	5.6, 1.8
	Control (n = 27)	7.2, 1.7	6.1, 1.6
	p value[a]	0.38	0.32

SD standard deviation, *TAP* transversus abdominis plane
[a]Adjusted for gender and operation
Table restructured using information from Oh et al. [21]

you see that no power calculation was performed. The authors state that they considered "a statistical power of 0.8", however, they did not perform a power analysis [21]. Using the information learned above, without performing a power calculation a priori we do not know if there was an adequate sample collected to properly detect a difference if one truly occurs. This discovery would be problematic as if inadequate sample size was used the study may not have enough power to detect a difference if one truly occurred. With inadequate sample size, and consequently, power, validity of results could be questioned and resources to perform the study could be potentially wasted.

Question 2: Was the sample size calculation detailed for the primary outcome?

The primary outcome for the Oh et al. [21] study was stated as pain following surgery, on coughing postoperative day 1 (POD 1). To measure pain, the authors used a numeric rating scale (NRS) on postoperative days (PODs) up to 3 days following surgery at rest, and on coughing [21].

Oh et al. [21] do not include their sample size calculation in the published article, instead the authors reference two previous studies [24, 25]. The first study referenced by Oh et al. [21] states that pain scores, at rest, 24 h following surgery was 4.3 [24]; the next resource states that pain when coughing was two points higher than it was at rest [25]. Oh et al. [21] use this previous information to determine that the pain score when coughing would be 6.3.

The authors then state that a 30% decrease in pain scores, which, would equal 4.4, would be considered "clinically significant". As the authors do not state where this 30% decrease was taken from you investigate and find that the Schwenk et al. [25] study mentions that their sample size was calculated to detect a 30% decrease in pain scores. The problem is that the Schwenk et al. [25] study uses a different pain score than Oh et al. [21] and therefore you are not convinced that this decrease in pain score would truly be clinically relevant for this sample, or pain measure.

Continuing on with their sample size calculation, Oh et al. [21] decide to set the alpha at 0.05 and set their power to 0.8, or 80%. Using these criteria, the authors determined that the study was required to have 25 individuals in each group. The authors then use a dropout rate of 10% and determined that 28 patients would be needed in each group.

In regards to the hypothesis statement, "investigating the effects of TAP blocks on pain after surgery", you feel that there is a lack of detail. For example, the hypothesis does not state where the expected difference would be seen, i.e., would the difference be seen between time points, within patients, or between the patient groups? Through a review of the methods section, you see that Oh et al. [21] are comparing the pain scores between groups at POD1 on coughing. Table 29.2 illustrates the time points that Oh et al. [21] used for their calculation. You feel that the authors should have stated the hypothesis as "expecting a 30%

Table 29.2 Comparing the mean pain scores between tap block and control patients across time points (analysis performed)

	NRS rest			NRS cough		
	TAP block	Control	Test	Tap block	Control	Test
PAR	*A*	*B*	*A* versus *B*	*C*	*D*	*C* versus *D*
POD1	*E*	*F*	*E* versus *F*	*G*	*H*	*G* versus *H*

Table 29.3 Comparing change in pain scores between groups at each time point (suggested analysis)

	NRS rest			NRS cough		
	TAP block	Control	Test	Tap block	Control	Test
PAR	*A*	*B*	–	*C*	*D*	–
POD1	*E*	*F*	–	*G*	*H*	–
POD1-PAR	$E - A = \Delta EA$	$F - B = \Delta FB$	ΔEA versus ΔFB	$G - C = \Delta GC$	$H - D = \Delta HD$	ΔGC versus ΔHD

difference in NRS pain scores between patient groups on coughing at POD1, represented as $[(H{-}G) * 100\%]/H$.

However, you also feel that a more appropriate null hypothesis would have been to hypothesize about the difference in change in pain on coughing between PAR and POD1 for the two groups, i.e., $\Delta HD - \Delta GC$ (see Table 29.3).

However, without information on the variability of the change in pain scores from PAR to POD 1 in this population, we are unable to calculate the appropriate sample size.

Question 3: Is the effect size clinically relevant?

While reading the Oh et al. [21] article, you realize that there is no effect size given in the article. Using the information that was provided by the authors, the predetermined effect size of this study would have been 0.76 or a "large" effect size. The calculation below was determined using information from the authors, for example, they assumed a mean pain score of 6.3 (standard deviation = 2.5) in coughing in the control group. They used a 30% decrease from 6.3 in the TAP group, therefore an estimated pain score of 4.4.

$$\mathrm{ES} = \frac{[\mathrm{Mean}(X_{\mathrm{initial}}) - \mathrm{Mean}(X_{\mathrm{Final}})}{\sigma_{\mathrm{baseline}}}$$

$$\mathrm{ES} = \frac{(6.3 - 4.4)}{2.5} = \frac{1.9}{2.5} = 0.76$$

Here, the sample size needed to detect this effect size is 29 in each group and with a 10% drop out rate, and the actual required sample size is 33 participants per group obtained using both GPower3.1 [18, 19] and PASS [17].

The actual post hoc effect size from the study on coughing at POD1 is calculated at 0.3125, closer to a small effect size:

$$\mathrm{ES} = \frac{[\mathrm{Mean}(X_{\mathrm{control}}) - \mathrm{Mean}(X_{\mathrm{TAPBlock}})}{\sigma_{\mathrm{control}}}$$

$$\mathrm{ES} = \frac{(6.1 - 5.6)}{1.6} = \frac{0.5}{1.6} = 0.3125$$

With the smaller observed effect size of 0.3125, a much larger sample size of 128 participants per group is needed to detect the difference in pain score of 0.5 observed on coughing at POD1. Adjusting for a 10% sample loss, the actual sample size needed is 143 participants per group.

Question 4: Would the difference in treatment effect result in a change in your practice?

The authors decided to use a 30% decrease in pain as the minimally clinically important difference, however, there was no reference given for this information and a 30% decrease in pain was not found [21]. Additionally, you do not believe that their hypothesis statement was correct (as stated in Question 2). As the hypothesis statement was ambiguous, you are not quite confident that the results can convince you to change your practice. The decision to change practice is subjective as introducing TAP blocks into a practice would also cause a delay in the treatment of the case. Therefore, each surgeon would have to weigh the pros and cons and determine if a possible decrease in pain is worth an increase in time and resources for the case.

Question 5: Is the effect size precise and consistent with your clinical experience and previously published trials?

Oh et al. [21] did not state an effect size, similarly, no reference was provided for the chosen 30% decrease in pain and therefore it is difficult to determine if the variables used by the authors are justified.

Question 6: If no power analysis was completed, are the results reported appropriately to estimate power?

While the authors did not calculate power, the results reported by Oh et al. [21] do allow you to conduct your own power analysis:

Using the mean difference of 0.5 in pain score on coughing at POD1, standard deviation of 1.6, alpha of 0.05 (two-sided test) and 28 patients per group, the trial post hoc power calculation is 0.231.

Question 7: Are confidence intervals included so that the estimation of the treatment effect can be determined?

Oh et al. [21] did not provide confidence intervals in their results or conclusions. Confidence intervals are used alongside p-values to describe the results seen in a study [23]. For example, while a *p*-value will indicate if the difference between two treatments is statistically significant, the confidence interval will indicate both the magnitude of the difference and give an idea of the interval of values where the true value is most likely to be found [23]. Confidence intervals are a very important part of research and help the reader to interpret the results of a study, for more information on confidence intervals please see Chap. 28.

Resolution of the Scenario

Based on the evidence presented in the Oh et al. [21] article, and her own appraisal of the article, the Fellow informed her program director that she is retracting her original recommendation. She recommends that they repeat the study but this time use robust methodology to find a more convincing answer. A more robust study could include some of the following changes:

- A clearly stated hypothesis that matches the research question and guides data analysis
  - e.g., To investigate the difference in change in pain scores on coughing between the control and TAP block from PAR to POD1.
- The authors should have performed a more appropriate literature search to determine criteria for clinically important differences and attrition rates. Criteria should be used that match the sample, the procedure, and the outcome measure being used.
  - i.e., the 30% decrease used by Oh et al. [21] originated in a study looking at a different intervention, and a different outcome measure
  - i.e., the 10% attrition rate seems to be chosen at random, there was no stated evidence to support that this attrition rate was applicable. The authors should have used previous literature or performed a feasibility study.
- The authors collect data for 24, 48, and 72 h following surgery, however, they report on the 24 h results as the primary outcome and consider the information for the other two time points as secondary outcomes
- The authors should have utilized a biostatistician to determine a proper sample size for the outcomes that they wanted to measure.

Appendix 1

Additional Information

Qualitative Research

This chapter only outlined how to assess power and sample size in a quantitative research study. A qualitative research study is dealt with in a different manner; the authors encourage the reader to access available resources [25–29].

Definitions for bolded terms

- *Reliable*:
  - The degree to which a specific instrument produces consistent results, and on multiple occasions, when no evidence of change exists [28].
- *Valid*:
  - The degree that an instrument measures what it is supposed to measure [28].
- *Responsive to change*:
  - The degree to which an instrument can detect change over time [28].
- Standard Deviation:
  - A measure of variability providing the "average distance" of a value from the mean. The units are always expressed the same as the original value [27].
  - The variation of a measure in a population can impact sample size, if the outcome being measured is similar across all members of the population than a smaller sample size is required. However, if the outcome is heterogeneous across the population, you would need a larger sample size to detect differences among the participants [5].

Additional Information:

- **One- or two-Tail test**
  - The tail refers to the end of the distribution of the test statistic.
  - A one-tail test means testing for the possibility of a relationship in only one direction and ignoring the possibility of a relationship in the other direction.
    A one-tail test enables us to test the difference in a single direction with more power because of the assumption of the direction of the difference [12].
    However, we also need to take into account the possibility of missing or failing to detect a difference in the other direction and hence the possibility of rejecting a promising intervention. So as tempting as it is deciding to go with a single tail test for the sole reason of having great power, it is not suggested [12].
  - A two-tail test, on the other hand, involves a bidirectional testing of the hypothesis and tests for the possibility of a relationship in both directions. This is because in most studies, we are not sure of the directionality of the relationship and hence two-sided test is almost universal [12].
- **Loss to follow-up**
  - This is an important issue in every study and more so in those comparing effects of different treatments.
  - Power decreases as the proportion lost to follow up (p) multiplied [16].
  - Thus, the effective sample size of the study (n) needs to be increased by a factor of $1/(1 - p)$ to give us a sample of size n'. That is, $n' = n/(1-p)$ [16].
    - where p is proportion lost, and n' is rounded up to the integer multiple of the number of arms in the trial.
- **Allocation Ratio** [5]
  - This term describes the ratio of participants that must be recruited into each group in a study (i.e., into the control group and into the treatment group).
  - As the ratio moves away from 1:1 (equal number of participants in each group), the sample size increases for the same power.
  - Power also decreases as the ratio moves from 1:1

Appendix 2: Using G*Power to Compute Power [30]

Figure 29.2a shows a screenshot of G*Power with the majority of the factors summarized in Table 29.1 highlighted. G*Power defaults to the most commonly selected effect size (δ), test statistic, Type I error rate (α), and Type II error rate (β, power = $1 - \beta$), but these can all be customized by the user as we have done. Additionally, the user must select the statistical test being performed and whether it is a one or two-tailed study. Figure 29.2–d gives examples of a G*Power calculation and how changing various factors impacts the required sample size. This chapter does not explain the three output

Fig. 29.2 **a** G*Power and required factors. **b** Example of sample size calculation [30] **c** Example of how changing effect size impacts sample size requirement [30]. **d** Example of how changing power impacts sample size requirement [30]

(a)

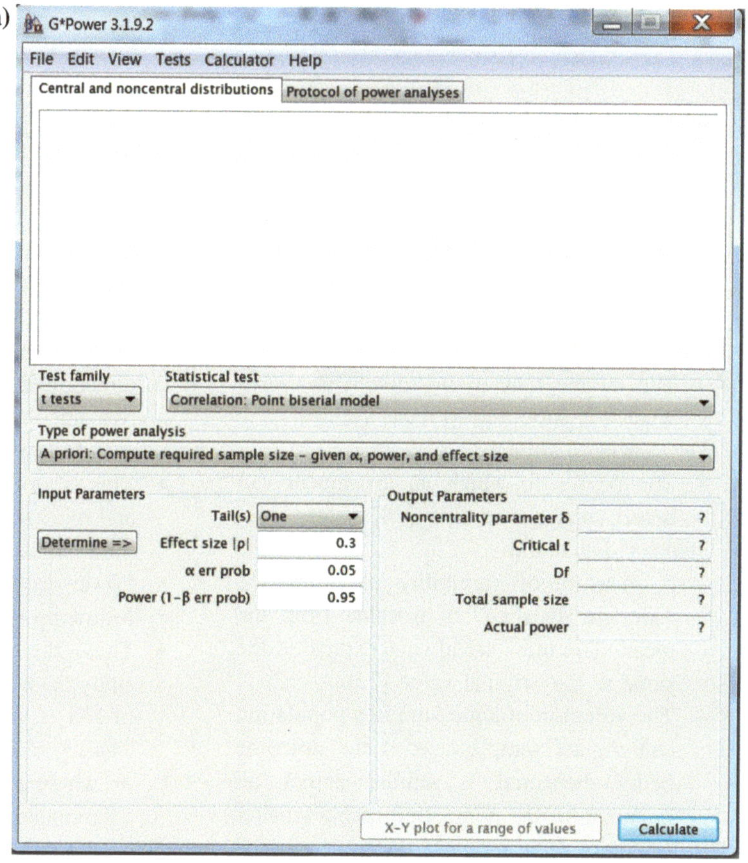

(b)

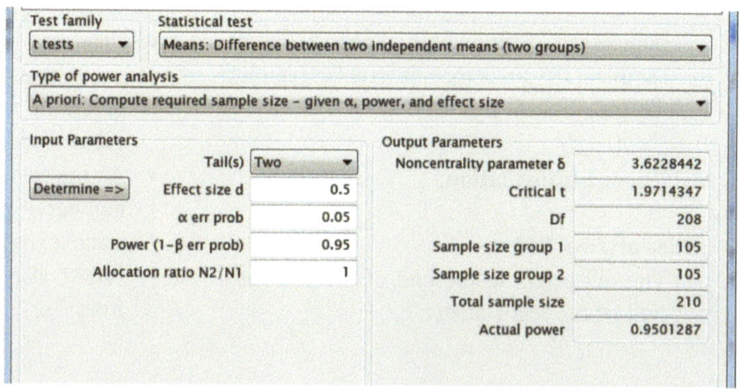

Fig. 29.2 (continued)

(c)

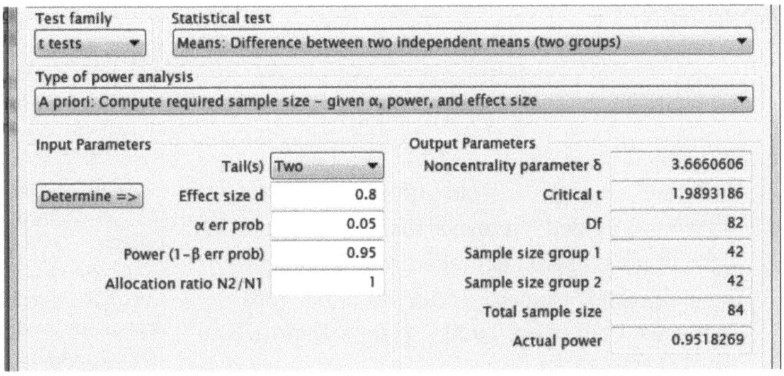

(d)

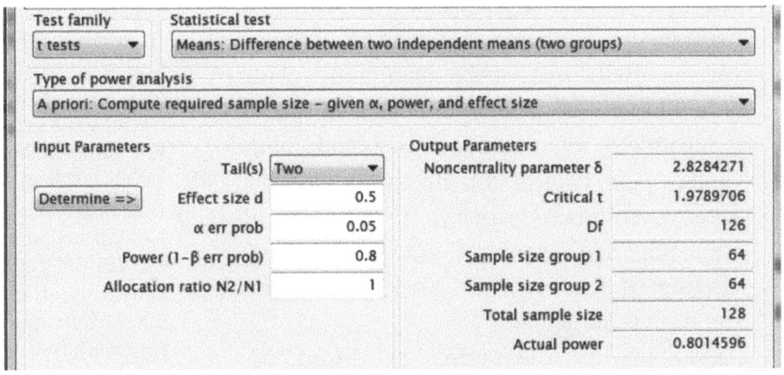

parameters—Noncentrality parameter δ, Critical t and Df; for more information, readers are redirected to the G*Power manual, available for download [30].

Figure 29.2b illustrates the required sample size for a two-tailed test, using a t-test to determine significant differences between two independent groups; an ES of 0.5 (medium), an alpha of 0.05, and a Type II error rate of 0.05 or power of 0.95 have been selected. Using this specific situation, a sample size of 210 (105 per group) would be required. In Fig. 29.2c, the ES has been changed to 0.8 with all other factors remaining the same; here you can see that the total required sample size has decreased to 84 (42 per group). The reason for the decrease in sample size is because we are indicating to G*Power that the expected difference in the outcome between the two groups is large. Therefore, it would take fewer participants to detect a large difference (0.8) than it would if the ES for that outcome between groups was smaller (0.2); an ES of 0.2 would have increased the required sample size. Last, in Fig. 29.2d, the power has been decreased to 0.80 or 80%; you can see here that keeping ES the same (0.5) and alpha the same 0.05 as in Fig. 29.2b, by decreasing power you have a smaller required sample size.

Appendix 3

For more information on calculating power and sample size in complex study designs, please see:

1. Wittes J. Sample size calculations for randomized controlled trials. Epidemiol Rev. 2002;24:39–53.
2. Whitley E, Ball J. Statistics review 4: sample size calculations. Crit Care. 2002;6:335–41.

Appendix 4

Literature Search Results:

1. Oh TK, Yim J, Kim J, Eom W, Lee SA, Park SC et al. Effects of preoperative ultrasound-guided transversus abdominis plane block on pain after laparoscopic surgery for colorectal cancer: a double-blind randomized controlled trial. Surg Endosc. 2017;31(1):127-24.
2. Lax E, Smithson L, Pearlman R, Damdi A. Comparison of therapeutic benefit of bupivacaine HCL transversus abdominis plane (TAP) blocks are part of an enhanced recovery pathway vs. traditional oral and intravenous pain control for elective minimally invasive colorectal surgery. In: Diseases of the colon and rectum. Conference: annual meeting of the American Society of Colon and Rectal Surgeons; 2018.
3. Pedrazzani C, Menestrina N, Moro M, Brazzo G, Mantovani G, Polati E et al. Local wound infiltration plus transversus abdominis plane (TAP) block versus local wound infiltration in laparoscopic colorectal surgery and ERAS program. Surg Endosc. 2016;30 (11):5117–25.
4. Park SY, Park JS, Choi GS, Kim HJ, Moon S, Yeo J. Comparison of analgesic efficacy of laparoscopic-assisted and ultrasound-guided transversus abdominis plane block after laparoscopic colorectal operation: A randomized, single-blinded, non-inferiority trial. J Am Coll Surg. 2017;225(3):403–10.

References

1. Spilker B, Cramer J. Patient recruitment in clinical trials. New York: Raven Press Ltd.; 1992.
2. Thoma A, Farrokhyar F, McKnight L, Bhandari M. Practical tips for surgical research: how to optimize patient recruitment. Can J Surg. 2010;53(3):205–10.
3. CONSORT. CONSORT glossary [Internet]. [cited 2018 Jun 12]. Available from: http://www.consort-statement.org/resources/glossary.
4. Jaeschke R, Singer J, Guyatt GH. Measurement of health status: ascertaining the minimal clinically important difference. Control Clin Trials. 1989;10:407–15.
5. Farrokhyar F, Reddy D, Poolman RW, Bhandari M. Why perform a priori sample size calculation? Can J Surg. 2013;56(3):207–13.
6. McGlothlin AE, Lewis RJ. Minimal clinically important difference: defining what really matters to patients. JAMA Guide Stat Methods. 2014;312 (13):1342–3.
7. Luiz RR, Almeida RMVR. On the measurement of change in medical research. Int J Stat Med Res. 2012;1:144–7.
8. Cohen J. Statistical power analysis for the behavioral sciences. 2nd ed. Hillsdale, NJ: Lawrence Erlbaum Associates; 1988.
9. LoBiondo-Wood G, Haber J. Research questions, hypotheses and clinical questions. In: Nursing education: methods and critical appraisal for evidence-based practice. 9th ed. Missouri: Elsevier MOSBY; 2018. p. 27–55.
10. Martinez-Mesa J, Gonzalez-Chica DA, Bastos JL, Bonamigo RR, Duqula RP. Sample size: how many participants do I need in my research? Bras Dermatol. 2014;89(4):609–15.
11. University of Leicester. Measures of variability: the range, inter-quartile range and standard deviation [Internet]. [cited 2018 May 29]. Available from: https://www2.le.ac.uk/offices/ld/resources/study-guides-pdfs/numeracy-skills-pdfs/measures-ariability-v0.1.pdf (2009).
12. Ruxton GD, Neuhäuser M. When should we use one-tailed hypothesis testing? Methods Ecol Evol. 2010;1:114–7.
13. The Centre for Evidence-Based Medicine (CEBM). Study designs [Internet]. University of Oxford; 2018 [cited 2018 May 29]. Available from: https://www.cebm.net/2014/04/study-designs/.
14. Duke University Medical Center Library & Archives. Introduction to evidence-based practice: types of studies [Internet]. Available from: https://guides.mclibrary.duke.edu/ebmtutorial/study-types (2018).
15. University of Ottawa. Society, the individual, and medicine: study designs [Internet]. [cited 2018 May 29]. Available from: https://www.med.uottawa.ca/sim/data/Study_Designs_e.htm.
16. Whitley E, Ball J. Statistics review 4: sample size calculations. Crit Care. 2002;6(4):335.
17. NCSS Statistical Software. PASS 16. [Internet]. 2018 [cited 2018 Jun 22]. Available from https://www.ncss.com/software/pass/.
18. Faul F, Erdfelder E, Lang A-G, Buchner A. G*Power 3: a flexible statistical power analysis program for the social, behavioral, and biomedical sciences. Behav Res Methods. 2007;39:175–91.
19. Faul F, Erdfelder E, Buchner A, Lang A-G. Statistical power analyses using G*Power 3.1: tests for correlation and regression analyses. Behav Res Methods. 2009;41:1149–60.

20. The R Foundation. *The R project for statistical computing [Internet]* [accessed 2018 Jul 24]. Available from: https://www.r-project.org/.
21. Oh T, Yim J, Kim J, Eom W, Lee S, Park S, et al. Effects of preoperative ultrasound-guided transversus abdominis plane block on pain after laparoscopic surgery for colorectal cancer: a double-blind randomized controlled trial. Surg Endosc. 2017;31(1):127–34.
22. Altman DG. Comparability of randomised groups. The Statistician. 1985;34:125–36.
23. Caddedu M, Farrokhyar F, Thoma A, Haines T, Garnett A, Goldsmith CH, et al. Users' guide to the surgical literature: how to assess power and sample size. Laparoscopic vs open appendectomy. Can J Surg. 2008;51(6):476–82.
24. Kang SB, Park JW, Jeong SY, Nam BH, Choi HS, Kim DW, et al. Open versus laparoscopic surgery for mid or low rectal cancer after neoadjuvant chemoradiotherpy (COREAN trial): short-term outcomes of an open-label randomised controlled tiral. Lancet Oncol. 2010;11:637–45.
25. Schwenk W, Bohm B, Muller JM. Postoperative pain and fatigue after laparoscopic or conventional colorectal resections. A prospective randomized trial. Surg Endosc. 1998;12:1131–6.
26. Malterud K, Dirk Siersma V, Dorrit Guassora A. Sample size in qualitative interview studies: Guided by information power. Innov Methods. 2016;26 (13):1753–60.
27. Sim J, Saunders B, Waterfield J, Kingstone T. Can sample size in qualitative research be determined a priori? Int J Soc Res Methodol. 2018; EPub Ahead of Print. https://doi.org/10.1080/13645579.2018.1454643.
28. Onwuegbuzie AJ, Leech NL. A call for qualitative power analyses. Qual Quant. 2007;41:105–21.
29. Centers for Disease Control and Prevention C. Health-related quality of life (HRQOL): measurement properties: validity, reliability, and responsiveness [Internet]. CDC; 2016 [cited 2018 Jun 12]. Available from: https://www.cdc.gov/hrqol/measurement.htm.
30. Bucher A, Erdfelder E, Franz F, Lang AG. G*Power: statistical power analysis for Windows and Mac. [Internet]; 2017. [cited 2018 Aug 12]. Available from http://www.gpower.hhu.de/.

Subgroup Analyses in Surgery

30

Alexandra Hatchell and Sophocles H. Voineskos

Introduction

As surgeons, we seek to ensure that we provide the best possible care to our patients. In doing so, we collect the highest level of available evidence from the published literature, such as randomized controlled trials (RCTs) . Although the available evidence is usually derived from more generalized patient populations, many surgeons attempt to make treatment decisions based upon specific individual patient factors. As a result, many published RCTs perform additional analyses on specific subgroups within the defined patient population.

A *subgroup* is subset of a trial group identified on the basis of a patient or intervention characteristic that is either measured at baseline or at randomization. A *subgroup analysis* is a statistical analysis that explores whether effects of an intervention (i.e., experimental versus control) differ according to the status of a subgroup variable. Although subgroup analyses may be helpful to individualize treatment decisions and plans, these analyses may also mislead clinicians due to lack of credibility [1, 2]. Specifically, surgeons may underestimate the influence of chance on treatment effects. For example, an apparent subgroup effect of zodiac sign was reported by the investigators of the Second International Study of Infarct Survival (ISIS-2) [3]. Specifically, patients born as a Gemini or Libra who presented with myocardial infarction did not experience the same reduction in vascular mortality attributable to aspirin as patients born under other zodiac signs. Despite a statistically significant finding ($p = 0.003$ for interaction), the investigators did not believe this to be a true subgroup effect, but reported these results to caution readers regarding the potential pitfalls of subgroup analyses. Therefore, when considering subgroup analyses, surgeons must be conscientious and critical in their appraisal to ensure the reported subgroup effect is meaningful and applicable.

The purpose of this article is to outline the criteria for rigorous subgroup analyses in methodologically sound RCTs. A clinical scenario, based upon a recent RCT in general surgery, will support these criteria throughout the text.

Clinical Scenario

A 65-year-old woman in your practice has recently been diagnosed with colon cancer, and more specifically involving the cecum. The current surgical plan is to perform a right hemicolectomy for surgical cure. The patient presents to your office to discuss the operative plan and

A. Hatchell · S. H. Voineskos (✉)
Department of Surgery, Division of Plastic Surgery, McMaster University, Hamilton, ON, Canada
e-mail: Sophocles.voineskos@medportal.ca

A. Thoma et al. (eds.), *Evidence-Based Surgery*,
https://doi.org/10.1007/978-3-030-05120-4_30

asks you about the planned method of surgical wound closure. Even though you have reiterated that the primary goal of this operation is to remove her cancer, she seems fixated on the potential postoperative cosmetic appearance of her surgical scar.

You have noticed that many of your plastic surgery colleagues frequently use subcuticular sutures to close surgical incisions and assume the cosmetic results of these wounds are likely to be quite good. Therefore, you wonder whether a subcuticular closure would result in a better surgical scar for this patient compared to closure with staples, while still minimizing the chance of infection or other wound complications. You decide to perform a literature search to answer this question.

Literature Search

As stated in previous chapters, the first step to finding the best available evidence is to formulate a research question based on the PICOT format (see Chap. 3):

- **P**opulation: Patients undergoing gastrointestinal surgery.
- **I**ntervention: Subcuticular sutures for skin closure.
- **C**omparative intervention: Staples for skin closure.
- **O**utcomes: Surgical scar, infection, and other wound complications.
- **T**ime: 6 months after surgery.

Using the PICOT format terms, your clinical research questions could be: "In patients undergoing gastrointestinal surgery, does skin closure using subcuticular sutures result in a better surgical scar, decreased infections, and decreased wound complications compared to skin closure using staples?"

Next, you use the above terms to perform a thorough literature search (See Chap. 4): "subcuticular suture AND staple AND gastrointestinal surgery AND infection AND scar". To ensure you only obtain reliable and valid evidence, you limit your search with "randomized controlled trials (RCT)". This search produces two articles (Appendix 1). As you review the titles of the articles, you notice that the first article contains "subcuticular sutures versus staples for skin closure after open gastrointestinal surgery" [4]. Since it appears this article will be directly comparing these two skin closure methods in gastrointestinal surgery, you believe it should provide some insight into your decision for your patient with the upcoming right hemicolectomy. You download the article for further reading and assessment.

Summary of the Appraised Article

The study by Tsujinaka and colleagues [4] was designed to compare the differences in rates of wound complications for gastrointestinal (GI) surgery, including superficial incisional surgical site infection and hypertrophic scar formation, depending on whether the surgical incision was closed with subcuticular sutures or staples. The authors sought to answer this question since no published studies have investigated the optimal method of skin closure for GI Class 2 (clean-contaminated) surgeries. From a total of 1080 enrolled patients, 562 patients were randomly assigned to subcuticular sutures (SC) and 518 to staples (ST). The primary outcome was the incidence of wound complications within 30 days of surgery. The secondary outcome was the incidence of hypertrophic scar formation within 6 months of surgery.

A total of 558 patients received subcuticular sutures, of which 382 patients underwent upper GI surgery and 176 underwent lower GI surgery (Table 30.1). A total of 514 patients received staples, of which 413 patients underwent upper GI surgery and 101 underwent lower GI surgery. The authors compared rates of the primary and secondary outcomes between the two treatment groups using Fisher's exact test. The authors also compared wound complications and hypertrophic scar formation between subgroups based

Table 30.1 Demographic characteristics and primary outcomes[a] of patients receiving skin closure with either subcuticular sutures or staples

	Subcuticular sutures (n = 562)	Staples (n = 518)	Odds ratio (95% CI)	p-value
Median age (years; IQR)	68 (61–75)	68 (61–74)		
Sex				
Male [n (%)]	388 (69.0)	365 (70.5)		
Female [n (%)]	174 (31.0)	153 (29.5)		
Surgery				
Upper gastrointestinal [n (%)]	385 (68.5)	417 (80.5)		
Lower gastrointestinal [n (%)]	177 (31.5)	101 (19.5)		
Wound complication rate [n (%)]	47 (8.4)	59 (11.5)	0.709 (0.474–1.062)	0.12
Surgical site infection [n (%)]	36 (6.4)	36 (7.0)	0.928 (0.558–1.543)	0.81
Nonsurgical site infection [n (%)]	11 (2.0)	23 (4.5)	0.435 (0.189–0.940)	0.0238
Hypertrophic scar formation [n (%)]	93 (16.7)	111 (21.6)	0.726 (0.528–0.998)	0.0429

[a]Adapted from Tsujinaka and colleagues [4]

upon the type of surgery performed (upper versus lower GI surgery). Significance of subgroup tests was set at alpha = 0.05.

Intention-to-treat analyses (Tables 30.1 and 30.2) revealed wound complications occurred in 8.4% of patients who received subcuticular sutures and 11.5% of patients who received staples ($p = 0.12$). In the subgroup of patients who had upper GI surgery, nonsurgical site infections were lower for patients with subcuticular sutures compared to staples (1.6% versus 4.6%, $p = 0.015$), but there were no differences in surgical site (superficial incision) infections between groups ($p = 0.53$). In the subgroup of patients who had lower GI surgery, significantly fewer patients who had subcuticular sutures experienced overall wound complications (10.2% versus 19.8%, $p = 0.03$) and specifically surgical site infections (7.4% versus 15.8%, $p = 0.04$) compared to those who had staples. Intention-to-treat analyses also revealed significantly lower hypertrophic scar rates in the subcuticular suture group compared to the staples group (16.7% versus 21.6%, $p = 0.043$). This finding was also mirrored in the subgroup of patients who had upper GI surgery (17.3% versus 23.7%, $p = 0.028$).

Appraisal of the Selected Article

You find articles by Sun and colleagues [5] and Dijkman and colleagues [6] that help you appraise the subgroup analysis in Tsujinaka and colleagues' RCT [4]. The credibility of their subgroup analysis can now be critically analyzed on a point-by-point basis (Box 1).

Box 1. Criteria to Assess the Credibility of a Subgroup Analysis

A. **Are the results valid?**

1. Was the subgroup analysis based on rationale indication?
2. Was the subgroup analysis predefined a priori or carried out post hoc?
3. Was the subgroup analysis one of a small number?

Table 30.2 Primary outcomes[a] of patients receiving upper or lower gastrointestinal surgery and skin closure with either subcuticular sutures or staples

	Upper gastrointestinal surgery				Lower gastrointestinal surgery			
	Subcuticular sutures (n = 382)	Staples (n = 413)	Odds ratio (95% CI)	p-value	Subcuticular sutures (n = 176)	Staples (n = 101)	Odds ratio (95% CI)	p-value
Wound complication rate [n (%)]	29 (7.6)	39 (9.4)	0.788 (0.459–1.339)	0.38	18 (10.2)	20 (19.8)	0.463 (0.217–0.978)	0.0301
Surgical site infection [n (%)]	23 (6.0)	20 (4.8)	1.259 (0.649–2.461)	0.53	13 (7.4)	16 (15.8)	0.425 (0.179–0.992)	0.0399
Nonsurgical site infection [n (%)]	6 (1.6)	19 (4.6)	0.331 (0.107–0.875)	0.0149	5 (2.8)	4 (4.0)	0.710 (0.149–3.666)	0.73
Hypertrophic scar formation [n (%)]	66 (17.3)	98 (23.7)	0.672 (0.465–0.965)	0.0282	27 (15.3)	13 (12.9)	1.226 (0.576–2.729)	0.72

[a]Adapted from Tsujinaka and colleagues [4]

4. Did the power calculation account for between-subgroup treatment effects?
5. Was randomization stratified for important subgroup variables?
6. Can chance alone explain the subgroup difference? Were interaction tests used for assessing subgroup treatment effect interactions?
7. Were the significance levels of treatment effect interactions adjusted for multiplicity?
8. Were subgroups checked for comparability of prognostic factors?

B. **What were the results?**

1. Are all performed subgroup analyses reported?
2. Are the subgroup analyses reported as relative risk reductions?
3. Does the emphasis of the discussion and conclusion remain on overall treatment effect?

C. **Will the results help me in caring for my patients in my practice?**

1. Is the subgroup difference consistent across other studies?
2. Is the subgroup effect or interaction clinically important?
3. Are the patients in the subgroup comparable to my patients?

A. **Are the results valid?**

1. *Was the subgroup analysis based on a rationale indication?*

When critically appraising a subgroup analysis, it is important to ensure that the analysis is based upon a logical rationale. If no logical rationale exists, it is difficult for a subgroup analysis to be of practical value regardless of whether the results are statistically significant [1, 7]. Certain patients may be expected to have different treatment effects due to the impact of differences in risk pertaining to a specific outcome or differences in pathophysiology. In these situations, it may be appropriate to separate these patients into subgroups. Unfortunately, Tsujinaka and colleagues [4] do not provide a rationale for the choice of separating patients into the upper and lower GI subgroups. The choice of subgroups would have been more justified if the authors had provided evidence-based hypotheses that the subgroups would differ due to certain characteristics, such as the potential differences in contamination of upper and lower GI surgical sites.

2. *Was the subgroup analysis predefined* a priori *or carried out post hoc?*

Subgroup analyses may be performed prior to or after the initiation of the study, but these analyses should be interpreted differently [1, 8]. Authors should identify and define specific subgroups in the protocol of the RCT a priori, including when the trial is initially registered. Furthermore, both the direction and magnitude of the hypothesized subgroups effect should also be reported a priori. These key steps avoid post hoc interpretations of the data that could bias the authors' conclusions and fit the data retroactively.

Although post hoc analyses may provide important clinical information and considerations, these analyses should be approached with caution [1, 9]. Usually, post hoc analyses may be performed due to the generation of new hypotheses if the original data analyzed produces unexpected results. Since subgroup analyses are generated by the trial data, the difference of treatment effect between subgroups may actually be due to the intervention rather than the subgroup characteristic [8, 9]. Therefore, the credibility of post hoc subgroup hypotheses is low [8, 9].

Tsujinaka and colleagues [4] did not clearly state in the article that they predefined the chosen subgroups. However, they must have defined the subgroups a priori given that they stratified according to the subgroup variable before randomization. This stratification is a useful way to reduce potential bias as it ensures, if the sample is large enough, that the patient characteristics would be balanced in the two trial arms within each subgroup stratum.

3. *Was the subgroup analysis one of a small number?*

The chance of type I error, or falsely obtaining significant subgroup effects and interactions, increases as the number of subgroup analyses increases [9–11]. The number of subgroup analyses is the product of the number of outcome analyses and the number of subgroups created. To mitigate the risk of chance and sampling error, the number of subgroups should be minimized. Furthermore, subgroup analyses should be restricted to the primary outcome of the main RCT as well as the secondary outcomes applicable to specific subgroups. Ensuring subgroup analyses are succinct and meaningful will also aid the authors in delivering a clear message to the readers regarding the findings of the study.

Tsujinaka and colleagues [4] repeat the main effect analyses of the primary (wound complications) and secondary (hypertrophic scar formation) outcomes on the subgroups of patients who had either upper or lower GI surgery. However, subgroups analyses are also applied to the six component outcomes of the overall wound complication rate which increased the number of outcomes analyzed from 2 to 8. Therefore, the results should be interpreted with caution given the increased risk of type I error from the multiple subgroup analyses.

4. *Did the power calculation account for between-subgroup treatment effects?*

The power of a trial is defined as the probability to detect a clinically important difference between two groups if one truly exists. Power is positively associated with the magnitude of the treatment effect as well as the sample size of the study. Usually, sample size calculations for RCTs are based upon a power of at least 80% to detect differences in treatment effect between the primary treatment groups. As a result, subgroup analyses are often underpowered to detect differences in treatment effect due to the much smaller number of participants within each subgroup [6, 7, 9, 12]. To detect interactions of the same size and with the same power as the overall effect, sample sizes should be inflated by four [13]. Furthermore, interaction effects are generally smaller than treatment effects, and thus even larger sample sizes would need to be obtained to demonstrate a statistically significant difference. The much larger sample sizes needed for reliable subgroup analyses are practically challenging to achieve in the clinical setting. When subgroup analyses are underpowered, the results might not be reliable and should be interpreted with caution.

In the trial by Tsujinaka and colleagues [4], the sample size was calculated for a power of 80% to detect an overall treatment effect, but this did not account for the subgroups. Since the authors applied the same statistical tests for each within-subgroup analysis, the same number of patients calculated for the subcuticular suture and staples groups (530) would have been needed for each subgroup to obtain 80% power. Additionally, more patients should have been included in each subgroup to account for the smaller interaction effect. These patient numbers were not achieved in the subgroups. Therefore, the probability of false-negative results was high for the subgroups and the results may not be considered as valid. As such, the conclusions drawn about differences in wound complications and hypertrophic scar formation between the upper and lower GI subgroups should be critically questioned.

5. *Was randomization stratified for important subgroup variables?*

When designing a RCT with predefined subgroups, it is important to stratify randomization by the important subgroups [8]. Stratified randomization maintains the randomization of known and unknown prognostic variables between treatment groups that may influence the treatment effect [14]. Therefore, both type I and II errors may be reduced with stratification. Stratification is especially important to consider in smaller trials, where the risk of differences in prognostic variables and type I error can be high [14]. Since subgroups are by definition smaller than the larger treatment arm groups, clinicians should not assume that prognostic variables between groups are similar at baseline unless stratification has taken place with randomization [14]. Since randomization ensures subgroups are similar with the exception of treatment, valid conclusions can be made about the treatment efficacy within subgroups. Tsujinaka and colleagues [4] performed stratified randomization according to the subgroup variable (e.g., upper or lower GI surgery).

6. *Can chance alone explain the subgroup difference? Were interaction tests used for assessing subgroup treatment effect interactions?*

Investigators and clinicians may be misled by the underappreciated potential of chance to influence the results of a trial [1, 9]. Tests for interaction can help determine whether the differences in effects may be explained by chance alone, where the null hypothesis of this test is that no difference exists in the true effect between subgroups. The lower the p-value, the more likely the null hypothesis can be rejected. Therefore, rather than just considering a threshold of significance (e.g., alpha < 0.05), clinicians may opt to consider the p-value where the null hypothesis is increasingly likely to be false as the criterion level of alpha gets progressively smaller [11].

Tsujinaka and colleagues [4] analyzed the subgroups with logistic regression to assess for statistical interactions between treatments.

7. *Were the significance levels of treatment effect interactions adjusted for multiplicity?*

There is an increased probability of detecting a positive finding caused by chance alone as the number of subgroup analyses increases [8, 11]. Therefore, it is important to adjust within-subgroup treatment effects for multiplicity when multiple subgroup analyses are performed concurrently. For example, the Bonferroni method adjusts for multiplicity by dividing the overall significance level (e.g., 0.05) by the total number of subgroup analyses (e.g., 10). As a result, a new significance level for each subgroup analysis is calculated (e.g., 0.005).

Tsujinaka and colleagues [4] did not make adjustments for multiplicity. Therefore, readers should be aware of the potential increase in type I error risk.

8. *Were the subgroups checked for comparability of prognostic factors?*

Despite randomization and stratification (if applicable), differences in prognostic variables may still exist between subgroups due to chance [6]. As such, it is helpful to evaluate the subgroups for differences in prognostic variables after randomization, especially if those prognostic variables are believed to bias the treatment effect. If subgroups are not similar with regards to specific prognostic variables, the investigators should clearly acknowledge this to caution readers regarding the interpretation of certain results.

Tsujinaka and colleagues [4] did not comment on differences in prognostic variables between subgroups. Therefore, this information is unknown.

B. **What were the results?**

1. *Are all performed subgroup analyses reported?*

Since the probability of a positive finding due to chance increases with the number of subgroup analyses performed [8, 11], the validity of a subgroup analysis is dependent on how many other subgroup analyses were performed but not reported [8]. Investigators may selectively report only statistically significant subgroup analyses [15]. As a result, clinicians may incorrectly conclude a difference in treatment effect due to believing the results are more reliable than what they actually are (see Chap. 6).

Tsujinaka and colleagues [4] registered their RCT with UMIN-CTR (a clinical trials registry; UMIN000002480). You enter the study number into the registry website in hopes that you can review the RCT protocol. Unfortunately, this type of detail is not available on the website, and therefore you cannot be sure that all subgroup analyses were reported.

2. *Are subgroup analyses reported as relative risk reductions?*

The magnitude of treatment effect can be presented via either absolute or relative risk reduction [6]. Absolute risk reduction (ARR) pertains to the difference in absolute risk for a particular outcome between the treatment groups being analyzed. Meanwhile, relative risk reduction (RRR) provides an estimation of risk that is removed by the treatment of interest.

RRR may be more appropriate to use when describing subgroup effects as RRR tends to be more similar across risk groups compared to ARR [16, 17]. For example, the ARR of a given treatment cannot be large if the patient already has a low baseline risk. Likewise, a patient with a high baseline risk may have a large ARR following a particular treatment. Therefore, although the ARR may be different for these two groups, the RRR may actually be similar in value for both groups. Clearly, readers may conclude that there is a significant treatment effect between subgroups if ARR is only considered, when, in fact, similar RRR between subgroups indicate that no difference exists.

In the study by Tsujinaka and colleagues [4], odds ratios were reported for the primary and secondary outcomes as well as for the subgroup analyses (Tables 30.1 and 30.2). No risk reductions are reported for the subgroups, but a calculation can be made by the reader using the percentages from the tables.

3. *Does the emphasis of the discussion and conclusion remain on overall treatment effect?*

Interestingly, industry-funded studies are more likely to perform and present subgroup analyses when the primary outcomes have null findings [15]. Tsujinaka and colleagues [4] performed an industry-funded study with a null finding that showed no differences in wound complications in patients receiving subcuticular sutures compared to staples in GI surgery. As suggested by Sun and colleagues [15], this null finding may have persuaded Tsujinaka and colleagues [4] to perform post hoc subgroup analyses to discover other potentially significant results.

The results of subgroup analyses are used in more than 25% of RCTs to support the conclusions of the studies [18]. However, due to the exploratory nature of subgroup analyses, discussions regarding these results should be limited and should not affect the conclusion of a trial [2]. Tsujinaka and colleagues [4] used nearly half of the text within the discussion to outline the results of the subgroup analyses. However, the authors remained true to the primary objective of their study and did not use the subgroup analyses to influence the conclusion. Instead, the conclusion is clear and the emphasis is placed on the fact that subcuticular sutures are not superior to staples in GI surgery.

C. **Will the results help me in caring for my patients in my practice?**

1. *Is the subgroup difference consistent across other studies?*

Subgroup analyses are far more credible when the subgroup interaction effect is consistent across multiple studies [9, 11]. However, it is difficult to compare subgroup analyses across studies. Since subgroups can be small, a lack of power and unreliable results may be an issue [6]. Furthermore, as it is common for surgical studies to vary greatly with regards to study design, populations, interventions, and outcomes, it can be very challenging to compare these studies and achieve meaningful results [6].

Tsujinaka and colleagues [4] report their RCT to be the first to evaluate subcuticular sutures versus staples for Class 2 (clean-contaminated) surgery. Your review of the literature did not find any additional studies regarding this particular topic.

2. *Is the subgroup effect or interaction clinically important?*

Readers may determine whether the observed subgroup effects or interactions are clinically important based on a variety of factors. For instance, the subgroup analysis should be based on a rational indication, the treatment or intervention being evaluated should be frequently provided to patients, the subgroup variables should be commonly used, and the outcomes presented should be clinically meaningful [6]. By ensuring these factors exist, subgroup analyses become clinically meaningful and applicable to the patient groups of the targeted audience (e.g., surgeons). Ideally, the results of similar subgroup analyses should also be replicated in future studies.

Tsujinaka and colleagues [4] selected the subgroups and performed the subgroup analyses with clinically important results. Subcuticular sutures and staples are both commonly used in multiple surgical specialties. Upper and lower GI surgeries are commonly performed by general surgeons throughout the world. Furthermore, wound complications and scarring are important patient outcomes in any surgical procedure. Therefore, the authors presented subgroup analyses that were clinically important to the intended audience of surgeons.

3. *Are the patients in the subgroup comparable to my patients?*

To determine whether a subgroup of patients presented in a study is comparable to your own group of patients, readers should critically assess the patient characteristics within the subgroup of interest [6]. These characteristics are usually defined within the presented patient demographics as well as the inclusion and exclusion criteria of the RCT. Due to the strict inclusion and exclusion criteria of RCTs, differences between patients from a RCT and the patients in a reader's practice are likely to exist. Therefore, readers must be cautious when making generalized conclusions from a particular study and applying these conclusions to their patients.

In the clinical scenario outlined at the beginning of this article, the patient is a 65-year-old woman recently diagnosed with cancer of the cecum who is planning to undergo a right hemicolectomy. The results of Tsujinaka and colleagues [4] subgroup analyses of patients with lower GI surgery could be applied to the patient in the clinical scenario if she was otherwise healthy with no major comorbidities, steroid use, or abdominal surgeries prior to her cancer diagnosis.

Resolution of the Scenario

After reading the article by Tsujinaka and colleagues [4], you conclude that although subcuticular sutures are not significantly different from staples with regards to wound complications in GI surgery, subcuticular sutures may be superior with regards to hypertrophic scar formation. You reach this conclusion based upon the overall study results, as it was a methodologically sound RCT with sufficient power to detect the overall treatment effect. However, you are uncertain with regards to the credibility of the subgroup analyses as these analyses were underpowered and had no adjustment for multiplicity. Therefore, you conclude that there is unlikely a difference in surgical scars, surgical site infections, and other wound complications between subcuticular sutures and staples in upper versus lower GI surgery.

Appendix 1

Search results for the following search strategy: "subcuticular suture AND staple AND gastrointestinal surgery AND infection AND scar AND randomized controlled trials".

1. Tsujinaka T, Yamamoto K, Fujita J, Endo S, Kawada J, Nakahira S, Shimokawa T, Kobayashi S, Yamasaki M, Akamaru Y, Miyamoto A, Mizushima T, Shimizu J, Umeshita K, Ito T, Doki Y, Mori M. Subcuticular sutures versus staples for skin closure after open gastrointestinal surgery: a phase 3, multicentre, open-label, randomized controlled trial. Lancet. 2013;382:1105–12.
2. Tanaka A, Sadahiro S, Suzuki T, Okada K, Saito G. Randomized controlled trial comparing subcuticular absorbable suture with conventional interrupted suture for wound closure at elective operation of colon cancer. Surgery. 2014;155(3):486–92.

References

1. Sun X, Ioannidis JP, Agoritsas T, Alba AC, Guyatt G. How to use a subgroup analysis: users' guide to the medical literature. JAMA. 2014;311:405–11.
2. Sun X, Briel M, Busse JW, You JJ, Akl EA, Mejza F, Bala MM, Bassler D, Mertz D, Diaz-Granados N, Vandvik PO, Malaga G, Srinathan SK, Dahm P, Johnston BC, Alonso-Coello P, Hassouneh B, Walter SD, Heels-Ansdell D, Bhatnagar N, Altman DG, Guyatt GH. Credibility of claims of subgroup effects in randomised controlled trials: systematic review. BMJ. 2012;344:e1553.
3. ISIS-2 (Second International Study of Infarct Survival) Collaborative Group. Randomised trial of intravenous streptokinase, oral aspirin, both, or neither among 17,187 cases of suspected acute myocardial infarction: ISIS-2. Lancet 1988;2: 349–60.
4. Tsujinaka T, Yamamoto K, Fujita J, Endo S, Kawada J, Nakahira S, Shimokawa T,

Kobayashi S, Yamasaki M, Akamaru Y, Miyamoto A, Mizushima T, Shimizu J, Umeshita K, Ito T, Doki Y, Mori M. Subcuticular sutures versus staples for skin closure after open gastrointestinal surgery: a phase 3, multicentre, open-label, randomised controlled trial. Lancet. 2013;382:1105–12.
5. Sun X, Briel M, Walter SD, Guyatt GH. Is a subgroup effect believable? Updating criteria to evaluate the credibility of subgroup analyses. BMJ. 2010;340:c117.
6. Dijkman B, Kooistra B, Bhandari M. Evidence-based surgery working group. How to work with a subgroup analysis. Can J Surg. 2009;52:515–22.
7. Oxman AD, Guyatt GH. A consumer's guide to subgroup analyses. Ann Intern Med. 1992;116: 78–84.
8. Rothwell PM. Treating individuals 2. Subgroup analysis in randomised controlled trials: importance, indications, and interpretation. Lancet 2005;365:176–86.
9. Guyatt G, Wyer P, Ioannidis J. When to believe a subgroup analysis. In: Guyatt G, Drummond R, Meade MO, et al., editors. User's guides to the medical literature: a manual for evidence-based clinical practice. 2nd ed. Toronto (ON): McGraw-Hill; 2008. p. 571–93.
10. Buyse ME. Analysis of clinical trial outcomes: some comments on subgroup analyses. Control Clin Trials. 1989;10:187S–94S.
11. Sun X, Heels-Ansdell D, Sprague S, Bandhari M, Walter SD, Sanders D, Schemitsch E, Tornetta P III, Swiontkowski M, Guyatt G. Is a subgroup claim believable? A user's guide to subgroup analyses in the surgical literature. J Bone Joint Surg Am. 2011;93:e8.
12. Yusuf S, Wittes J, Probstfield J, Tyroler HA. Analysis and interpretation of treatment effects in subgroups of patients in randomized clinical trials. JAMA. 1991;266:93–8.
13. Brookes ST, Whitely E, Egger M, Smith GD, Mulheran PA, Peters TJ. Subgroup analyses in randomized trials: risks of subgroup-specific analyses; power and sample size for the interaction test. J Clin Epidemiol. 2004;57:229–36.
14. Kernan WN, Viscoli CM, Makuch RW, Brass LM, Horwitz RI. Stratified randomization for clinical trials. J Clin Epidemiol. 1999;52:19–26.
15. Sun X, Briel M, Busse JW, You JJ, Akl EA, Mejza F, Bala MM, Bassler D, Mertz D, Diaz-Granados N, Vandvik PO, Malaga G, Srinathan SK, Dahm P, Johnston BC, Alonso-Coello P, Hassouneh B, Truong J, Dattani ND, Walter SD, Heels-Ansdell D, Bhatnagar N, Altman DG, Guyatt GH. The influence of study characteristics on reporting of subgroup analyses in randomised controlled trials: systematic review. BMJ. 2011;342:d1569.
16. Furukawa TA. From effect size into number needed to treat. Lancet. 1999;353:1680.
17. Schmid CH, Lau J, McIntosh MW, Cappelleri JC. An empirical study of the effect of the control rate as a predictor of treatment efficacy in meta-analysis of clinical trials. Stat Med. 1998;17:1923–42.
18. Assmann SF, Pocock SJ, Enos LE, Kasten LE. Subgroup analysis and other (mis)uses of baseline data in clinical trials. Lancet. 2000;355:1064–9.

Introduction to Clinical Practice Guidelines

31

Christopher J. Coroneos, Stavros A. Antoniou, Ivan D. Florez and Melissa C. Brouwers

Introduction

Clinical practice guidelines (CPGs) are systematically developed statements aimed to optimize patient care and experience; they are informed by a systematic review of evidence and an assessment of the benefits and harms of alternative care options [1, 2]. In addition to supporting the clinical encounter, CPGs can inform clinical policy and access to care options (e.g., equipment and technology to support surgical procedures, support quality improvement activities, or to fund drugs). By condensing a large body of evidence into a high-yield resource, CPGs can serve as useful educational tools for trainees and established clinicians wanting to keep their knowledge current. CPGs can identify where research gaps exist by identifying areas where the quantity of evidence is insufficient or where the quality of evidence is so weak that additional studies are warranted to enable clear actionable recommendations. And just as important, they can promote collaboration and build capacity among the interdisciplinary teams involved in their development. CPGs are not simply technical research documents that signal clinical actions that surgeons should perform; the processes of CPG development, evaluation, and implementation are social ones that contribute to establishing and sustaining an evidence-informed culture [3].

The promise of CPGs is only as good as their quality [4, 5]. Poor quality CPGs can be biased and lead to recommendations that are of poor quality, not effective, potentially harmful, or difficult to implement; this is particularly relevant to surgical guidelines [6]. In assessing the quality of CPGs in surgery, a number of unique factors are considered. External validity often cannot be assessed because of poor reporting of personnel and material resources that impact implementation (e.g., surgeon experience, institutional resources, healthcare infrastructure). Subsequently, authors rarely provide guidance on how

C. J. Coroneos (✉)
Division of Plastic Surgery, McMaster University, Hamilton, ON, Canada
e-mail: coronec@mcmaster.ca

S. A. Antoniou
Department of Surgery, Royal Devon and Exeter NHS Foundation Trust, Exeter, UK

I. D. Florez
Department of Pediatrics, University of Antioquia, Medellin, Colombia

I. D. Florez
Department of Health Research Methods, Evidence and Impact, McMaster University, Hamilton, ON, Canada

M. C. Brouwers
School of Epidemiology and Public Health, University of Ottawa, Ottawa, ON, Canada
e-mail: mbrouwer@mcmaster.ca

M. C. Brouwers
Department of Oncology, McMaster University, Hamilton, ON, Canada

A. Thoma et al. (eds.), *Evidence-Based Surgery*,
https://doi.org/10.1007/978-3-030-05120-4_31

CPGs can be implemented into practice [5, 6]. The lack of RCTs in surgery poses a methodological challenge to quality requiring developers to use and risk overrating, observational studies. Furthermore, potential conflicts of interest and sources of funding are not reported in as many as 90% of surgical CPGs [6].

What is the current status of surgical CPGs? The 2018 report on the appraisal of English-language CPGs produced by surgical societies using the AGREE II instrument revealed that while there are successes there are many opportunities for improvement [7]. Specifically, using the AGREE II (a tool used to assess the quality of CPGs that we will describe later in the chapter), 67 eligible CPGs were evaluated. A total of 27 CPG (40%) were considered not suitable for use. Most of the domains evaluated by the AGREE II got scores of less than 50% of the maximum possible score. CPGs that were developed by groups who produced more than 9 documents within a 10-year period, that were developed in a committee structure, and that used GRADE (Grading of Recommendations Assessment, Development and Evaluation approach) [8, 9] operational methods were more apt to be recommended or achieve scores above 50% [7].

To help mitigate the risk of poor quality CPGs, interdisciplinary teams of the AGREE Enterprise (Appraisal of Guidelines, REsearch and Evaluation), an international program of CPG research, have used evidence-based methods to produce a collection of tools to support the development, reporting and evaluation of CPGs and their recommendations [4, 10, 11]. In this chapter, we provide a practical snapshot of the AGREE II and the AGREE REX, two of the tools in the portfolio, and describe how the surgical community can use these tools to differentiate the quality of existing CPGs, to help prioritize relevant CPGs for adoption, and to inform the development and reporting of their own CPGs. We will use the questions posed in these tools to help structure the discussion.

Clinical Scenario

You are a general surgeon practicing breast surgical oncology at a midlevel center. You are comanaging a patient with breast cancer with your colleagues in plastic and reconstructive surgery. The patient is 45 years old, with Stage I disease. She is planned for skin-sparing mastectomy, sentinel lymph node biopsy, and immediate abdominally based tissue free flap reconstruction. The total length of surgery is expected to be 8 h. She has normal body weight, and otherwise healthy with the exception of a family history of venous thromboembolism (VTE) and known Factor V Leiden mutation discovered after multiple miscarriages. To support your decision-making process, you decide to review the literature to find guideline recommendations on the most effective and safest surgical management as it relates to her risk of VTE.

Literature Search

You proceed with a PubMed search, entering terms “VTE prophylaxis surgery cancer”, and selecting the “guideline” article type filter, “5 years” publication dates filter, and “English” language filter. Your search yields five reports. Two of the results focus on Asian patient populations [12, 13] and two other results focus on head and neck cancer [14] and gynecology patient populations [15]. You select the article by Lyman et al. entitled “*Venous Thromboembolism Prophylaxis And Treatment In Patients With Cancer: American Society Of Clinical Oncology Clinical Practice Guideline Update*”, an updated CPG [16]. In contrast to the other options, the ASCO CPG is current, its questions and scope align with your clinical questions, and ASCO has a reputation of being a credible and high-quality source of information [16]. You also find the website of the American Society for Clinical Oncology (ASCO), as directed in the paper, to look up supporting materials to this publication [17].

Appraisal of Clinical Practice Guidelines: AGREE II and AGREE-REX Tools

The AGREE II is reliable and valid CPG evaluation tool, and a foundation for CPG development and reporting (Table 31.1) [4, 10, 11]. Comprising of 23 items in six domains, the AGREE II targets the whole CPG process—the "who", the "what", the "how", and the "where". Each item is scored on a 7-point score with higher scores for CPGs reflecting more of the quality criteria that define the time. Domain scores are calculated by adding all the scores of the individual items in a domain (or the consensus score) and by scaling the total as a percentage of the maximum possible score. When consensus methods are not used to arrive at an agreed-up score, four independent raters should be used to optimize inter-rater reliability (r's across domains >0.7) [10]. The AGREE II successfully differentiates among CPGs of varying quality [4].

The AGREE-REX is a tool in the final stages of development that comprises nine items in three themes (Table 31.2) [18]. The AGREE-REX focuses specifically on the quality of the CPG *recommendations*. The AGREE II and AGREE-REX are complementary resources. As with the AGREE II, each item is scored on a 7-point scale. There is also an optional scale to assess the suitability of the recommendations for use in another setting. The scoring system of the AGREE-REX mirrors that of the AGREE II. AGREE II can be used to determine if a CPG or set of CPGs meets the minimum standards of

Table 31.1 AGREE II—High-quality CPGs features [4, 8, 9]

AGREE II domain	AGREE II item
Scope and purpose	1. The overall objective(s) of the guideline is (are) specifically described 2. The health question(s) covered by the guideline is (are) specifically described 3. The population (patients, public) to whom the guideline is meant to apply is specifically described
Stakeholder involvement	4. The guideline development group includes individuals from all relevant professional groups 5. The views and preferences of the target population (patients, public) have been sought 6. The target users of the guideline are clearly defined
Rigour of development	7. Systematic methods were used to search for evidence 8. The criteria for selecting the evidence are clearly described 9. The strengths and limitations of the body of evidence are clearly described 10. The methods for formulating the recommendations are clearly described 11. The health benefits, side effects, and risks have been considered in formulating the recommendations 12. There is an explicit link between the recommendations and the supporting evidence 13. The guideline has been externally reviewed by experts prior to its publication 14. A procedure for updating the guideline is provided
Clarity of presentation	15. The recommendations are specific and unambiguous 16. The different options for management of the condition or health issue are clearly presented 17. Key recommendations are easily identifiable
Applicability	18. The guideline describes facilitators and barriers to its application 19. The guideline provides advice or tools on how the recommendations can be put into practice 20. The potential resource implications of applying the recommendations have been considered 21. The guideline presents monitoring or auditing criteria
Editorial independence	22. The views of the funding body have not influenced the content of the guideline 23. Competing interests of guideline development group members have been recorded and addressed

Table 31.2 AGREE-REX—High-quality recommendations features [4]

AGREE-REX domain	AGREE-REX item
Clinical applicability	1. Evidence 2. Clinical relevance 3. Patients/population relevance
Values	4. Target user 5. Patient/population 6. Policy 7. Guideline developer
Implementability	8. Purpose 9. Local applicability and adoption

methodological quality. The AGREE-REX can be used to determine if a recommendation or set of recommendations meets the minimum standards of clinical quality, appropriateness, and implementability. The appraisal of a CPG involves evaluating its validity, interpreting the results, and applying study findings clinically (Box 1). In Box 2, readers can find a short list of useful resources and websites with more information and tools related to Guidelines development and evaluation.

Box 1: Framework for the Appraisal of Surgical Clinical Practice Guidelines

I. **Are the Results Valid?**
   i. What is the scope and purpose of the CPG?
   ii. Is stakeholder involvement considered?
   iii. Is the CPG methodologically rigorous?
   iv. Is the CPG development process independent?

II. **What Are the Results?**
   i. Are quality recommendations presented?
   ii. How is the CPG presented?

III. **How Can I Apply the Results to Patient Care?**

Box 2: Additional Resources for Readers

AGREE collaboration	https://www.agreetrust.org
GRADE Working Group	http://www.gradeworkinggroup.org
Guidelines International Network	https://www.g-i-n.net/home
The National Academies of Science Engineering and medicine book: "Guidelines we can trust"	http://www.nationalacademies.org/hmd/Reports/2011/Clinical-Practice-Guidelines-We-Can-Trust.aspx

Are the Results Valid?

i. **What is the scope and purpose of the CPG?**

When evaluating or developing a guideline, readers should look for a concise statement of its aim, what specific health questions will be addressed, and the patient populations for whom it is meant to apply. This is particularly important if your goal is to use an existing guideline to help in your own clinical practice or to inform clinical policies that might be relevant to you and your colleagues. Is the particular guideline you are considering relevant to your clinical challenge? PICOH (patient(s), intervention(s), comparison (s), outcome(s), health care setting) framed questions can inform this decision. It is important for all clinicians to think about the CPG questions and patient populations not solely with the lens determining if there is a direct alignment with the clinical activities they might perform but rather with the lens if the scope aligns with patients with whom they might be involved with somewhere in the course of the care trajectory. For example, when considering the surgical ablative and reconstructive aspects of breast cancer, surgeons must consider the timing of neoadjuvant/adjuvant chemotherapy and adjuvant radiotherapy. Procedures must be timed with the consideration of the entire scope of cancer management, and adjuvant therapy if indicated may have a negative effect on immediate reconstruction. In our ASCO CPG scenario, Lyman et al. address questions on the role of anticoagulation for VTE prophylaxis in different clinical contexts (hospitalized patients, ambulatory patients, patients undergoing surgery) but also on the timing and duration of the regimen and patients' knowledge [16].

ii. **Is stakeholder involvement considered?**

This AGREE II quality domain focuses on who is involved in the development of the guideline, who is the guideline designed for, and how patients are involved in the process. A multidisciplinary guideline development team comprised of clinicians, methodologists, and patients ensures appropriate methodological, content, and experiential perspectives are "at the table". This serves as a strategy to mitigate bias, and enable debate and the thoughtful contextualization of the evidence to inform the recommendations. Patient involvement is of great importance; authors rarely report patient-important outcomes in systematic reviews [19]. Having surgeons involved in guideline generation is important to the group. While opinion leaders have a small but measurable effect on physicians [20], it is magnified among surgeons [21]. Thus, surgeons' participation can play a key role for the development of the CPG but also for the adoption of the recommendations. In our ASCO CPG example, Lyman et al. [16] cite a multidisciplinary panel composed of medical oncology, surgery, community oncology, patient/advocacy representation, and guideline implementation under the ASCO Clinical Practice Guidelines Committee (CPGC). A linked supplement discusses the role of specific members, content experts, and patient representatives.

iii. **Is the CPG methodologically rigorous?**

This is often seen as the most important CPG quality dimension in the AGREE II tool. High-quality guidelines use systematic review as an evidentiary foundation. Chapter 15 discusses the key issues and methodological steps of systematic reviews. High-quality study designs such as randomized controlled trials (RCTs) can make the development of CPG recommendations more straightforward. However, RCTs are not required to make CPGs. Most important are the methods by which the evidence base is constructed—how studies are searched, selected, appraised, and synthesized. Methods to reduce bias and provide the guideline team a valid and credible source of information on which to make judgments are key, even in the absence of RCTs. High-quality methods to interpret the evidence and come to consensus on final recommendations ensure that the results are transparent, credible, and fair. In the absence of high level evidence provided by RCTs, CPG developers may be tempted to lower the threshold for providing strong recommendations. Guideline users need to assess the link between recommendations and supporting evidence before clinical implementation. GRADE strategies to evaluate the body of evidence and the Evidence to Decision Framework are popular methods that reflect the quality expectations and criteria in the "Rigour" domain [8, 22]. In the ASCO CPG example, Lyman et al. describe a thorough methodology, including literature search, rigorous study selection criteria, specific data abstraction, evaluation of study quality, and summarized data tables [16, 17]. For example, RCTs and systematic reviews of RCTs including at least 50 patients per intervention were included in the development of this evidence-base.

iv. **Is the CPG development process independent?**

Editorial independence from the funding body and being explicit about the competing interests of CPG authors are essential to maintaining the credibility of the document and reducing real or perceived conflicts of interest. Interest groups may differ in their motivations, and subsequently in their interpretation of a body of evidence [23]. For example, a patient-focused cancer interest group may support the introduction of a new population screening program, whereas public health interest groups do not believe it is cost-effective [7]. CPG panels should not only declare all the potential interests related to the interventions or topics addressed in the CPG but also they should make explicit the way the identified conflicts were analyzed and handled. Lastly, the potential impact of the CPG funding organization may have on the content of the guideline.

The ASCO CPG program has a publicly available Competing Interests Policy [17]. The Lyman et al. [16] CPG provides links to the policy and provides a complete listing of author competing interests. While there are not gold standards for managing competing interests, the transparency provides users with information from which to make judgments. Conflicts of interest for individual authors are listed at the end of the Lyman et al. [16] CPG: none were employed by, or owned stock with a relevant corporation, five authors acted in a consulting or advisory role, three authors received honoraria, and five authors received research funding.

What Are the Results?

i. **Are quality recommendations presented?**

High-quality recommendations are those that are clinically relevant, consider the values of stakeholders, and that are implementable. Recommendations will be relevant if they address a clinical/health problem that is important to the target user (e.g., physicians, nurses), provide actionable guidance appropriate to their scope of practice and the patients they see, and will result in clinical changes that are important to their patients. In the ASCO CPG [16], the recommendations specified the patient population and only considered research evidence that addressed the primary outcome, prevention of VTE.

Consideration of the values of different stakeholders is a defining feature of high-quality recommendations. Stakeholders include a broad range of actors including target users (e.g., clinicians), patients, policy makers, and the CPG developers themselves (see Table 31.2, Values domain). For example, patients' values and preferences can influence the acceptability of the recommended action, and the role of the patient in the shared decision-making process. Understanding CPG developer values provides users information about the relative importance of different factors (e.g., the priority of different outcomes) and how CPG developers managed situation when values between other parties did not align. This aspect was not explicitly addressed by Lyman et al. [16].

Finally, the benefits of CPGs will only be realized if recommendations are put into practice. The implementability of CPG recommendations requires an alignment between the actual recommendations and the goal(s) of the CPG. For example, are the recommendations intended to be adopted immediately or are they to be used to leverage clinical policy or funding decisions with the goal of eventual access to the care option. Tools to support their adoption also reflect high-quality recommendations. The ASCO CPG has derivative products such as slide decks (for clinicians and consumers), patient information page, example order sets, and the like. These tools facilitate the operationalization of the recommendations in practice.

Lyman et al. [16] provide relevant recommendations addressing our clinical scenario, including: (i) "*3.1: All patients with malignant disease undergoing major surgical intervention should be considered for pharmacologic thrombopro-phylaxis with either UFH or LMWH unless contraindicated because of active bleeding or high bleeding risk*", (ii) "*3.2: Prophylaxis should be commenced preoperatively*", (iii) "*3.4: A combined regimen of pharmacologic and mechanical prophylaxis may improve efficacy, especially in the highest-risk patients*", and (iv) "*3.5: Pharmacologic thromboprophylaxis for patients undergoing major surgery for cancer should be continued for at least 7–10 days. Extended prophylaxis with LMWH for up to 4 weeks postoperatively should be considered for... additional risk factors*".

ii. **How is the CPG presented?**

Presentation is not a quality dimension intended to make guideline "look pretty"; information and recommendations should be easily identifiable, transparent, and explicit. Ensuring guideline users know what actions to take, for what patients, in what circumstances, and with what caveats and qualifying factors provide the foundation for optimized care. For example, the use of "Bottom Line" section in the ASCO CPG provides users with concise advice that is comprised of easy to find recommended clinical actions [16, 17]. For example, *"Patients undergoing major cancer surgery should receive prophylaxis starting before surgery and continuing for at least 7–10 days*", and "*Extending postoperative prophylaxis up to 4 weeks should be considered in those with high-risk features*". The full report also provides a summary of original and updated recommendations for each question so that the reader can more clearly understand where changes to current clinical practices are required.

How Can I Apply the Results to Patient Care?

Appropriate engagement, sound methods, and evidence-informed recommendations are important but not sufficient to facilitate adoption. Understanding factors that may impede or facilitate uptake and the provisions of resources and tools to enable adoption are part of an overall quality agenda; a point often overlooked in surgery [24]. Recommendations should be structured for both academic or community level practice, stratified for risk, and integrated into normal workflow across different settings and context [25–28]. Adapting guidelines to a local setting is important in overcoming surgeon behavior [29]. These considerations are especially true when considering VTE prophylaxis [30]. Finally, readers should remember that structured processes exist to modify and tailor to an existing guideline to a local setting [31]. The entire CPG does not need to be adopted; the guideline can be adapted to answer specific questions, and suit needs and resources of a different setting without undermining its validity. The ASCO CPG provides recommendations that are transferable to a variety of practices that do not require specific settings, resources, or additional personnel to implement. The interventions described, both mechanical and pharmacologic, are available at any center [16, 17].

Resolution of Clinical Scenario

You appraise the CPG by Lyman et al. and discuss it with your colleagues at your next multidisciplinary clinic [16, 17]. You believe that the guideline is suitable for its use and the specific recommendations are applicable to your patient. As per the recommendations, you decide to use preoperative low molecular weight heparin as is routine at your institution, but add concomitant mechanical prophylaxis with intraoperative lower extremity sequential compression device. You intend to continue your patient's DVT prophylaxis while admitted postoperatively, again, as is routine at your institution. However, you also plan to refer your patient for a hematology consultation with the Thrombosis service specifically to manage DVT prophylaxis after hospital discharge for a total of four weeks. You intend to discuss the guideline at your hospital's next quality improvement rounds, with the intention of adapting it locally for breast reconstruction patients in the future, including predefined criteria for hematology/thrombosis consultation, preoperative dosing timing, specific pharmacologic prophylaxis medications and dosing, and predefined duration of pharmacologic prophylaxis in routine patients.

Conclusions

Considerable effort has been dedicated to creating tools to support clinicians' efforts to differentiate between high and low-quality CPGs and recommendations and to be able to create high-quality CPGs. Surgeons need to remember that CPGs are distinct from the compulsory steps in more familiar clinical pathways. Practically, they should be used as tools to facilitate surgical decision-making, by interpreting the evidence for options, and balancing risks and benefits. From a broader system perspective in surgery, CPGs influence policy by demonstrating strengths and limitations in the evidence base, and defining cost effective interventions, resource allocation, and quality indicators. In this chapter, we apply two internationally recognized tools designed to achieve this goal—the AGREE II and the AGREE-REX. The surgical community is encouraged to take advantage of the existing tools and to create opportunities for improvement as they continue to build a strong evidence-informed culture.

References

1. Steinberg E, Greenfield S, Wolman DM, Mancher M, Graham R. Clinical practice guidelines we can trust. National Academies Press; 2011.
2. Qaseem AF, Frode; Macbeth F, Ollenschläger G, Phillips S, van der Wees P. Guidelines international network: toward international standards for clinical practice guidelines. Ann Intern Med. 2012;156 (7):525–31.
3. Browman GP, Brouwers M, Fervers B, Sawka C. Population-based cancer control and the role of guidelines-Towards a "systems" approach. Cancer control. 2010;1.
4. Brouwers MC, Kho ME, Browman GP, Burgers JS, Cluzeau F, Feder G, et al. Development of the AGREE II, part 2: assessment of validity of items and tools to support application. Can Med Assoc J. 2010;182(10):E472–8.
5. Brouwers MC, Rawski E, Spithoff K, Oliver TK, McGlynn, Schuster, et al. Inventory of cancer guidelines: a tool to advance the guideline enterprise and improve the uptake of evidence. Expert Rev Pharmacoeconomics & Outcomes Res. 2011;11(2):151–61.
6. Antoniou SA, Tsokani S, Mavridis D, López-Cano M, Antoniou GA, Stefanidis D, et al. Guideline assessment project: filling the GAP in surgical guidelines. Ann Surg. 2018, https://doi.org/10.1097/SLA.0000000000003036 (Epub ahead of print).
7. Shaneyfelt TM, Mayo-Smith MF, Rothwangl J. Are guidelines following guidelines?: The methodological quality of clinical practice guidelines in the peer-reviewed medical literature. JAMA. 1999;281 (20):1900–5.
8. Guyatt GH, Oxman AD, Vist GE, Kunz R, Falck-Ytter Y, Alonso-Coello P, et al. GRADE: an emerging consensus on rating quality of evidence and strength of recommendations. BMJ (Clin Res ed). 2008;336(7650):924–6.
9. Guyatt G, Oxman AD, Akl EA, Kunz R, Vist G, Brozek J, et al. GRADE guidelines: 1. Introduction—GRADE evidence profiles and summary of findings tables. J Clin Epidemiol. 2011;64(4):383–94.
10. Brouwers MC, Kho ME, Browman GP, Burgers JS, Cluzeau F, Feder G, et al. Development of the AGREE II, part 1: performance, usefulness and areas for improvement. Can Med Assoc J. 2010;182 (10):1045–52.
11. Brouwers MC, Kho ME, Browman GP, Burgers JS, Cluzeau F, Feder G, et al. AGREE II: advancing guideline development, reporting and evaluation in health care. Can Med Assoc J. 2010;182(18):E839–42.
12. Liew NC, Alemany GV, Angchaisuksiri P, Bang S-M, Choi G, De DS, et al. Asian venous thromboembolism guidelines: updated recommendations for the prevention of venous thromboembolism. Int Angiol: J Int Union Angiol. 2017;36(1):1–20.
13. Bang S-M, Jang MJ, Kim KH, Yhim H-Y, Kim Y-K, Nam S-H, et al. Prevention of venous thromboembolism: Korean society of thrombosis and hemostasis evidence-based clinical practice guidelines. J Korean Med Sci. 2014;29(2):164–71.
14. Robson A, Sturman J, Williamson P, Conboy P, Penney S, Wood H. Pre-treatment clinical assessment in head and neck cancer: United Kingdom National multidisciplinary guidelines. J Laryngol Otol. 2016;130(S2):S13–22.
15. Piróg MM, Jach R, Undas A. Thromboprophylaxis in women undergoing gynecological surgery or assisted reproductive techniques: new advances and challenges. Ginekol Pol. 2016;87(11):773–9.
16. Lyman GH, Bohlke K, Falanga A. Venous thromboembolism prophylaxis and treatment in patients with cancer: American society of clinical oncology

clinical practice guideline update. J Oncol Pract. 2015;11(3):e442–4.
17. American Society of Clinical Oncology. Venous Thromboembolism Prophylaxis and Treatment in Patients With Cancer Update, 2018 [July 30, 2018]. Available from: https://www.asco.org/practice-guidelines/quality-guidelines/guidelines/supportive-care-and-treatment-related-issues#/9911.
18. Brouwers MC, Spithoff K, Florez ID, Kerkvliet K, Alonso-Coello P, Burgers J, et al. The development of the AGREE-REX (Appraisal of Guidelines Research and Evaluation—Recommendations excellence). A tool to assess the credibility, trustworthiness and implementability of guidelines recommendations. TBD. 2018;Manucript in preparation.
19. Agarwal A, Johnston BC, Vernooij RW, Carrasco-Labra A, Brignardello-Petersen R, Neumann I, et al. Authors seldom report the most patient-important outcomes and absolute effect measures in systematic review abstracts. J Clin Epidemiol. 2017;81:3–12.
20. Rogers EM. Diffusion of innovations. Simon and Schuster; 2010.
21. Young JM, Hollands MJ, Ward J, Holman CAJ. Role for opinion leaders in promoting evidence-based surgery. Arch Surg. 2003;138(7):785–91.
22. Alonso-Coello P, Schünemann HJ, Moberg J, Brignardello-Petersen R, Akl EA, Davoli M, et al. GRADE Evidence to Decision (EtD) frameworks: a systematic and transparent approach to making well informed healthcare choices. 1: Introduction. bmj. 2016;353:i2016.
23. Coulter I, Adams A, Shekelle P. Impact of varying panel membership on ratings of appropriateness in consensus panels: a comparison of a multi-and single disciplinary panel. Health Serv Res. 1995;30(4):577.
24. Browman GP. Improving clinical practice guidelines for the 21st century: attitudinal barriers and not technology are the main challenges. Int J Technol Assess Health Care. 2000;16(04):959–68.
25. Pai M. Electronic strategies to enhance venous thromboprophylaxis in hospitalized medical patients: a randomized controlled trial. 2012.
26. Lloyd NS, Douketis JD, Cheng J, Schünemann HJ, Cook DJ, Thabane L, et al. Barriers and potential solutions toward optimal prophylaxis against deep vein thrombosis for hospitalized medical patients: a survey of healthcare professionals. J Hosp Med. 2012;7(1):28–34.
27. Heit JA, O'Fallon WM, Petterson TM, Lohse CM, Silverstein MD, Mohr DN, et al. Relative impact of risk factors for deep vein thrombosis and pulmonary embolism. Arch Intern Med. 2002;162(11):1245–8.
28. Burgers JS, Grol RP, Zaat JO, Spies TH, van der Bij AK, Mokkink HG. Characteristics of effective clinical guidelines for general practice. Br J Gen Pract. 2003;53(486):15–9.
29. Guadagnoli E, Soumerai SB, Gurwitz JH, Borbas C, Shapiro CL, Weeks JC, et al. Improving discussion of surgical treatment options for patients with breast cancer: local medical opinion leaders versus audit and performance feedback. Cancer Res Treat. 2000;61(2):171–5.
30. Lau BD, Haut ER. Practices to prevent venous thromboembolism: a brief review. BMJ Qual Saf. 2013:bmjqs-2012-001782.
31. Fervers B, Burgers J, Voellinger R, Brouwers M, Browman G, Graham I, et al. Guideline adaptation: an approach to enhance efficiency in guideline development and improve utilisation. BMJ Qual Saf. 2011:qshc. 2010.043257.

Index

A
Absolute risk reduction (ARR), 57, 109, 110, 333
Accelerated surgery, 21
ACCESSSS, 28, 34, 35
Accuracy, 204
ACP Journal Club, 28, 32
Actual response rate, 272
Acute scaphoid fracture, 145–146
Acute symptomatic meniscal tear, 85
Adenocarcinoma, 183
Adhesive small bowel obstruction (aSBO), 160
guide to interpretation of, 160
potential source of bias, 163–164
results
interpreting, 167–168
meaning of, 165–166
validity, 161–162
statistical analysis, 164–165
Age of scientific information overload, 279
AGREE (Appraisal of Guidelines, REsearch and Evaluation)
AGREE Enterprise, 338
AGREE II tool, 193, 338, 339, 344
high-quality CPGs features, 339
AGREE-REX tool, 338, 339, 344
high-quality recommendations features, 340
Allocation ratio, 55, 121, 315, 321
American College of Surgeons (ACS), 194, 196, 268
American Medical Association, 232, 266, 268, 269, 273
American Shoulder and Elbow Surgeons (ASES) scale, 142
American Society for Clinical Oncology (ASCO), 338
CPG scenario, 341, 342, 343
American Society of Anesthesiologists (ASA) scale, 58, 186, 258, 259, 285, 317
American Society of General Surgeons, 268
American Thyroid Association (ATA), 212
Analysis of variance (ANOVA), 137
Analyzed response rate, 272, 273
Annals of Surgery, 184
Anti-arrhythmic medications, 87
Anticoagulant therapy, 88, 89, 91, 221
Aortic stenosis (AS), 218, 219
Appraisal
of an article, 53–55, 62, 94
based on harm, 258
evaluating surgical interventions, 52
with HRQL, 94, 95
of cohort studies in surgery, 160–161
critical appraisal, 11, 34, 35, 47, 147
of an article, 258–260
framework for non-inferiority randomized controlled trial, 127–128
diagnostic test, 41
of selected article, 32, 33, 173, 329–330
of surgical article, 10
of surgical case series, 184–185
surgical clinical practice guidelines, 340
of surgical literature on prognosis, 95
of surgical survey, 266–267
Appraisal skills, 6
Appraisal tool, 5, 179, 197, 338, 339
Area under the receiver operating characteristic (AUROC) curve, 161, 166
Arthroscopic knee surgery, 88, 243

B
Background questions, 18, 24
Bariatric program/surgery, 23, 24, 25, 27, 28, 280
Bethesda System for Reporting Thyroid Cytopathology, 208, 209, 211, 212
diagnostic categories, 208, 209
Bias, 6, 34, 38, 40, 51, 52, 172, 218
blinding, 54
detection bias, 202
HRQL issues, 96
information bias, 163, 167, 183, 186
interviewer bias, 163, 270
observer bias, 163
intentional bias, 65
language bias, 147
measurement error and, 75
per-protocol analysis versus intention-to-treat analysis, 108
potential sources of, 163
selection bias, 54, 105, 140, 148, 163, 167, 183, 185, 186, 270, 303
publication bias, 147, 148–149
referral bias, 220

A. Thoma et al. (eds.), *Evidence-Based Surgery*,
https://doi.org/10.1007/978-3-030-05120-4

Risk of Bias tool, 149
Biomarkers, 85 *See also* Surrogate endpoints
Biomedical research, 305
Blinding, 30, 41, 43, 48, 54, 103, 106, 121, 129, 168
blind comparison, 210
double-blinding, 149, 278, 316
outcome assessment, 187
Body mass index (BMI), 14, 24, 58, 85, 90, 107, 247, 252, 317
Boolean function, 52
Boolean operators, 24, 26, 27, 88, 302
Boolean search strategy, 67
Breast-conserving therapy, 265, 266, 273
Breast Evaluation Questionnaire, 76
Breast implant-associated anaplastic large cell lymphomas (BI-ALCL), 187
BREAST-Q, 72, 73, 74, 75, 76, 77, 78, 79
Breast Reduction Assessment Severity Scale, 76
Breast-Related Symptoms Questionnaire, 76
British Journal of Cancer (BJC), 116
British Journal of Obstetrics and Gynaecology (BJOG), 116
British Journal of Surgery (BJS), 116
British Medical Journal (BMJ), 9, 116
BMJ Best Practice, 28, 31
BMJ Evidence-based Medicine, 33

C
California Office of Statewide Health Planning and Development (OSHPD) datasets, 220
Canadian Association of General Surgeons, 268
Canadian Journal of Surgery, 2
Canadian Medical Association Journal (CMAJ), 2
Canadian occupational performance measure (COPM), 62
Canadian Task Force on Periodic Health Examination (CTFPHE), 2
LOE, 2, 3, 37
Cancer risk, 171, 207
Capture-Mark-Recapture (CMR) techniques, 148
Cardiac arrhythmias, 87
Carpal tunnel syndrome symptom severity scale (CTS-SSS), 62
Case-control design, 39, 42, 45, 176, 218, 219
Case-control studies, 171, 256
applicability
benefits of exposure, 178–179
exposure to second surgery, 177
GATE framework, 179
homogeneous patients, 179
long-term follow-up, 177
magnitude of risk, 177–178
meaning of different OR, 178
resolution of the scenario, 179
appraisal of selected article, 173
comparison with cohort, 172
meaning of results
exposure and outcome, 175
matched case-control study, 176
odds ratio, 175
preciseness of estimate of risk, 176–177
univariable analysis, 176
unmatched case-control study, 176
PICOT format, 172–173
result validity, 174
circumstances and methods, 174
correct temporal relationship, 174
dose-response relationship, 174–175
homogeneous case–control, 174
Case series, 183
appraisal of surgical case series, 184–185
framework for, 185
common study design, 190
key characteristics of, 184
meaning of results
appropriate outcome, 187–188
complete outcomes, 188
resolution of scenario, 189–190
results changing practice
applying results, 189
homogeneous patients, 188–189
results validity
appropriate intervention, 187–188
clear objectives, 185
consecutive patient recruitment, 186
outcome assessment, 186–187
prospective study designs, 185–186
Centers for Medicare and Medicaid Services (CMS), 196
Centre for Evidence-Based Medicine, 37
Centre for Reviews and Dissemination at York University, 5–6
CHEERS (Consolidated Health Economic Evaluation Reporting Standards) guideline/statement, 6, 252
Chi-square test, 56, 150, 151, 287, 288, 289, 292, 294, 295
analysis, 137
distribution, 290, 291
p-value, 166
reference distribution, 291
sensitivity analysis, 297–298
statistics, 290, 291, 295
Chi-square Test for Association, 290
CHORUS trial, 126, 127, 128, 129
baseline characteristics of participants, 130, 132
investigators, 130
selection of non-inferiority margin, 131
overall survival in, 131
study flow of, 128
Chunk sampling, 268
Chylothorax, 172, 173, 174, 175, 176, 177, 178, 179, 180
CIA (statistical software), 291, 293
Circulation, 116
Classical test theory (CTT), 77
Clinical data, 87–88
Clinical decision-making, 51, 165, 225
adequate sample size, 55
appraisal of article, 53

follow-up, 54
intention to treat principle, 54–55
outcomes, 55
binary versus continuous outcomes, 55
multivariable regression, 56
univariable and multivariable analyses, 56
resolution of clinical scenario, 59
treatment effect, 57
applicability of results, 58
comparing patient population, 58
estimate of, 58
evaluating surgical skill, 59
measured outcomes, 59
precision of, 57
Clinical epidemiology, 76, 179, 180
Clinical knowledge, 281–282
Clinically important difference (CID), 56, 64, 65, 66, 67, 77, 287, 317, 320, 331
Clinical measurement, 67
Clinical Practice Guidelines (CPGs), 197, 198, 337
applicability of results, 343
appraisal of
AGREE II tool, 339
AGREE-REX tool, 339–340
framework for, 340
ASCO CPG. 338, 341, 342, 343
independent development process, 342
meaning of results
CPG presentation, 343
high-quality recommendations, 342–343
methodologically rigorous CPG, 341–342
poor quality CPGs, 337
resolution of clinical scenario, 343–344
results validity
scope and purpose of CPG, 340–341
stakeholder involvement, 341
surgical CPGs, 338
Clinical Practice Guidelines Committee (CPGC), 341
Clinical question, 9–10, 23–24, 37, 77, 104, 120, 137, 161, 163, 167, 168, 218, 235, 338
adequate sample size, 55
art of formulating, 17
background questions, 18
boundary of knowledge, 17
broken into PICO(T), 24, 301
clinical research project, 17
foreground questions, 18, 21
importance of question, 24
keywords from, 146
sensible clinical question, 147
specific clinical question, 31
statistical significance, 142
ClinicalTrials.gov database, 5
Clinician-based outcome (CBO) measures, 61, 63
Clinician-reported outcomes, 95
Cochrane Central Register of Controlled Trials (CENTRAL), 28, 32, 33
Cochrane Collaboration, 4, 5, 6
Risk of Bias tool, 149, 298
Cochrane Controlled Trial Register, 148
Cochrane Database, 10, 11, 12, 94, 244
Cochrane Database of Systematic Reviews (CDSR), 26, 28, 33, 234, 286
Cochrane evidence summary, 32
Cochrane Library, 6, 11, 173, 202, 316
Cochrane review, 285
Cochrane's Q test, 150
Cochrane Systematic Review, 167
Cohort studies, 159, 163, 164, 165, 218
aim of, 167
comparison with case-control studies, 171, 172
diagnostic, 41
inception, 44, 47, 48
interpretation of, 160
limitation of, 168, 256
longitudinal studies, 256
prospective, 41, 43, 159, 161, 256, 257
retrospective, 38, 43, 44, 159, 162, 219, 256
Colon cancer, 10, 21, 327
Colonoscopy, 285
COMET (Core Outcome Measures in Effectiveness Trials) initiative, 5, 6, 153, 269
Computer simulation models (CSM), 44, 46
Computing
associated *P*-vales, 288, 290–293
confidence intervals, 293
multiplicity, 294–295
sensitivity analysis, 293–294
software, 293
test statistic, 290
mean, 290
Confidence interval (CI), 19, 56, 57, 58, 126, 165, 166, 167, 178, 221, 222, 226, 286, 287, 301
calculating, 307
CIA software, 291, 293
factors impacting width of, 307
getting to estimation, 304
and heterogeneity, 150, 151
hypothesis testing, 305–306
interpreting results, 286, 287, 306
literature search, 302
demographics of patients, 303
need for using, 307–308
and OR estimate, 176
and *p*-values, 303–304
questions about article validity and applicability, 308
research questions, 301–302
and sample size, 118
to test null hypothesis, 288, 295
two-tailed, 289, 293
uncertainties, 227
understanding, 302
SD, 302
selection bias, 303
Confounder, 53, 55, 88, 103, 165
Confounding, 51, 53, 88, 91, 163, 168, 174, 175
directed acyclic graph, 164
measured confounding, 164, 167

multivariable model, 176
unmeasured confounding, 164, 167
Congenital heart surgery, 172
database, 178
Risk Adjustment for Congenital Heart Surgery (RACHS-1) score, 175
COnsensus-based Standards of health status Management INstruments (COSMIN), 5, 6, 76, 77, 269
CONsolidated Standards Of Reporting Trials (CONSORT), 6
checklist, 119, 120–122
extension, 115, 119, 120
reporting guideline, 119
Constructing research question
answerable question, 15
relevant questions, 9, 10, 11
Construct validity, 75, 76, 271
Content validity, 61, 74, 75, 78, 271
Continuous process improvement (CPI), 195
Controlled vocabulary, 25, 27, 30, 35
for gastric bypass in PubMed, 26
Core Outcome Measures in Effectiveness Trials (COMET), 5, 6, 153, 269
Core outcome sets (COS), 5, 153, 269
Cost analysis (CA), 240, 241
Cost–benefit analysis (CBA), 240, 241, 243
Cost-effectiveness acceptability curves (CEAC), 247
Cost-effectiveness analysis (CEA), 240, 241, 245, 251
Cost–utility analysis (CUA), 232, 240, 242–243
CRAN (Comprehensive R Archive Network), software, 293
Criterion validity, 75
Critical evaluation, for reporting RCTs, 286–288
risk of bias tool, 287
summary of findings, 287
validity checklist, 286
Cronbach's alpha coefficient, 76, 77
Cryptorchidism, 193
resolution of scenario, 198
Culture of change and safety, 198
Culture of shame and blame, 197

D

Danish Colorectal Cancer Group database, 257, 258
Decision analysis, 79, 225
applicability
probability estimates, 236
results to be generalized, 235
value on decision outcomes, 236
background, 225–226
components of
clinical application, 229
decision tree, 226–227
outcomes, 227–228
treatment modalities, 229
literature search, 225
PubMed, 225
meaning of results
clinically important gain for patients, 234
difference between strategies, 234
strong evidence in analysis, 234–235
uncertainty in evidence change, 235
resolution of scenario, 236–237
results validity, 230–231
explicit and sensible process, 231–232
potential impact of any uncertainty, 233–234
strategies and outcomes, 231
utilities obtained from credible sources, 232–233
users' guide, 229–230
disabilities, 230
probabilities, 230
questions to appraise, 229
utilities, 230
Decision analytic model, 230, 235
Decision-making, clinical, 165, 225
benchmarks, 64
in health care, 4
and outcome, 226
process, 51, 217, 338
shared, 71, 72, 79, 342
in surgery, 51, 280, 344
uncertainty, 233
Decision pathway, 227
Decision tree, 226–227
bad outcome, 226
disutility, 227
good outcome, 226
parts of, 227
utility, 227
Deep Inferior Epigastric Perforator (DIEP) flap, 18, 241, 242
Deep vein thrombosis (DVT), 85
Degree of confidence, 304, 307 *See also* Confidence interval (CI)
Degrees of freedom (DF), 288, 290, 291, 292, 293, 297, 298
Delphi technique, 269
Detection bias, 202 *See also* Bias
Deterministic analysis, 234, 245
Diagnostic research, 41
Level I evidence, 41–43
case-control design, 42
case series design, 42, 43
prospective cohort design, 41, 42
RCT study design, 41, 42
retrospective cohort design, 42
Level II evidence, 41, 43
Level III evidence, 41, 43
Level IV evidence, 41, 43
Level V evidence, 41
Diagnostic study in surgery, 201–202
diagnostic testing and true results in cancer diagnosis, 205
evaluating literature, 209–210
primary guides, 209
results validity, 210
secondary guides, 209–210

flow chart of study design, 203
important aspects of, 204
false negative, 204
false positive, 204
likelihood ratio, 204
true negative, 204
true positive, 204
nomogram for result, 207
study summary, 202–203
Diagnostic tests, 41, 201, 202, 208
characterizing, 207
understanding, 204
Directed acyclic graph (DAG), 164
Disability arm shoulder and hand (DASH), 62, 64
Quick(DASH), 64
Distal radius fracture (DRF), 61, 66
post-DRF, 67
Document(ation), 1, 73, 194, 259, 278, 280, 337, 342
PRISMA flow diagram, 150, 155
Duke Clinical Research Institute (DCRI), 2
DynaMed Plus, 28, 32, 34

E
EASY trial, 94, 99
EBSCO CINAHL, 30
Economic analysis, 95, 239, 244
Economic evaluation, 6, 46, 98, 227 *See also* Surgical techniques, economic evaluations
Economic research, 37, 46, 47
EMBASE, 10, 26, 28, 30, 32, 33, 148, 219, 302, 308
Emotional functioning, 99, 100
Endoscopic Carpal Tunnel Release (ECTR) technique, 21
End Result Idea, 194
Enhanced Recovery after Surgery (ERAS) program, 255, 261
EORTC trial, 97, 132
overall survival in, 131
QLQ-C30, 98, 99, 100, 101
QLQ-CR29, 98, 99, 100, 101
quality of life questionnaire, 131
questionnaires, 96
Epistemonikos, 28, 34
ePROVIDE (database), 63
EQ-5D (EuroQOL 5-Dimension), 62, 63, 96
EQ-5D-5L (EuroQOL 5-Dimension 5-Level), 98
EQUATOR (Enhancing the QUAlity and Transparency Of health Research) Network, 5, 6, 252
Equivalent-forms reliability, 76
Essential Evidence Plus, 28, 32
Estimation, 286, 304, 305, 317, 320
horizon estimation, 148
interval estimates, 104
OR estimation, 176
outcomes and, 122
point estimates, 104
of true values, 163
Ethical, 18, 19, 119, 120, 122, 171, 194, 211, 256
European Organization for Research and Treatment of Cancer Scales, 76 *See also* EORTC trial
Evaluating, literature on diagnostic test, *see* Case series; Surgical intervention, evaluating; Surgical research, evaluating surveys and questionnaires in
Evidence-based medicine (EBM), 1, 9, 24, 37, 103, 194
of CPGs, 197
expert opinion on, 278
in surgery, 2, 4
Evidence-Based Medicine (EBM) Working group, 180
Evidence-based resources, 31
Evidence-based surgery (EBS), 1, 2, 9, 37, 47, 93, 143
basis for decision making, 2
cohort studies in, 159 *See also* Cohort studies
definition, 9
evidence-based approach, 9, 10
construction of clinically relevant, answerable question, 9–10, 11
critically appraising literature, 10, 14–15
applying evidence to clinical practice, 11, 15
evaluating effectiveness and efficiency, 11, 15
planning and carrying out literature search, 10, 11–14
expert opinion in, 278
LOE, 2, 3
overall philosophy of, 6
Expert opinion, 51, 74, 76, 197
application, 280
in context of
evidence-based medicine and surgery, 278
surgical literature, 280
limitations of, 279
mechanism-based reasoning, 40
questions to appraise, 281
trusting, 281
value of, 278–279
Expertise-based randomized controlled trial (EBRCT), 136
block randomization, 139
concealment of allocation, 139–140
considering learning curve, 138
equally skilled surgeons, 139
guidelines to assess, 136
ITT analysis, 141
minimizing bias, 140
prognostic factor, 140
time to treatment, 140
research validity, 137–138
resolution of scenario, 144
stratification, 140–141
sufficient level of expertise, 138–139
sufficient number of surgeons, 139
trial results, 141
applicability to practice, 142–143
measurement, 141–142
overweighing risks and costs, 143
patient-important outcomes, 143

recurrent instability, 142
treatment effect, 142
External responsiveness, 97
External validity, 52, 58, 152, 154, 167, 183, 186, 190, 245, 258, 273, 278, 337

F
Face validity, 271, 272
Fagan nomogram, 212, 213
FAITH trial, 104, 105, 106, 108, 109, 110, 111
False negatives (FN), 53, 55, 204, 205, 314, 332
False positives (FS), 53, 58, 148, 150, 166, 204, 205, 314
Feasibility investigation, 115
Feasibility studies, 115, 116
Feasibility trial, 115, 119, 122
Feasible, interesting novel, ethical, relevant (FINER), 18, 22
ethical, 19
feasible, 18
interesting, 18–19
novel, 19
relevant, 19
Federated Search Tools, 33–34
Femoral neck fracture, 103, 106, 110, 111
avascular necrosis, 104
reoperations, 104
Fine-needle aspiration biopsy (FNAB), 202, 210, 211, 213
US-guided, 203, 208, 212
Fixation using Alternative Implants for the Treatment of Hip fractures (FAITH) trial, 41, 104, 105, 106, 108, 109, 110, 111
Follow-up, 14, 48, 52, 54, 79, 131, 177, 183
appointment, 153–154
follow-up interval, 101
IDEAL framework, 117, 119
immortal person-time bias, 163
intermediate follow-up period, 21
loss to follow-up (LTFU), 137, 141, 188, 220, 221, 321
minimizing loss to, 129
postoperative follow-up, 72
sample size calculation and, 108–109
sufficiently complete, 259
sufficiently long, 177, 219
time-frame for, 38
Food and Drug Administration (FDA), 5, 72, 95
Kefauver-Harris Act, 1
PROM development, 73–74
steps in development of PRO instrument, 74
Foreground questions, 81, 21, 24
Forest plot, 131, 150, 151

G
G*Power to compute power, 322–323
required factors, 322–323
G*Power version 3.1, 316
Generalizability, 51, 90, 110, 116, 147, 208, 229, 235, 236, 245, 268, 272, 273, 302
Generalization, 314
Glaucoma, 87
Glenohumeral instability, 135
Global rating of change (GRC), 62
Google, 34
Google Scholar, 34
GRADE (Grading of Recommendations Assessment, Development and Evaluation), 4, 6, 31, 197, 338, 340, 341
GRADEpro, 4
quality of evidence, 4
Graduated compression stockings (GCS), 88–89
Graphical Appraisal Tool for Epidemiological studies (GATE) framework, 179, 180
Guides
primary guides, 95
important aspects of HRQ, 96–97
measuring aspects of patients' lives, 95–96
valid, reliable and responsive HRQL instruments, 97
secondary guides, 95
appropriately timed HQRL, 98
quantity and quality of life, 98
users' guides, 2
Guyatt, Gordon, 1

H
Hazard ratios (HR), 110, 131, 166, 222
Health Information Research Unit (HiRU), 31
Health-related quality of life (HRQL/HRQoL/HRQOL), 63, 72, 75, 93, 94, 95, 313, 315
disease-specific, 96
generic instruments, 96
magnitude of effect, 98–101
QLQ-C30, 100, 101
QLQ-CR29, 100, 101
SF-36 scores, 99, 101
primary guides, 95
aspects omitted, 96–97
aspects patients consider important, 95–96
reliability, 97
responsive, 97
validity, 95, 97
resolution scenario, 101–102
results help informing patients, 101
secondary guides, 98
assessments appropriately timed, 98
quantity and quality of life, 98
Health utility index (HUI), 62, 96, 98
Heart surgery, 172
redo heart surgery, 177
Hernia repair, 52, 54, 93, 240, 245
Heterogeneity, 153
chi-square test, 151
degree of, 150
I squared statistic (I^2), 151
Hierarchy of evidence, *see* Levels of evidence (LOE)
Highly reliable organizations (HROs), 196
Hip fracture, 21, 105, 115
Homogen(e)ous patients, 106, 141, 150, 219, 307
Human Factors Engineering, 197

Hypothesis testing, 286, 287, 303, 304, 305

I
IDEAL (Idea, Development, Exploration, Assessment, and Long-term follow-up), 117, 119, 120
Identifying concepts, 24, 35
Identifying search terms, 25
Ileostomy, 93, 94
Incremental cost-effectiveness ratio (ICER), 241, 242, 246, 247, 248, 251, 252
Incremental cost-utility ratio (ICUR), 98, 243, 246, 247, 248, 251, 252
Information bias, 163, 172, 183, 185, 186, 298
Institute for Healthcare Improvement (IHI), 195
Institute of Medicine (IOM), 195
Intention to treat principle, 54–55
 hazard ratio (HR), 131
 ITT analysis, 107–108, 129, 131, 141, 289, 329
Internal consistency reliability, 76, 271
Internal responsiveness, 97
Internal validity, 52, 154, 258
International Society for Pharmacoeconomics and Outcomes Research, 73
Internet-derived expertise, 201
Interrater reliability, 76, 271
Intervention, *see* Outcome measure, information on; PICOT format; Randomized controlled trials (RCTs); Surgical intervention, evaluating
Intra-class correlation coefficient (ICC), 76, 77
Intraocular pressure (IOP), 87
Invasive lobular breast carcinoma, 71
Item response theory (IRT), 77

J
Joint Commission on Accreditation of Hospital Organizations (JCAHO), 196
Journal of Bone and Joint Surgery (JBJS), 37, 38, 41, 46
Journal of Clinical Oncology, 72
Journal of the American Medical Association (JAMA), 2, 116

K
Keywords, 25, 26, 27, 30, 52, 94, 146, 219
Knee arthroscopy, 88, 90, 91
Knowledge
 clinical knowledge, 281–282
 technical knowledge, 281, 282
 translation, new advances in surgery, 6

L
Lancet, 116, 126
Laryngoscopy, 202
Level I evidence, 38, 41–43, 45, 46–47
 case-control design, 42
 case series design, 42, 43
 prospective cohort design, 41, 42
 RCT study design, 41, 42
 retrospective cohort design, 42
Level II evidence, 38, 41, 43, 45, 46
Level III evidence, 38, 40, 41, 43, 46
Level IV evidence, 40, 41, 43, 46
Level V evidence, 41, 43, 46
Levels of evidence (LOE), 2, 37
 CTFPHE's LOE, 3
 for diagnostic research, 41–43
  clinical example, 43
 for economic research, 44–46
  clinical example, 46–47
 Oxford Centre for Evidence-Based Medicine, 48
 for prognostic research, 43–44
  clinical example, 44
 Sackett's LOE, 3
 for therapeutic research, 37–41
  clinical example, 41
Lichtenstein tension-free method, 59
Likelihood ratio (LR), 204, 210, 211
 calculated, 211
 for each category, 206
 of negative test (LR–), 204, 205
 of positive test (LR+), 204, 205
Likert scale, 269, 270
Limits and search filters, 30–31
Lind, James, 1
Literature search, 71–72, 88–89, 94, 104, 116–117, 125–126, 137, 160, 172–173, 184, 193, 202, 219, 225, 265–266, 277–278, 285–286, 302, 328, 338
 applying to patients, 79
 appraising on prognosis, 219–222
 within cardiac surgery, 178
 decision analysis literature, 229
 existing literature, 167
 expert opinion in surgical literature, 280
 reporting statistical findings in, 296
Low-molecular-weight heparin (LMWH), 89, 90, 91, 343

M
Mann–Whitney *U* tests, 166, 272
Marfan syndrome, 218
McGill pain questionnaire (MPQ), 62, 64
McMaster-Toronto Arthritis Patient Preference Disability Questionnaire (MACTAR), 78
Mechanism-based reasoning, 40
Medial epicondylectomy, 232
Medical Subject Headings (MeSH), 52, 71, 72, 193
 non-MeSH, 52
MEDLINE, 30, 32, 33, 148, 219, 279
MedSelect, 268
Meta-analyses (MA), 38, 51, 145, 233 *See also* Systematic reviews (SR)
 of continuous outcome measures, 152
 limitation of, 153, 154
Michigan hand questionnaire (MHQ), 62, 64

Micromedex, 32
Minimal detectable change (MDC), 64, 65, 66, 67
Minimal important change (MIC), 79
Minimal important difference (MID), 79
Minimum Clinically Important Difference (MCID), 305
Miniopen technique, 152
Minitab 18 (software), 290, 291, 292, 293, 297
Model-based economic evaluation, 240–241
Modern psychometric test theory, 77
Monte Carlo simulation, 44–45
Multiplicity, 294–295
Multivariable regression, 56, 165
Myocardial infarction (MI), 88
Myocardial injury after noncardiac surgery (MINS), 87
Myocardial necrosis, 87

N
National Health Services (NHS), 196
National Institute for Health and Clinical Excellence (NICE), 28, 251
National Institutes of Health (NIH), 5, 103
  NIH Toolbox (database), 63
National Library of Medicine (NLM), 5, 104
National Surgical Quality Improvement Program (NSQIP), 194
NCSS Statistical Software, 316
Negative predictive value (NPV), 204, 207, 208
Negative pressure wound therapy (NPWT), 117
New England Journal of Medicine (NEJM), 116
Nodules, 202
Non-displaced scaphoid waist fracture, 146
Non-inferiority randomized controlled trial, 127–128
Nonoperative approaches, 251
Non-preappraised research, 31
Non-steroidal anti-inflammatory drugs (NSAIDs), 255
Novel, 18, 19
Null hypothesis, 314, 315
Number needed to harm (NNH), 261
Number needed to treat (NNT), 109, 110, 261
Numeric(al) rating scale (NRS), 62, 316, 317, 318

O
Observer-reported outcomes, 95
Odds ratio (OR), 56, 165, 175, 178, 305
OMERACT (Outcome MEasurements in Rheumatoid Arthritis Clinical Trial) initiative, 4
One-tail test, 315, 321
One-way sensitivity analysis, 233
Open carpal tunnel release (OCTR) technique, 21
Open-ended questions, 269
Open reduction and internal fixation (ORIF), 277
Oral contraceptive pill (OCP), 85
OrthoEvidence, 31, 33
Orthopedic scores (database), 63
Outcome measure, information on, 61
  adaptive measures, 64
  applications, 66–67
    assessing hand function, 67
    assessing joint function, 67
    distal radial fracture management, 66
  cautions to be exercised, 66
  CBOs, 63
  ceiling or floor effects, 64
  choosing proper measure, 64–65
  defining the concept, 61
  interpreting the score, 66
  MDC, 65
  measurement error, 65
  measurement parameters, 62
  measurement threats, 65
  PROs, 63
  reliability, 65
  sources of, 63
Ovarian cancer-specific quality of life questionnaire, 131
Overestimate risk, 56
Ovid MEDLINE, 30, 34, 148
Oxford Centre for Evidence-Based Medicine, 48

P
Pare, Ambroise, 1
PASS software, 316
Patient-important outcome measures, 71
  patient-reported outcome, 72, 73
    conceptual framework of, 73
  PROM, 72
  searching the literature, 71–72
    evaluating PROs, 72
    patient perceptions of outcomes, 72
Patient-rated elbow evaluation (PREE), 64
Patient-rated ulnar nerve evaluation (PRUNE), 62, 64
Patient-rated wrist evaluation (PRWE), 62, 64, 67
Patient-reported health instruments (database), 63
Patient-reported outcome measure (PROM), 72
  BREAST-Q, 72, 74, 75, 76, 77, 79
  CLEFT-Q, 74
  developing, 73–74
    adjusting conceptual framework, 74
    collecting, analyzing, and interpreting data, 74
    confirming conceptual framework, 74
    hypothesizing conceptual framework, 73–74
    modifying instrument, 74
  evaluating
    reliability, 76–77
    validity, 75–76
  implant-based versus autologous breast reconstruction, 79
  interpreting results, 79
  types of, 77–78
    dimension specific, 77, 78
    disease or condition-specific instruments, 77–78
    generic, 77, 78
    individualized, 77, 78–79
    region or site-specific, 77
    utility measures, 77, 79
Patient-reported outcomes (PROs), 95

measures, 61, 63 *See also* Patient-reported outcome measure (PROM)
disease-specific, 64
patient-specific, 64
symptom-specific, 64
Patient-Reported Outcomes Measurement Information System (PROMIS) scores, 79
Patient-Reported Outcomes Measurement Information System-29 (PROMIS-29), 78, 79
Patient-specific functional scale (PSFS), 62, 64
P-D-S-A (Plan, Do, Study, Act) concept, 195
Pearson method, 290, 297, 298
PEPID, 32, 34
Percutaneous fixation, 152
Performance outcomes, 95
Per-protocol analysis, 108
Personalized care, 194
PICOH (patient(s), intervention(s), comparison(s), outcome(s), health care setting), 340
PICO, 125
PICOT format, 15, 18, 19–20, 22, 23–24, 28, 28, 94, 104, 137, 146, 147, 202, 301, 316
clinical question, 24, 146
comparative intervention or control, 10, 11, 20
intervention, 10, 11, 20
outcome, 10, 11, 20–21
patient or population, 10, 11, 20
PICO, 125
time horizon, 10, 11, 21
Pilot study, 115
Pilot trials, 115
criteria of success, 118–119
current practice in, 116–117
definition, 115–116
importance of, 116
key considerations for designing, 117
key resources for further references, 119, 120
methods of analysis, 118
objectives, 117
outcomes, 118
learning curves, 118
reporting, 119
sample size, 118
study rationale, 117
Pilot work, 115
Population, 314
Positive predictive value (PPV), 204, 207, 208
Post-test probability, 212, 213
Power, 314–314
clinically relevant effect size, 319
difference in treatment effect, 319–320
effect size precise and consistent, 320
to estimate power, 320
estimation of treatment effect, 320
key questions to assess, 317
mean pain scores, 319
pain outcomes, 318
performing power analysis, 317–318
power calculation a priori, 314
resolution of scenario, 320
Preappraised research, 31
Preferred Reporting Items for Systematic reviews and Meta-Analysis (PRISMA), 149, 155
Pre-syncope, 217
Pre-test probability, 205, 213
Primary chemotherapy, 125, 131 *See also* CHORUS trial
Primary surgery, 125, 131 *See also* CHORUS trial
Probabilistic analysis, 240
Prognostic study, 217
applicability, 222
appraising surgical literature, 219
biased prognostic studies, 220
sample representative, 219–220
important clinical implications, 221
literature survey, 219
long-term follow-up, 220–221
objective outcome, 221
patient-important outcomes, 220
preciseness, 221–222
reasons for measuring, 217–218
repeatability, 221
resolution of clinical scenario, 222
study designs for, 218–219
case–control design, 218, 219
RCTs, 218
unbiased outcome criteria, 221
user's guide to surgical literature, 219
PROMIS (database), 63, 64
Prophylactic ureteric catheter placement (PUCP), 301, 302, 303, 305
PROSPECT (PRObiotics: prevention of Severe Pneumonia and Endotracheal Colonization Trial), 116
Prospective cohort studies, 159
guide to interpretation of, 160
interpreting results
clinically important outcomes, 167
context of clinical question, 167
existing literature, 167
limitations of the study, 167–168
resolution of clinical scenario, 168
meaning of results
baseline characteristics, 165
effective size, 165–166
issue of multiple testing, 166
planned sensitivity analyses, 166
preciseness, 165–166
relevant statistics, 165
subgroup analyses, 166
outline of, 161
potential source of bias, 163
confounding, 164
directed acyclic graph, 164
information bias, 163
selection bias, 163
and randomized controlled trials, 168
result validity, 161
data collection method, 162

justifiable definitions of outcome, 162
reliable data source, 162
study population, 161–162
statistical analysis, 164–165
study's research question and clinical relevance, 161
result validity, 162
PROSPERO, International prospective registrar of systematic reviews, 5, 6, 149
Proximal humerus fracture, 277
PsycINFO, 30
Publication bias, 148
Published evidence, 87–88
PubMed database, 11, 13, 14, 23, 30, 32, 33, 34, 88, 94, 104, 125, 202, 219, 225
for gastric bypass in, 26
search, 257, 338
PubMed MEDLINE, 148
PubMed.gov, 184, 265
Pulmonary embolism (PE), 89
Purposive sampling, 268
P values, 286, 288–289, 290–293
chi-square distribution, 290
confidence intervals, 293
CRAN network, 293
Minitab 18 (software), 291
multiplicity, 294–295
relative risk, 291, 292
sensitivity analysis, 291, 293–294, 297–298
Pyramid of EBM resources, 24, 28, 28, 31, 32
non-preappraised research, 32
preappraised research, 31
summaries and guidelines, 32

Q
QLQ-C30, 96, 97, 98, 99, 100, 101
QLQ-CR29, 96, 97, 98, 99, 100
Qualitative research, 321
reliable, 321
responsive to change, 321
valid, 321
Quality-adjusted life years (QALYs), 45, 46, 96, 98, 227, 234, 242, 248
Quality improvement (QI), 195
research, 195–196
Quality improvement and patient safety (QIPS), 193, 194, 195, 196, 198
Quality of life (QoL), 63, 72, 93, 94
Questions, evidence finding, 23
importance of, 24
background questions, 24
foreground questions, 24
(Quick)DASH, 64
Quota sampling, 268

R
Randomization, 53, 105
Randomized controlled trials (RCTs), 38, 44, 94, 103, 115, 126, 135, 159, 171, 218, 233, 256, 286, 311, 317, 327
application, 132
comparative analysis, 132
patient-important outcomes, 132
patient inclusion criteria, 132
computing test statistic, 290
critical evaluation of reporting, 286–287
bias tool, 287
for diagnostic studies, 42
evaluating, 104–105
expertise-based, 136 *See also* Expertise-based randomized controlled trial (EBRCT)
meaning of results
clinical relevance, 110–111
generalizability, 110
to healthcare provider, 111
hypothetical hypertensive drug trial, 110
impact from treatment, 109
ITT analysis, 131
measuring quality of life, 131
preciseness, 110
pros and cons, 131, 132
non-inferiority design, 126
critical appraisal framework for, 127
justifying, 128
observed treatment differences for adverse outcomes, 127
play of chance, 289–290
randomization, 129
resolution of clinical scenario, 111, 295–296
results validity, 128
analyzing patients, 129–130
justify margin, 130–131
prognostic balance, 129
unwarranted conclusion, 129
for therapeutic research, 39–40
things relevant to outcome
baseline characteristics, 287
complications, 288
main outcome, 287
mean SD by group, 287
prehabilitation, 288
presentation of data, 287
relative risk, 287
sample size justification, 287
secondary outcomes, 287
severity, 287
statistical tests, 287
study elements, 287
validity, 104–105
allocation concealment, 105
blinding, 106
homogeneous patients, 106
intention-to-treat analysis, 107–108
learning curve and expertise-based RCTs, 105
participant attrition, 109
patient baseline characteristics, 107
patient randomization, 105
sample size calculation and follow-up, 108–109
treatment standardization, 108
Rasch Measurement Theory (RMT), 77
RCTs, *see* Randomized controlled trials (RCTs)

Real-world effectiveness, 183
Rectal cancer, 94, 96, 98
Redo surgery, 175, 176, 177, 180
Regression, 220
Rehabilitation outcome measure database, 63
Relative risk (RR), 109, 110, 287, 291
Relative risk reduction (RRR), 109, 110
Reliability, 271
Renaissance humanists, 278
Repeatability reliability, 76
Retrospective cohort studies, 159
  guide to interpretation of, 160
  interpreting results
    clinically important outcomes, 167
    context of clinical question, 167
    existing literature, 167
    limitations of the study, 167–168
    resolution of clinical scenario, 168
  meaning of results
    baseline characteristics, 165
    effective size, 165–166
    issue of multiple testing, 166
    planned sensitivity analyses, 166
    preciseness, 165–166
    relevant statistics, 165
    subgroup analyses, 166
  potential source of bias, 163
    confounding, 164
    directed acyclic graph, 164
    information bias, 163
    selection bias, 163
  and randomized controlled trials, 168
  result validity, 161
    data collection method, 162
    justifiable definitions of outcome, 162
    reliable data source, 162
    study population, 161–162
  statistical analysis, 164–165
Retrospective patient assessment, 185
Retrospective study*See also* Retrospective cohort studies
  bias, 218
Return to work (RTW) outcomes, 146
Review articles, 145
Risk of bias, 129, 159, 220, 298
  tool, 149, 287, 298
Risk ratios (RR), 56, 57, 166
Robotic-assisted prostatectomy, 21
Roux-en-Y surgery, 23, 24, 26, 27, 28, 34
Rule in, 213
Rule out, 213

S
Sackett, David, 37
Sample, 314
Sample size, 312–314
  clinically relevant effect size, 319
  difference in treatment effect, 319–320
  effect size, 313
    precise and consistent, 320
  to estimate power, 320
  estimation of treatment effect, 320
  factors informing, 312
  mean pain scores, 319
  pain outcomes, 318
  resolution of scenario, 320
  sample size calculation, 318–319
  standard deviation units, 313
  and study design, 315
Sampling element, 267
Sampling frame, 267
Sampling strategy, 268
Scientific Advisory Committee of the Medical Outcomes Trust, 73
SCOPUS, 148
Search strategy
  access to resources, 34
  applying Boolean operators, 27
  choosing appropriate resources, 31
  complex search, 29–30
    list of resources for, 28
  controlled vocabulary, 25–26
  creating, 28
  developing, 24
  identifying
    concepts, 24
    search terms, 24, 25
  keeping current, 34
  limits, 30, 31
  search concepts
    identifying, 24, 25
    selecting, 28
  search filters, 30
  search terms
    generating additional terms, 25
    identifying, 25
  searching for clinical practice guidelines, 28
  simple strategy, 28–29
    list of resources for, 28
Second International Study of Infarct Survival (ISIS-2), 327
Selection bias, 54, 105, 140, 148, 163, 165, 167, 168, 172, 183, 186, 270, 298
  sources of, 303
Sensitivity, 204, 206
Sensitivity analysis, 233, 293–294, 297–298
Shared decision model, 194
Short Form 12/36, 76, 78
Short Form Health Survey 36 (SF-36), 96, 97, 99, 101
Short musculoskeletal function assessment (SMFA), 62
Single Assessment Numerical Evaluation (SANE), 63
6S Pyramid, 24, 28, 28, 32
  summaries and guidelines level, 32
  synopses
    of single studies, 33
    of syntheses, 32
  syntheses, 32–33
  systems, 32

Small bowel obstruction, 161, 167
SMLTREE, 231
Snowball sampling, 268
Specificity, 204, 206
SQUIRE guidelines (Standards for QUality Improvement Reporting Excellence), 195, 196
Standard deviation (SD), 287, 302, 303, 321
Standard error of measurement (SEM), 65, 67, 79
Standardization, 108
Standardized difference, 165
Stanford University Center for Clinical Research (SCCR), 3
Statistical inference, 314
Statistical tests, 285, 288–289
  chi-square test, 287, 289
  confidence intervals, 293
  CRAN network, 293
  degrees of freedom, 287
  multiplicity, 294–295
  PICOT format, 285, 296
  PubMed, 285
  reporting statistical findings, 296
  sensitivity analysis, 293–294, 297–298
Stratification, 106, 140–141
Student's *t* test, 287, 288, 292, 293
Studies reporting harm in surgery, 256
  applicability
    benefits associated, 261–262
    magnitude of the risk, 261
    similar results, 260–261
  meaning of results
    exposure and outcome, 260
    risk estimation, 260
  PICOT, 256–257
  primary study designs, 257
  results validity, 258
    correct temporal relationship, 259
    dose-response gradient, 259–260
    homogeneous patients, 258
    patient characteristics, 259
    similar circumstances and methods, 259
    standard follow-up, 259
  study appraisal, 257–258
Subgroup, 327
Subgroup analysis, 327
  applicability
    clinically important effect, 334
    comparability, 334–335
    consistent differences, 334
    resolution of scenario, 335
  to assess credibility of, 329–330
  demographic characteristics, 329
  intention-to-treat analyses, 329
  obtained results
    overall treatment effect, 334
    relative risk reductions, 333
    reporting analyses, 333
  PICOT format, 328
  primary outcomes, 330
  results validity
    between-subgroup treatment effects, 331–332
    comparability of prognostic factors, 333
    predefined a priori, 331
    rationale indication, 330–331
    small number analysis, 331
    stratified randomization, 332
    subgroup treatment effect interactions, 332
    treatment effect interactions adjusted for multiplicity, 332–333
    within-subgroup analysis, 332
Submuscular transposition, 232
Subtotal gastrectomy, 183
Successful surgical outcome, 93
SumSearch, 34
Supercharged jejunal flap, 183
Surgery, opinion pieces in, 277–278
  clinical knowledge, 281
    relevant clinical training, 281–282
    relevant training, 281
  conflict of interest, 282
  expert opinion in, 278
    applicability, 280
    flawed results, 279
    limitations of, 279
    in surgical literature, 280
    trusting, 281
    value of expert opinion, 278–279
  MEDLINE, 277
  perception as expert, 282
  PICOT format, 277
  resolution of case, 282
  technical knowledge, 281, 282
Surgical intervention, evaluating, 51
  clinical scenario, 52
  randomization process, 53
  resolution of clinical scenario, 59
  search strategy, 52
    external validity, 52
    internal validity, 52
    results, 52
  treatment effect, 57
    applicability of results, 58
    comparing patient population, 58
    estimate of, 58
    evaluating surgical skill, 59
    measured outcomes, 59
    precision of, 57
Surgical proficiency, 59, 118
Surgical research, evaluating surveys and questionnaires in, 265, 274
  breast-conserving therapy, 265, 266
  meaning of results
    appropriate conclusions, 273
    appropriate statistical methods, 272
    sufficient response rate, 272
    transparent results, 272
  resolution of scenario, 273
  results in practice

generalizable results, 273
survey changing practice, 273
results validity
primary guides, 267–270
secondary guides, 270–271
surgical survey
appraisal of, 266–267
evaluating, 267
key characteristics of, 266
Surgical Research Methodology (SRM), 4
Surgical survey
primary guides
administration of questionnaire, 270
appropriate development of questionnaire, 269–270
research question and objective, 267
selection of sampling frame, 267–269
secondary guides
clinical sensibility testing, 271
performing pilot testing, 270–271
reliability testing, 271
validity assessment, 271
Surgical techniques, economic evaluations, 239
applicability
cost and benefits, 251
costs, 252
patients expectation on health outcomes, 252
CHEERS statement, 252
clinical scenario, 243–244
cost-effective, 239
EQUATOR network, 252
finding evidence, 244
Cochrane, 244
PICOT format, 244
PubMed, 244
formulas, 241–244
cost analysis, 241
cost–benefit analysis, 243
cost-effectiveness analysis, 241–242
cost–utility analysis, 242–243
meaning of results
allowance for uncertainties, 248
cost effectiveness plane, 251
incremental costs and outcomes, 247–248
net-benefit regression analysis, 249–250
possible outcomes, 250
new innovations in, 239
resolution of scenario, 252
results validity
accurate measuring of costs, 246
clinical effectiveness, 245–246
costs and outcomes integration, 246–247
economic comparison of healthcare strategies, 244
estimates of costs and outcomes and baseline risk, 247
relevant clinical strategies, 245
relevant viewpoints, 244–245
uncertainties in analysis, 247
terminologies used, 240–241
types of economic evaluations, 240
cost analysis, 240
cost–benefit analysis, 240
cost-effectiveness analysis, 240
cost–utility analysis, 240
Surrogate endpoints, 85–86
clinical scenario, 90–91
easier and cheaper, 86
more objective and precise, 86
proof-of-concept, 86
reducing the sample, 86
results
applicability, 90, 91
meaning of results, 89–90, 91
validity, 89, 91
risk–benefit balance, 86
Surrogate outcome measures, *see* Surrogate endpoints
Swiss cheese model, 197
Symptom severity scale, 64
Systematic reviews (SR), 38, 145, 197
applicability
interpreting to patients. 152
patient-important outcomes, 153
finding evidence, 146
MEDLINE database, 146
LOE hierarchy, 145
meaning of results
degree of heterogeneity, 150
overall results review, 151
preciseness, 151
random-effects models, 150, 151
similar results, 150
potential costs and risks, 153, 154
result validity
addressing sensible clinical question, 147
assessing publication bias, 148–149
exhaustive search, 147–148
methodological quality, 149
reproducibility, 149–150
users' guide for, 147

T

Technical knowledge, 281, 282
Test–retest reliability, 76
Three-item Jadad score, 149
ThyroSeq ver3, 201, 212, 213
Time-honoured process, 201
Time trade-off techniques, 232
TIRADS (Thyroid Imaging Reporting And Data System), 43, 202, 203, 206, 207
applicability, 212
change managing patients, 212–213
patients be better off, 213
grouping categories, 208
meaning of results, 211
likelihood ratios, 211
reproducibility of test results, 211
satisfactory interpretation, 211–212
results validity

appropriate spectrum of patients, 210
blind comparison with reference standard, 210
decision to perform reference standard test(s), 210–211
permitting replication, 211
risk of malignancy associated, 209
Transcatheter aortic valve replacement (TAVR), 218, 219
Transverse Rectus Abdominis Myocutaneous (TRAM) flap, 241, 242
Transversus abdominis plane (TAP) blocks, 21, 311
Trial-based economic evaluation, 240, 241
TRIP database, 28, 34, 35
TRIP PRO, 34
Troponin, 87
True negatives (TN), 204, 205
True positives (TP), 204, 205
12-item MINORs score, 149
Two-tail test, 321
Type I error, 55, 314, 322
Type II error, 55, 314, 315, 322

U
Ulnar neuropathy, 225
Upper limb functional index (ULFI), 64
UptoDate, 28, 31, 32
Ureteric catheters (UC), 301
Ureteric injury (UI), 301
US Food and Drug Administration, 5, 72, 95, 126
See also Food and Drug Administration (FDA)
Users' Guide for Surgical Literature, 137

V
Validity, 271
construct validity, 75, 76, 271
content validity, 61, 74, 75, 78, 271
criterion validity, 75
external validity, 52, 58, 152, 154, 167, 183, 186, 190, 245, 258, 273, 278, 337
face validity, 271, 272
internal validity, 52, 154, 258
validity assessment, 271
validity checklist, 286
Value-based care, 194
Variance, 55, 76, 289, 290, 291, 307
variance estimates, 117, 303
variance homogeneity, 292, 293
Venous thromboembolism (VTE), 85, 89, 338
Ventilator-associated pneumonia (VAP), 116
Virgin surgery, 180
Visual Analog Scale (VAS), 62, 313

W
Well-defined research question, 104
Welsh *t* test, 292
Wilcoxon tests, 287
WOMAC index (Western Ontario and McMaster Universities Osteoarthritis Index), 246, 247, 248
Work limitations questionnaire (WLQ), 62

Kolibri 360 GmbH
Ferdinand-Jühlke-Straße 7
99095 Erfurt, Deutschland
produktsicherheit@kolibri360.de